W9-ACQ-699

NURSING
WITHIN A
FAITH
COMMUNITY

NURSING
WITHIN A
FAITH
COMMUNITY

Promoting Health in
Times of Transition

Margaret B. Clark
Joanne K. Olson

Sage Publications, Inc.
International Educational and Professional Publisher
Thousand Oaks ▪ London ▪ New Delhi

147325

For information:

Sage Publications, Inc.
2455 Teller Road
Thousand Oaks, California 91320
E-mail: order@sagepub.com

Sage Publications Ltd.
6 Bonhill Street
London EC2A 4PU
United Kingdom

Sage Publications India Pvt. Ltd.
M-32 Market
Greater Kailash I
New Delhi 110 048 India

Printed in the United States of America

Library of Congress Cataloging-in-Publication Data

Clark, Margaret B. (Margaret Beckwith), 1946-
Nursing within a faith community: Promoting health in times of transition / by Margaret B. Clark and Joanne K. Olson.
p. cm.
Includes bibliographical references and index.
ISBN 0-7619-1210-X (cloth: acid-free paper)
ISBN 0-7619-1211-8 (pbk.: acid-free paper)
1. Parish nursing. I. Olson, Joanne K. (Joanne Kaye), 1950- II. Title.
RT120.P37 C56 2000
610.73'43—dc21   00-008369

This book is printed on acid-free paper.

00   01   02   03   04   05   06   7   6   5   4   3   2   1

Acquisition Editor:	Rolf Janke and Dan Ruth
Editorial Assistant:	Heidi Van Middlesworth
Production Editor:	Sanford Robinson
Editorial Assistant:	Cindy Bear
Typesetter:	Barbara Burkholder
Indexer:	Molly Hall
Cover Designer:	Michelle Lee

CONTENTS

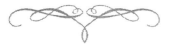

PART II: THEORETICAL FOUNDATIONS

PART IV: PROMOTING HEALTH
IN TIMES OF TRANSITION

PART V: THE PROCESS OF NURSING CARE WITHIN A FAITH COMMUNITY

PART VI: FAITH COMMUNITIES PROMOTING
IMAGES OF HEALTH

FOREWORD

From a Theological Educator

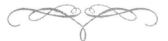

The idea for this book was conceived long ago when the authors—one a nurse, the other a theologian—heard the clarion call to a mission: "Tell the people I love them! Tell the people I want them to be healthy!" Thus began a collaborative exploration into the realm of parish nursing—nursing within a faith community. Joanne K. Olson and Margaret B. Clark, augmented by Pauline Paul's insightful essay, argue cogently that health is more than the absence of disease, and healing more than the cure of an illness. Drawing from a wide range of disciplines, they integrate psychological, sociological, and physiological dimensions of health with the spiritual quest for harmony and wholeness. A bevy of models for theological reflection and cultural analysis are presented as tools for assessing the spiritual and health needs of a congregation. The McGill Model of Nursing is afforded special attention as a conceptual framework for delineating the nurse's role as a health promoter. Without being obscure or esoteric, Margaret and Joanne have courageously and skillfully addressed the thorny question of the relationship between faith and wellness, a dilemma too often encumbered by the church's obsession with sin and guilt. They envision the religious community as a unique "place of seeking" for health and faith. In addition to an enriched understanding of parish nursing, the discerning reader will capture the potential and excitement of faith communities as "places of belonging and dialogue, where we can discover that we can grow in love, find healing for our hearts, and do something worthwhile for others" (Vanier, 1998). In the words of T. S. Eliot (1943/1971), "With the drawing of this Love and the voice of this Calling, / We shall not cease from exploration."

—The Reverend William E. Cantelon, B.A., M.Div.
Pastor, Riverbend United Church
Instructor in Christian Scriptures, St. Stephen's College
Edmonton, Alberta

References

Eliot, T. S. (1971). *The four quartets.* New York: Harcourt Brace Jovanovich. (Original work published in 1943.)
Vanier, J. (1998). *Becoming human.* Toronto, Ontario: Anansi.

FOREWORD

From a Nurse Educator

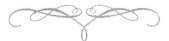

Nurses are skilled observers and assessors of people's healthful living, health risks, and health concerns. They gather information by means of a breadth of knowledge and skill, and are able to draw on this information in promoting the health of individuals, families, and groups in diverse settings. While competent and caring nurses can be found in recognized health institutions, such as hospitals and clinics, a growing number of nurses are moving outside these structures to another type of health care setting: local faith communities. These communities may exist within diverse faith traditions and draw on a variety of cultural as well as religious practices, but they have in common the understanding that health is a valued dimension of humanity.

The time is right for a book that focuses on health care in faith community settings, with the correlate potential for expanding nursing roles. A profession grows only as it examines itself, and nursing is no exception. This book, *Nursing Within a Faith Community: Promoting Health in Times of Transition*, invites nurses to look at their potential as

xvi NURSING WITHIN A FAITH COMMUNITY

promoters of health within local faith community settings. The coauthors recognize the influence of a growing body of literature on spiritual care as integral to nursing care. They contend that faith communities need to say, "We are here," to make known their presence alongside health-promoting initiatives, and they need to move with those initiatives into homes, schools, ambulatory clinics, industry, shopping malls, and churches—where people's lives are multidimensional.

Finally, they suggest that *faith community nurses*—that is, "registered professional nurses who are hired or recognized by a faith community to carry forward an intentional health promotion ministry"—can stand at the crossroads of change and serve as integrators of faith and health through their presence and collaborative skills.

This innovative, well-written book has several strengths. One is the combination of its authors' disciplines—that is, the knowledge bases of both nursing and theology. As linkages between faith and health are recognized anew, and as the people who provide health care from various disciplines become less suspicious of one another, horizons of thought expand, and true interdisciplinary collaboration becomes possible. This is richly apparent in the collaborative work of coauthors Margaret B. Clark, a clinical theological educator, and Joanne K. Olson, a nurse educator. By working together, they have broken new ground for both of their professional disciplines. Using broad definitions of faith, ministry, community, and their respective professions, they appeal to a wide audience of nurses, religious leaders, and educators. I recommend this book as a resource that can enhance understanding across disciplines, and can identify ways in which collaboration between nurses and faith group leaders can improve the health and faith care they offer others.

—Eleanor J. Sullivan, R.N., Ph.D., FAAN.
Professor, School of Nursing
University of Kansas
Lawrence, Kansas

PREFACE

Several years ago, while teaching our first course on promoting well-being in faith communities, the idea of writing a book about nursing in the context of a faith community was conceived. Over the past five years, we have learned a great deal about this topic. Now our book is born. It draws from a growing body of information on the parish nurse movement developing not only in North America, but also in other parts of the world.

The innovative idea of hiring parish-based nurses to form a bridge between churches and the health care system by emphasizing both wellness and wholeness was put forward by Granger Westberg (1987, 1990a, 1990b, 1999). Westberg was a Lutheran clergyperson and retired clinical professor in the Department of Preventive Medicine at the University of Illinois College of Medicine until his death in February, 1999. Soon after Westberg introduced the concept of parish nursing, a resource center was established in Park Ridge, Illinois, now under the direction of Ann Solari-Twadell. This center, known as the International Parish Nurse Resource Center,[1] publishes references on parish nurse education and practice development. In addition, nursing faculties at a number of colleges and universities in the United States and Canada have designed courses to prepare nurses for working within faith communities. The groundswell of interest in parish nursing underscores a shift in nursing practice from institutional health care facilities to community agencies, and signals the importance of considering faith communities as settings for health promotion activities.

In writing this book, we seek to expand on literature in the field of parish nursing. We are broadening the concepts of *parish* and *parish nursing* to those of *faith community* and *faith community nursing* in order to include the rich diversity of faith traditions existing in our world. Each faith tradition includes practices that have health promoting potential. It is our intention to highlight this potential by means of both theoretical and practical considerations. The uniqueness of this text is its focus on theoretical underpinnings for faith community nursing written from the perspectives of two disciplines: theology and nursing. We believe that sound professional practice emerges from an understanding of theory, and is sustained by continuous reflection on how the theory informs and guides one's professional practice. We have included in our emphasis on theoretical foundations information on nursing theory and theories of transition, development, theological reflection, and health promotion as these occur within the context of faith communities.

This book is divided into seven sections. In *Part I*, we provide introductory reflections on faith seeking and health seeking as parallel processes. These processes occur within individuals, across a variety of social groupings, and among faith communities informed by rich and diverse faith traditions. In *Part II: Theoretical Foundations*, we draw attention to the faith community as a context for nursing practice, developing conceptual foundations with input from both nursing and theological knowledge bases.

In *Part III: Nurse as Health Promoter*, focus is on the nurse as an agent of health promotion. We counter some stereotypical nursing images with images of nursing that more appropriately portray the full nursing potential. We consider the seven parish nursing functions enumerated in Holstrom (1999)—the nurse as (a) health educator, (b) personal health counselor, (c) referral agent and liaison with congregational and community resources, (d) developer of support groups, (e) trainer of volunteers, (f) integrator of faith and health, and (g) health advocate—in relationship with the McGill model of nursing developed by Moyra Allen and colleagues at McGill University in Montreal, Quebec, Canada.[2] Within this model, nursing is viewed as the "science of health promoting interactions" and as "a professional response to a person's natural search for healthful living" (Ford-Gilboe, 1994, p. 117). *Part IV: Promoting health in times of transition* discusses concepts related to living in times of transition, and provides information on both the types and characteristics of transitions.

In *Part V: The process of nursing care within a faith community,* our attention returns to the nurse and, in particular, to the process of nursing care. Nursing care, according to the McGill model, is directed by certain core concepts: health, family, learning, and collaboration. We demonstrate how the nurse can employ a "situation-responsive" (Kravitz & Frey, 1989) way of relating to events arising within faith communities. *Part VI: Faith communities promoting images of health* is a place where we draw together the conceptual frameworks introduced in earlier sections of the book, and consider these by means of interdisciplinary and reflective dialogue. In *Part VII,* we provide concluding remarks on how to bring a vision of faith to bear on health—and a vision of health to bear on faith—and we highlight the important role that faith communities can play as contexts for the promotion of health.

Margaret B. Clark

Joanne K. Olson

Notes

1. You can contact the International Parish Nurse Resource Center at 205 W. Touhy, Suite 124, Park Ridge, Illinois, 60068 (telephone, 1-800-556-5368; e-mail, *parish.nurse.resource.center@worldnet.att.net*).

2. We wish to acknowledge the depth of discussions still occurring with regard to the labeling of this approach to nursing. In their collection of writings titled *Perspectives on Health, Family, Learning and Collaborative Nursing: A Collection of Writings on the McGill Model of Nursing* (1997), Laurie Gottlieb and Helene Ezer list the following names given to this approach over the past 20 years of its existence: situation-responsive nursing, complemental nursing, the McGill Model of Nursing, the Allen Model, the Developmental Health Model, and the Strengths Model. For purposes of our book, we use the name *the McGill Model of Nursing,* because it provides readers with an academic location where additional information can be acquired. Furthermore, this label reflects the values of colleagueship and collaboration held by Moyra Allen, who "often commented how fortunate she was to have around her, people who stimulated and challenged her to think differently" (Gottlieb & Ezer, 1997, p. xii). As coauthors of the current text on faith community nursing, we believe deeply in these values ourselves, and see them to be integral to the development of ministry partnerships between faith group leaders and faith community nurses.

Acknowledgments

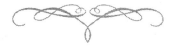

From the moment of its inception right through to its published form, this book has involved the generosity and dedication of many. As coauthors, we wish to express our special thanks to the following people. First we thank Dr. Jane Simington, who was there with us in the beginning, and who has accompanied this project from year to year as our coursework continued. To Reverend Hal Paulson, we say thanks for sharing the discoveries and struggles of our first year together. Special appreciation is also expressed to Dr. Pamela Brink, who first introduced us, and who expressed belief in the idea of this book by encouraging us to submit our proposal to Sage Publications. Finally, special thanks to Dan Ruth, Jim Nageotte, Rolf Janke, Sanford Robinson, and all of those at Sage Publications who have brought the drafts of our manuscript forward into print.

In addition to the support and encouragement we have received in working together, each of us has been sustained in the endeavor of writing this book through the wellsprings of love and encouragement in our personal support networks. Margaret Clark expresses abundant thanks to her older sister and closest friend of heart and soul, Mary Clark. Likewise, deepest thanks go to her faithful pilgrim friend of many adventurous years, K. C. Young. Margaret is blessed to have a circle of "sophia sisters," whose love and encouragement is an enduring gift. Thanks to Lorraine Nicely, Yvette Plessis, Barb Purin, and Jean Waters for being there in colleagueship, true friendship, and as her caring circle. Furthermore, Margaret gives special thanks to those family, friends, and mentors who have nurtured her spirit in so many important ways: Emily and Tom Baril, and the whole "Baril Bunch"; Cathleen and Fred Bleidorn, and all their family; Solomon Delver; Bonnie and Al Donahue; Aldona Ewazko; Helen Finley and many wonderful cousins; Dolores Fruiht; Dolores Helbling; Dolores Kueffler; Sol Levin; and Florence Leone Poch. Loving thanks and heartfelt gratitude go to Angela Merici and her followers, both living and deceased, religious and lay, who have gifted Margaret with spiritual roots that are deep, thriving, and continue to foster her life of ministry. Last, but not least, Margaret's contributions to this book are dedicated with deepest gratitude to her parents, sisters, and their families: Beckwith and Catherine Clark (both deceased); Mary Clark and her son John Barbachano; and Catherine and Steve Nessier, and their sons, Matthew and Blair Nessier.

Realizing that none of us becomes who we are in isolation, Joanne Olson acknowledges the enduring love, support, and encouragement she has received from those closest to her. First, she thanks her husband and best friend, David Olson, for his love and constant belief in her potential. Thanks go as well to her daughters, Erica and Kristen, for being the unique and special people they have become. Joanne further acknowledges Fiona Macpherson for being as loving and supportive as any daughter by birth could be. Thanks go to Joanne's siblings, James Thompson, Mary Collins, and Marna Kallevig; to her parents-in-law, Paul and Joyce Olson; and to sister-in-law Barbara Bunk. All have contributed their love and encouragement from a distance. Furthermore, Joanne thanks her friend, Carroll Iwasiw, for being a constant companion through life's many adventures. Joanne thanks friends at Riverbend United Church for their encouragement and belief in her ability to complete this project. Joanne feels deep gratitude for the abiding love of her aunt Dorothy Freese. She thanks her grandparents, Sam and Myrtle Skindelien, and Martin and Martha Thompson (all now deceased), for their love early in her life. Finally, Joanne offers her most heartfelt thanks to her parents, Verona and Hubert Thompson, for their unconditional and ever enduring love. She thanks them especially for always encouraging her to be who she is, even when doing so has taken her geographically far away from them.

W e also take this opportunity to acknowledge three special groups of people who have contributed time and expertise to the development of this book. Each kind deed, word of encouragement, and type of involvement in this endeavor has made the work not only a creative adventure, but also a product of enthusiasm and joy. For your support, critique, and patience, we say a heartfelt thanks.

First we acknowledge and thank each of the students in the "pioneer" theory and practicum courses at the University of Alberta, Faculty of Nursing. Likewise, we are grateful to those who participated in the first clinical pastoral education course for parish nurses offered through Pastoral Care Services at the University of Alberta Hospital, Edmonton, Alberta. You have contributed a great deal to this book through your questions, feedback, and openness to learn. We also acknowledge the faith group leaders and preceptors who guided our students and dialogued with us as we developed our ideas about faith community nursing. We sincerely appreciate the mentorship and encouragement of Rosemarie Matheus and Phyllis Ann Solari-Twadell as we were taking our first steps in education for faith community nursing in Canada. We thank Alberta Pasco for her assistance with the research project that captured the thoughts of these students, faith group leaders, and preceptors.

Second, we appreciate the contributions of colleagues, mentors, and friends who reviewed sections of this manuscript as it was being developed. To Marion Allen, Pamela Brink, Bill Cantelon, Bill Close, Elaine Domning, Evelyne Forbes, Kathleen Gilchrist, Reg Graves, Laveryne Greene, Frank Henderson, Joe Holland, Joanne Kinoshita, Kris Lund, Orlow Lund, Don Mayne, Fiona Macpherson, Don Misener, Anne Neufeld, Carol Pierce, Barb Purin, Peter Rutter, Case Vink, Margie Warner, Jean Waters, Wynn Weist, Lee Wollery, and K. C. Young, we say a sincere thanks. Likewise, we are grateful to Peter Jeremy and Christine Plican, in the Graphic Design Department at the

University of Alberta Hospital, for sharing their expertise in preparing figures for this publication.

Finally, we express heartfelt gratitude to the people within our work environments who have supported us so generously. Margaret acknowledges with deepest thanks the following current and former employees at the University of Alberta Hospital: Dan Alexis, Ruby Brown, Gwen Buschau, Elaine Cole, Janet Davidson, Priscilla Edwards, Donald Gray, Bonnie Herring-Cooper, Meg Jordan, Jane Mealey, Nasreen Omar, Marcel Peltier, Marj Pettinger, Neal Roehl, Adele Roy, and Jane Smith-Eivemark, as well as several groups of Chaplain Residents and Interns. Your kindness, affirmation, and encouragement have kept me going from start to finish. Joanne acknowledges members of the Faculty of Nursing at the University of Alberta, and, in particular, Lillian Douglass, Pauline Paul, and Marilynn Wood. Your encouragement to begin this project and your interest in its progress have kept me motivated throughout. Joanne also acknowledges specific Sigma Theta Tau colleagues who have believed in her, been an inspiration to her, and have, by their example, shown the results of effective leadership and commitment to excellence: Fay Bower, Nancy Dickenson-Hazard, Melanie Dreher, Joan Gilchrist, Angela Barron McBride, Annabel Sells, and Eleanor Sullivan.

PART I

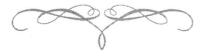

INTRODUCTION

1 ᘛ

Faith Seeking and Health Seeking as Parallel Processes

Margaret B. Clark
Joanne K. Olson

With the drawing of this Love and the voice of this Calling
We shall not cease from exploration
And the end of all our exploring
Will be to arrive where we started
And know the place for the first time.

—T. S. Eliot

Nursing within the context of a faith community is about exploration. The faith community nurse responds to an allure that exists within both faith and health.[1] She or he then goes on to give practical shape to this response by means of professional knowledge and skills. In this book, a *faith community nurse* is defined as a registered professional nurse who is hired or recognized by a faith community to carry forward an intentional health promotion ministry. With the voice of this calling, faith community nurses find themselves involved in both health-seeking and faith-seeking processes. Their exploratory endeavors occur in a network of rich and diverse ministry relationships, which may include associations with faith group leaders, faith community members across the life span, various aggregates or associated groupings, sacred traditions and texts, and congregational structures and polity.

In this chapter, we will provide introductory reflections on the two underlying themes of our book: First, there is the theme of *exploration*, which we are calling faith seeking and health seeking; second, there is the theme of getting to know the *explorers*, whom we believe will be the main readers of this text. These include nurses pursuing faith community nursing or seeking to integrate spiritual care into their practice in a more intentional manner, faith group leaders interested in learning about faith community nursing and the theoretical implications for this type of nursing, and educators from the fields of both nursing and theology interested in the concepts, models, and theories that may support interdisciplinary learning among nursing and faith group ministry professionals.

Our belief is that a rich dialogue on matters of faith and health will flourish as theologically prepared ministry professionals and professional registered nurses work collaboratively in a variety of faith community settings. This collaboration may lead nurses to seek theological education and ministry leaders to pursue education in the health sciences. Whatever the result, we hope our book will contribute to the ongoing enrichment of this kind of interdisciplinary exchange.

Furthermore, we believe there is wisdom to be found in Eliot's suggestion that the outcome of exploration is "to arrive where we started / And know the place for the first time" (Eliot, 1943/1971). It may seem like a paradoxical approach, but we see the process of coming home to a faith community, whether it is one's own or another's, as a process that begins with departure from what is familiar. This can sometimes be discomforting, and can lead exploring cominsters along a path of uncertainty. What any one of us knows, however, is not all that there is to know. Rather, with the benefit of fresh vision and the added insight of different points of view, faith seeking and health seeking can expand our knowledge, and contribute to a wonderful journey of shared discovery. We have experienced just this through our own interdisciplinary dialogue and learning. Indeed, the process of writing a book for diverse audiences has been a challenge. We are aware, for example, that terminology in certain chapters will appeal more to some readers than to others. We encourage all readers, however, to start with those chapters that are most appealing and professionally familiar. Then, we suggest that you progress toward chapters that are less familiar with an attitude of exploration, openness, and discovery. We believe this approach will give practical shape to Eliot's paradoxical wisdom as both nurses and faith group leaders arrive at well-known ministry activities and discover them anew, as if "for the first time," with the expanded awareness of interdisciplinary vision.

∽ Faith Seeking and Health Seeking as Parallel Processes

Faith communities provide unique settings for health promotion. Originally seen as centers for hospitality, learning, and growth among seminomadic peoples, today's faith communities are often identified in relationship with buildings, such as churches, mosques, synagogues, and temples. Such identification has left a number of people spiritually hungry and with a truncated understanding of faith and spirituality. Their hunger can be seen as a natural search for *health* and wholeness. In fact, the popular groundswell inviting our return to more participative involvement with faith as a mysterious relationship between divine and human existence may be a positive sign as we move into the third millennium. Rather than reacting to this shift as a crisis, we should look to these changes as spiritual health indicators. Decreased attendance at structured faith community activities may have less to do with religious disaffiliation than with a natural search for spiritual health. This phenomenon is evidenced by popular literature, the proliferation of workshops on spiritual themes, and a corporate drive to include spirituality in the workplace. Seeking spiritual meaning in one's life outside of traditional religious communities underscores the timeliness of revisiting ties between faith and health. This text represents one genre of inquiry into the possibility that faith seeking and health seeking are parallel processes inviting innovative response as well as committed professional participation.

Connections between faith and health have long been recognized within the professions of both nursing and faith community ministry. From the primitive emergence of spiritual healers in societies throughout the world, to detailed guidelines for assessing spiritual needs and spiritual distress in clinical practice, a partnership between nurses and faith group representatives is visible. We envision the current time of transition to be an opportunity for learning and for continuing inter-disciplinary dialogue. Our collaborative reflection is born out of a belief that nurses and faith community leaders will be better able to transcend role stereotyping and to grow creatively as colleagues when we can learn from one another about the similarities and differences between our unique professions. In this way, we envision the nurse and the faith leader to be companions on a journey of inquiry that seeks health as an integral part of faith.

Although there are many nursing models to choose from in formu-lating connections between faith and health, we have found the McGill model approach to nursing to be compatible with the revisioning of hospitality, learning, and growth in faith communities. Likewise, we believe there are linkages between this nursing model and theological reflection models that have evolved from faith-renewing initiatives in various faith community settings. At a time when technological inno-vations are contributing to the deinstitutionalization of many service industries, and when we observe a return to the home as locus for business and learning, there is need to consider the family as a primary context in which both health and faith are learned. We believe our text will contribute to a dialogue that examines connections between the McGill model of nursing and faith-seeking activities. Furthermore, we see a potential outgrowth of this dialogue being stronger linkages between faith and health. Finally, as these linkages are better under-stood, we envision collaborative undertakings within families, faith communities, and society at large that are both health promoting and faith renewing.

We describe the faith seeking and health seeking that occur through interdisciplinary dialogue between faith community nurses and faith group leaders as parallel processes. What do we mean by this? Metaphorically speaking, just as train tracks run parallel to one another in such a way that trains can depart as well as return to the sta-tion, faith seeking and health seeking are companion processes that transport faith community members in a twofold movement of depar-ture and homecoming. Departure, in our metaphor, signals the move-ment away from what is familiar. It occurs in response to the allure, draw, or attraction of both faith seeking and health seeking. Homecoming, in turn, represents the new integration that results as faith and health issues are brought together in practical experience. Between the going-out and the coming-home, there is an interlude, a "time of transition." In such times, change and response to change transpire. We believe it is crucial for faith communities to be able to provide their members with both health and faith resources during these transitional times. The many developmental and situational transitions that occur in the course of a lifetime can, with the benefit of both types of resources, become occasions for growth and well-being. Thus, faith communities become community health centers that foster wholeness through the integration of both faith and health within the lives of individuals, families, groups, and our broader society.

Nursing within the context of a faith community, then, is an opportunity to respond to people in their times of departure, transition, and integration. The faith community nurse is a registered professional who knows how to connect health resources with faith resources. She or he carries forward an intentional health promotion ministry through collaborative exploration, learning, and discovery in tandem with faith group leaders and faith community members. The faith community nurse is there when others commence their journeys into what is unfamiliar, discomforting, or uncertain; she or he is also there at the times of return and homecoming to celebrate experiences of physical, mental, and spiritual integration. Such ministry fosters wholeness.

✍ Choosing Language That Recognizes Multifaith Exploration

In writing this text, we have struggled with ambiguities in language surrounding both the multifaith and interdisciplinary nature of nursing within a faith community. Our first concern has been to find a name to use in describing a faith community as the context for health promotion activities and as a setting for nursing practice. Likewise, we have struggled with the question of what to call a registered professional nurse who functions as a member of a ministerial team, combining health and nursing expertise with theological concepts to facilitate the healing mission of a faith community.

To date, *parish, parish nurse,* and *parish nursing* are terms found in the literature on this topic. Although we support the benefits of establishing specific terminology to identify the unique nursing functions under consideration (Holstrom, 1999; Westberg, 1999), we believe the focus on *parish* limits the scope of nursing practice being discussed. In a world where multiple faith traditions intermingle in every country and at every level of society, *parish* is predominantly associated with the Christian faith. Being of Christian faith backgrounds ourselves, and we do not wish to minimize this rich heritage; at the same time, however, we believe that nursing within a faith community need not be limited to the Christian context. Health seeking and health promotion exist in all faith traditions. Likewise, nursing through the seven functions of health educator, personal health counselor, referral agent and liaison with congregational and community resources, developer of support groups, trainer of volunteers, integrator of faith and health, and health advocate (Holstrom, 1999; Westberg, 1999) can be just as beneficial to the Jew, Sikh, Muslim, or Baha'i as it is to the Christian.

We propose that the broader and more inclusive terminology needed for this type of community health nursing is *faith community, faith community nurse,* and *faith community nursing.* This is the language we will use most often. It is not, however, terminology that we will use exclusively. Thus, when referring to the unique functions developed through the International Parish Nurse Resource Center we will use *parish nursing* (Holstrom, 1999; Solari-Twadell & McDermott, 1999; Westberg, 1990b, 1999). At other times, when referring to faith communities as they are contextualized by differing faith traditions, we will use such terms as *parish, church, synagogue, mosque, temple,* and *congregation.*

Rooted in our own faith traditions and practices, we do not pretend to comprehend the rich nuances of faith, spirituality, theology, and religious heritage as they exist in other cultures and traditions. We do, however, respect this diversity. Furthermore, we are eager to hear from nurses and faith group leaders within other faith traditions regarding how the dialogue of faith and health is expanded through the introduction of nursing activities currently described as parish nursing (Solari-Twadell & McDermott, 1999). Writing articles for professional journals and adding multifaith perspectives to materials available through the International Parish Nurse Resource Center would be two ways for nurses and faith group leaders of many faith traditions to foster this dialogue. Finally, we hope that any language used in this book that is inaccurate, restrictive, or disagreeable to members of diverse faith traditions will be brought to our attention by means of direct correspondence.

⌒ Choosing Language That Recognizes *Interdisciplinary Exploration*

In addition to the ambiguities of language concerning multiple faith experiences, we are aware of the linguistic difficulties arising from the interdisciplinary nature of faith community nursing. Such nursing is carried forward in a network of relationships through which the nurse interacts with other members of a ministerial team. Thus, our question: What shall we call those theologically and/or professionally educated faith group leaders who have been ordained, licensed, certified, or commissioned by means of recognized standards within differing religious traditions?

Christianity, for example, designates the office of leadership with such words as *priest, pastor, clergy, reverend,* and so forth. In Judaism, *kohen, hakham,* and *rabbi* are terms that have evolved in meaning over the years. For Muslim congregations there is the leadership role of an *imam.* In other faith community settings, the term *priest* has been applied to *mullahs* in Islam, as well as to Sikh *granthi,* Hindu *brahmans,* and Taoist *tao-shih.* The differences in order, duties, appointment, and role are extreme, however, and need to be respected within the unique traditions from which they emanate (Bowker, 1997).

Likewise, in addition to the designation of office, there are terms that indicate unique ministry functions, such as *teacher, music minister, religious educator, preacher, youth minister, pastoral counselor, social justice coordinator,* and so forth. These, too, have their parallels in a variety of traditions. In other words, the language of ministry is a very complex one. Indeed, even our use of the word *ministry* may not be appropriate outside of Christian nomenclature. For purposes of our book, however, we will use the terms *faith group leader, ministry leader, congregational leader,* and *pastoral leader* to speak about those in offices of leadership within various religious traditions. When referring to Christian ordained men and women, we will sometimes use the term *clergy.* In identifying other unique or specific ministry functions, we will draw from the descriptive terms outlined here.

The question of how to identify various ministry professionals introduces a topic that is far more complex than distinguishing between *office* and *function*. An assumption we make about faith community nursing is that it is a ministry profession. Bringing the words *ministry* and *profession* together invites our consideration of ministry as an inclusive term. That is, the meaning of *ministry* is both broad and specific. According to McBrien (1987), ministry takes four major forms. First, there is a universal call to ministry that is rooted in our humanity. In this sense everyone is called to minister to the needs of others. Second, there is a type of ministry that derives not only from one's humanity, but also from certain competencies that are publicly certified or validated in one way or another, such as through registration or licensing. McBrien situates helping professions, including nursing, here. Of note is the fact that neither of these first two types of ministry is intrinsically religious. In the third and fourth forms of ministry, however, religious motivation enters in. In the third form, any general service rendered to others that flows out of a person's religious convictions can be seen as a form of ministry. Here we have people who donate 10% of their earnings to charities, or nurses who spend several years of their lives caring for others in foreign service. Finally, there are those who serve in the name of and for the sake of a particular faith tradition or community. This fourth type of ministry is rooted in some form of designation, recognition, or commissioning by the faith group. It is here that we find the ordained and lay ministries described earlier under the distinctions of office and function.

When referring to faith community nursing as a ministry profession, we are viewing it in keeping with McBrien's fourth category. In our book, therefore, we define *ministry* as an orientation to serve others that is both representative of and carried out in relationship with a faith community's reason for being. Furthermore, ministry is endowed with and accountable to a public trust. In this definition, there are three major components to ministry. First, it is representative; the one who ministers reveals the human face of a faith community's mission or purpose. Second, ministry is carried forward in direct relationship with a particular faith community. Ministering persons do not act in isolation, but rather as part of a larger whole; that is, they are part of the faith community's reason for being as it gives practical shape to values emanating from spiritual and religious traditions. Third, ministry is endowed with the trust of those being served. The one who ministers, therefore, is accountable to that public trust.

This definition applies not only to faith community nurses, but also to everyone who functions as a member of the ministry team in a faith community. We recognize, therefore, that ministry is a form of service that integrates both *vocational* and *professional* elements. As a vocation, ministry gives expression to one's sense of call and free response. As a profession, ministry gives practical shape to this response by means of a unique body of knowledge, such as nursing or theological knowledge, and its related skills.

Although it is probably unintended, a line in the Eliot poem quoted at the beginning of this chapter captures what we see to be the twofold movement toward integration occurring in ministering persons. Eliot writes, "With the drawing of this Love and the voice of this Calling / We shall not cease from exploration" (Eliot, 1943/1971). The vocational dimension of ministry occurs in response to the attraction or "draw" of some principle, value, or aspiration. The professional dimension of ministry occurs as a person gives "voice" to their principles, values, and aspirations by means of particular competencies and publicly recognized standards of behavior. To speak of the faith community nurse as a ministry professional, therefore, is to speak of a person who (a) has been drawn to nursing within the context of a faith community, (b) gives voice to health-promoting values by means of registered professional nursing standards of practice and a familiarity with the unique functions associated with the parish nursing role (Solari-Twadell & McDermott, 1999), and (c) carries forward his or her ministry activities in relationship with a faith community's mission or purpose.

Before leaving the topic of ministry identity, we draw attention to one additional area of distinction worth reflecting on: the distinction between ministry identity and ministry relationships. Among those in designated faith group ministries, there is broad debate about whether or not one should identify oneself as a "professional." Undergirding this debate is a significant question: What makes a *person* a *professional*? Responses to this question highlight the different ways in which the nature of ministry and the identity of ministering persons are defined and valued. Such a debate about ministry identity needs to flourish. When approaching the topic of ministry relationships, however, the issue is not so much one of debate as of clarification. Since ministry relationships are endowed with and accountable to the public trust of those being served, they are professional by their very nature. What, then, makes a *relationship* professional?

Literature on this topic makes a distinction between professional and social relationships. Social relationships serve the interests of both parties, are for the purpose of mutual benefit and pleasure, and are the responsibility of both parties involved (Alberta Association of Registered Nurses, 1997). In contrast, professional relationships emanate from role differences: One person seeks assistance, and the other provides a service. In ministry relationships, the person serving an individual or community is guided by a set of principles that help to maintain the professional integrity of the relationship. These principles, adapted from Irons (1991), instruct that ministry relationships (a) respect human dignity, (b) avoid personal gratification by the minister at the expense of those ministered to, (c) do not interfere with the personal relationships of those ministered to, (d) promote autonomy and self-determination on the part of those ministered to, (e) promote fiduciary (or trust-based) interchange, and (f) are self-regulating in accord with the standards of practice and codes of professional conduct developed by missioning and professional associations. With the support of such principles, interdisciplinary exploration by faith group leaders and faith community nurses along paths of faith and health seeking will realize the potential for both integration and relational integrity.

∽ Summary

This chapter has provided introductory reflections on the underlying themes of our book. We discussed the idea of faith community nursing as a form of exploration. We also looked at those who are explorers in this new field of nursing. Central to our reflections has been the idea that faith seeking and health seeking are parallel processes in the pursuit of wholeness.

We have drawn attention to ambiguities existing in language surrounding both the multifaith and interdisciplinary nature of nursing within a faith community. In this regard, we discussed terminology related with the identification of faith communities, faith community nurses, and faith group leaders. Finally, we explored the concepts of ministry, ministry identity, and ministry relationships.

Throughout the pages of this book, we will return to these themes, concepts, and ambiguities on a number of occasions. Our desire is to deepen both learning and dialogue with regard not only to faith community nursing and parish nursing, but also to the theoretical underpinnings within both nursing and theology that can contribute to this new field of nursing, and to the benefits of interdisciplinary collaboration for furthering faith and health integration. As authors, readers, learners, and practitioners, let us "not cease from exploration" (Eliot, 1943/1971), but rather let us move onward in this journey of discovery with confidence in the allure of both faith seeking and health seeking.

Note

1. Use of the words *allure* and *allurement* in this text draw their meaning from the insights of Brian Swimme, a specialist in mathematical cosmology. He points to the "basic binding energy found everywhere in reality" as a "cosmic allurement," in which all beings participate (Swimme, 1984, p. 45). He then goes on to say that "love is a word that points to this alluring activity in the cosmos" (p. 49), and, further, that the primary result of all allurement is an "evocation of being" and "the creation of community" (p. 49). In keeping with Swimme's ideas, we believe that responsiveness to "the magnificence of the cosmic allurement of love" can foster individual and communal "life enhancing" potentialities (pp. 50-51). Thus, we see cosmic allurement as something integral to both faith seeking and health seeking.

PART II

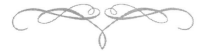

THEORETICAL
FOUNDATIONS

2 ✍

Characteristics of Faith Communities

Margaret B. Clark

Faith community nursing is situated within the broader context of community health nursing. The nurse within a faith community emphasizes health promotion by drawing attention to the relationship between faith and health (Achterberg, 1985; Sanford, 1977). This relationship reveals itself in a variety of ways through the beliefs, customs, clothing, dietary practices, rituals, and religious observances of all cultures and all faith traditions (Germain, 1992; Sampson, 1982; Turner, 1995; Wenger, 1993). Processes for promoting health within faith communities require that a nurse gain familiarity with a knowledge base that draws on the disciplines of nursing and theology, as well as the sciences of anthropology, sociology, and psychology.

An initial task facing the registered nurse who enters a faith community is that of "getting one's bearings." It is important to listen to questions that may arise from bringing key nursing theory concepts to bear on a particular and unique faith community. In this light, a nurse will benefit by asking herself or himself the following questions: How is the *person* appreciated within this setting? What degree of emphasis is being placed on the broader *environment* within which the faith community is situated? How do members of the faith community speak of *health*? and, What perceptions of *nursing* are operative here? Listening to the individual and collective stories of a faith community will enable the nurse to gain considerable insight into the values, beliefs, perceptions, memories, images, and assumptions that exist in this community. These can be appreciated as cultural and faith *filters* (Burley-Allen, 1995; Jones, 1989, 1992), through which the community attends to and discerns its meaning and purpose. We wish to stress the importance of using, in the process of listening, the community assessment skills learned in nursing courses. These skills will contribute to the quality and depth of a nurse's ability to observe and to describe the faith community as a setting within which to provide nursing care (Anderson & McFarlane, 1988; Rice, 1994; Trocchio, 1994).

In addition to the theories and models derived from community health nursing, the person who seeks to practice nursing within a faith community will benefit from a review of the literature exploring such concepts as *spirituality, religion, faith,* and *theology.* Nurses have already made significant contributions in this area by reflecting on the terms *spirit, spiritual,* and *spirituality.*[1] The concepts *religion, religious,* and *religiosity* have received considerably less attention,[2] with other related ideas, like *faith* and *theology,* receiving only passing mention or referred to theological literature (Barnum, 1996; Carson, 1989; Stuart, Deckro, & Mandle, 1989). Nurses who read the articles and books that discuss these various terms will discover a wide range of understandings about each concept informed by research, philosophy, sacred texts, theoretical constructs, and the behavioral sciences. Insights emanating from various approaches to the concepts address such concerns as how to connect with the sacred in oneself and in others; how to provide spiritual care; and how to identify and assess the spiritual dimension of persons; the importance of recognizing and responding to a person's spiritual needs; and how to explore the concepts of spiritual distress and spiritual well-being.[3]

To expand on this blend of ideas in a manner pertinent to the topic of this book, we spend the remainder of this chapter discussing faith, spirituality, theology, and religion as constitutive elements undergirding the practice of nursing in a faith community. Each concept will be described rather than defined, and following each description we will consider nuances in meaning related to the original concept. This "teasing out" of the meaning will accomplish two purposes: First, it will expand our understanding of the original concept through reference to information and insight derived not only from nursing but also from theology and its related disciplines; second, it will provide pathways through which we will be able to connect each concept, seeing how the parts contribute to a whole. The whole we speak of is the sum of persons, environments, structures, and practices that constitute a faith community. Although they may be called by a variety of names, including parish, congregation, synagogue, mosque, or temple, each faith community manifests characteristics of faith, spirituality, theology, and religion in a manner that can be recognized and assessed. As such, further consideration of each term will be of value to those who practice nursing in a faith community.

⌒ Faith: Being in Relationship With

For purposes of our text, *faith* is described as *being in relationship with*. This description is compatible with, but not identical to, a number of definitions found in both secular and theological sources (Bowker, 1997; Buttrick, 1962; Rahner & Vorgrimler, 1965; Vine, 1966; *Webster's*, 1991). These texts speak of faith as an allegiance, commitment, trust, or loyalty. They situate faith in relationship with one's duty or promises, as well as in relationship with a person, deity, or style of life. Each definition makes an assumption of *relationship*. We choose to describe faith by cutting through all of these assumptions, and to speak about the relational core existing in and fundamental to each definition. A sense of being in relationship with is a universal baseline common to all cognitive, affective, and behavioral expressions of faith. Indeed, some would say that without faith one cannot be authentically human, inasmuch as being human rests on a condition of incompleteness, and requires "existential openness toward transcendence" (Panikkar, 1971, p. 244). Simply stated, to be human means that one is not alone; it is in our relationships that we "live and move and have our being" (Acts 17:28 NRSV). Seen in this light, humans are endowed by their very nature with the impetus toward being in relationship with, which we describe as faith.

Individuals can engage this description, expanding from the word "with" to include a special person, deity, or some object of meaning. There is a great deal of room for discussion here as to whether faith is a noun or a verb, a disposition or an intuition, personal or inspired knowledge, given or developed, religious or human.[4] Faith has been studied through a variety of disciplines, including anthropology, philosophy, theology, sociology, and psychology. It is a rich and far-reaching concept, and each discipline provides a point of entry through which to deepen and broaden its meaning. Using the description of faith as being in relationship with invites further exploration, reflection, dialogue, and action by those who may choose to consider the term faith in relationship with other equally expansive terms, such as *health, healing,* and *wholeness.* These latter terms are important in the development of later chapters.

If a nurse accepts the description of faith as being in relationship with, she or he can draw on this information, observing and assessing the broad range of relationships that exist within a faith community. The following questions will guide one's observations within the wide variety of faith traditions, including those of Aboriginal peoples, Baha'is, Buddhists, Christians, Druzes, Hindus, Jews, Muslims, Sikhs, Taoists, Wiccans, Zoroastrians, and others. To begin with, a nurse may ask herself or himself the following questions: Is this community's faith expressing relationship with a deity, revered human beings, entities found in nature, or a combination of such beings? What names are given to the deity, legendary heroes, or revered objects? What images are used to represent those who are held in reverence by the community? What are the ways through which members of the community express their relationships with the deity or revered beings? What are the stories, sacred texts, rituals, and symbols that the faith community draws on to describe and relate with esteemed persons or objects?

In another vein, the nurse may want to look at how members of the faith community act in relationship with one another. What are some of the shared beliefs, values, and attitudes of this community? How are these beliefs, values, and attitudes expressed in such concrete relationships as teaching, supporting, guiding, affirming, correcting, and encouraging? What structures, rituals, and disciplines in the faith community, such as classes, committee work, sacred actions, sacraments, worship, fasting, and social outreach, serve to foster these relationships? How does the community look beyond itself and relate to the larger environment within which it is situated?

As faith community nurses explore the broad spectrum of "being in relationship with" through a process of inquiry, they will acquire a solid base of knowledge that will assist them in understanding the cultural and faith filters through which people in the community view health, life, suffering, self-care, and social responsibility.

∽ *Spirituality: Experiences of Being in Relationship With*

We now turn to a second elemental concept characteristic of faith communities, that of *spirituality*, which we describe as *an experience of being in relationship with*. Here, we make a distinction between the neutral state of being, and the more engaged notion of experience. For example, I may *be* in relationship with a friend who is several hundred miles away, but I have an *experience of being* in that relationship when I answer the telephone and hear my friend's voice speaking to me. Likewise, a person may be in relationship with God and not know it until there is some form of awakening or enlightening experience. Recognizing the difference between *being* and *experience of being* undergirds the distinction between faith and spirituality.

Experiences of being in a relationship can take many forms. Thus, we read about spirituality motivating a person "to choose meaningful relationships and pursuits," connecting him or her with the "whole of life" or with the "inner resources" needed to find answers to questions about the meaning of life. We also read about experiences of detachment, well-being, and interconnectedness that are expressions of spirituality.[5]

When professional nurses listen to experiences of being in relationship shared by the members of a faith community, they are connecting with the concept of spirituality. At such times, the inquiry will need to focus not so much on *what* as *how*: How do members of this faith community act in relationship with one another? How often do they gather for worship? How do they communicate with the divine? How do they act in relationship with revered persons or objects? How do they speak of their origins, significant historical events, beliefs, and practices? How do they speak of the connectedness of their children with the community and with the divine? How do they speak of death as related to the divine? How are people welcomed and sent forth by this community? How and to what extent does the community reach beyond itself in relating with other people in the surrounding environment? Each of these questions provides an inroad for the nurse to learn about not only the faith, but also the spirituality of a community. The nurse not only learns about the community's sense of being in relationship with, but also hears stories, questions, and lore about how individuals and groups experience themselves being in relationship with God, one another, the broader community, the planet, and the cosmos. Spirituality is thus a broadening concept that opens one to great plurality of expression.

In this regard, we have much to learn about differences in spiritual traditions manifest through major world religions. These differences exist not only from religion to religion, but also within the unique spiritual heritage of each religion. Thus, while one can notice that many spiritual traditions include the major stages or movements of awakening, purification, illumination, and unification (James, 1961; Underhill, 1911/1961), the diversity of experience giving rise to each tradition reveals itself through different schools and lineages of spirituality. Each tradition has been influenced by context, time and space. Thus, we may speak broadly of Buddhist spirituality, and more specifically of *theravada* and *mahayana* lineages. We may speak broadly of Jewish spirituality, but more specifically of orthodox, cabalistic, or Hasidic schools. Likewise, within the broad field of Christian spirituality one will find the variations of Benedictine, Franciscan, and Ignatian spiritualities, along with schools of quietist, apostolic, and lay spirituality. Finally, among many of the above named faith groups one will discover traditions of monasticism and mysticism, as well as specific disciplines or techniques related with meditation.

Each spiritual tradition amplifies the language that surrounds spirituality, and underscores the richness of describing it as an experience of being in relationship with. Again, we make only brief reference to a topic and body of knowledge that has generated—and continues to generate—an abundance of written material. This literature continues to need contributions by the disciplines of nursing, medicine, theology, philosophy, history, the behavioral sciences, and the humanities. Anyone seeking a career in faith community nursing will benefit from ongoing learning about personal spirituality and the spiritualities of others.

↬ Theology: Reflection on Experiences of Being in Relationship With

Both being in relationship with (*faith*) and recognizing experiences of being in relationship with (*spirituality*) are important antecedents to consideration of our third concept, *theology*. This term is not readily associated with nursing. There is benefit to be gained, however, from a greater effort on the part of nurses to include theology as a dialogue partner when generating literature pertinent to the field of faith community nursing.

The word *theology* derives from the Greek *theos* ("god") + *logos* ("discourse"). Its original usage was in poetic discourse about the gods, goddesses, heroes, and heroines of ancient civilizations (Bowker, 1997, p. 970). Thus, deep stories evolved containing mysterious and elusive truths, and reflecting human communities linked by their shared knowledge of both divine and human figures. These stories are often referred to as "myths," from the Greek word *muthos*, meaning "story" (Bowker, 1997; Campbell, 1968, 1988; Eliot, 1976; Hamilton, 1940; Leeming, 1990). Among all cultures, myths are still recognized as vehicles through which religious affirmations and beliefs are expressed. The universal mythic themes of cosmology (e.g., creation, floods, the underworld, and afterlife), theism (e.g., god and goddess figures, personifications of evil), heroism (e.g., origins, journeys, quests, and accomplishments of legendary figures), and sacred places or objects (e.g., mountains, cities, trees, rocks, gardens, caves, and temples) are included in the sacred texts of most world religions, and can be traced back to the oral tradition of theology as poetic, narrative discourse (Bowker, 1997, p. 869).

During the period of Greek cultural influence within western civilization, certain veins of philosophical thought and reasoning began to dominate the storylike expression of theology. This imposition of philosophical overlays on oral traditions radically changed the way theology functioned within the emerging religion of Christianity. Wisdom derived through narrative discourse was replaced with disciplined reflection on the nature of reality (metaphysics); methods of inquiry that previously included intuitive ways of knowing were altered by greater emphasis on logical reasoning. Studies into the nature of being (ontology), knowing (epistemology), and the wonders of our universe (cosmology) became increasingly complex as these topics were elucidated through a precise and detailed use of classical languages. Socrates, Plato, and Aristotle figured prominently in the development of systems of thought that began to undergird theological reflection. It must be noted, however, that this arrangement of making theology dependent on philosophical and logical reasoning within Christianity was not paralleled in the cultures of other major world religions (Bowker, 1997, p. 970).

By the Middle Ages, western theology had become systematically organized, categorized, and rationalized. It lost its poetic and narrative connection with the experiences of everyday life. Theology as a conversational activity of ordinary people was replaced with theology as a scholarly discipline. Prerequisites for theology included a study of the classics, philosophy, and Greek and Latin languages. In this manner, theology became somewhat isolated and elitist as an academic discipline. More importantly, theology lost sight of its relationship with spirituality, insofar as it is theology's role to be at the service of spirituality in the same way that reflection is at the service of experience (Hellwig, 1992). Although there is a definite need for university courses and degree programs in theology, there is also a need for an exploration of narrative theology emanating from personal experience. Thus, just as everyone has spiritual experiences to reflect on, everyone has the potential for putting these experiences into words through belief statements and expressions of meaning. This can form a person's personal theology, and it is a kind of theology to which the nurse working within a faith community can listen. Likewise, it is a theology that arises not only from within members of the faith community, but also from within the nurse herself or himself.

For purposes of this text, we suggest that theology be described as *reflection on and celebration around experiences of being in relationship with.* This description continues to expand one's awareness beyond being and experiencing, to include the cognitive activity of *reflection* and the embodied activity of *celebration* around experience. Although reflection and celebration may include philosophy, it is not restricted to the one discipline alone. Rather, tools for reflection are available through the theories and methodologies of such disciplines as anthropology, archaeology, history, psychology, social analysis, and even quantum physics. Likewise, celebration and worship can be facilitated through art, dance, song, instrumentation, and the use of symbols.

Theology can no longer afford to be treated as a discipline isolated from the experiences of everyday life. Nor can it remain separated from a faith community nurse's professional practice. Thus, the nurse might ask who the community's storytellers are; what experiences are shared by the community through its oral tradition; how these experiences are being reflected on; and what types of worship, memorials, ceremonies, rituals, and other kinds of celebration exist in relationship with the community's experience of itself as well as its faith traditions.

With care and courage, theology as poetic narrative discourse needs to be reclaimed and integrated into various courses on nursing within faith communities. Although a number of Christian groups are making some effort in this regard, in matters of faith and health, nurses need to be included further as dialogue partners within a multitude of faith traditions. Nurses, likewise, will benefit from both academic and clinical courses that call for the learning of theological reflection skills (Holland & Henriot, 1986; Killen & deBeer, 1994; Whitehead & Whitehead, 1995).

✎ Religion: Community Contexts Within Which to Share Reflection and Celebration

The fourth element for consideration at this time is *religion*. This concept receives mixed reviews in nursing literature; it is perceived as more restrictive than spirituality (Barnum, 1996; Carson, 1989), and is often associated with people coming together to share common beliefs, observances, diet, clothing, symbols, and rituals (Sampson, 1982). For purposes of our text, we describe religion as *a community within which to share reflection and celebration around experiences of being in relationship with*. Once again, we are moving and expanding on the earlier descriptions; moving beyond being, experiencing, reflecting, and celebrating, we arrive at the dimension of *sharing*. Our description underscores that people, as an integral part of their faith, need to have and belong to a community. A person's faith community may be small or large, formal or informal, socially recognized or unnoticed; but whatever form it takes, the faith community can provide both a context and a container for sharing (Graham, 1992; Rutter, 1993; Thistlethwaite & Engel, 1990). What religion achieves, then, is an environment for shared reflection and celebration. Central to every world religion is the phenomenon of being in relationship (*faith*) and the diverse experiences of being in that relationship (*spiritualities*): It is the work of *religion* to encircle both faith and spirituality with an environment for sharing. As we shall see, this environment needs to foster reverence, provide connection, and enable deepening levels of commitment.

Too often, the word *religion* has been identified with one or another of its component parts; an example of this is the identification of religion with a system of beliefs or a combination of ethical and legal practices. Although many religions include beliefs and practices, the whole of a religion cannot be reduced to these elements. According to *Webster's Ninth New Collegiate Dictionary* (1991), the word *religion* is derived from the Latin noun *religio*, or "reverence." The etymology of *religio*, however, is difficult to determine, because this noun may be pointing to one of three root verbs: *relegere*, meaning to gather things together or to pass over the same ground repeatedly; *religare*, meaning to bind things together; and *re-eligere*, meaning to choose again (Bowker, 1997; McBrien, 1981). Each verb is valued for its nuance of interpretation, and, although there appears to be consensus favoring *religare* (*Webster's*, 1991), we suggest remaining open to the linguistic richness surrounding the possible etymologies of *religion*. By describing religion as a community within which to share reflection and celebration, we are emphasizing the way religion acts as a container or holding environment within which we can foster reverence, provide connections, and nurture deepening levels of commitment. Such an approach to religion envisions reverence as something active, animating, and engaging, and situated within one's everyday life experiences. Seen in this light, religion is more than something to join or practice: It can become the glue that connects and sustains a person's network of relationships.

Although traditional understandings of religion might seem to be at odds with these reflections, this is far from true. Traditional understandings enable people around the world to associate the word religion with Buddhism, Christianity, Hinduism, Islam, Jainism, Judaism, Sikhism, and Zoroastrianism, among others. In this regard, world religions serve as large, formal, and socially recognized communities within which people share and celebrate their faith. Most religions include a variety of subgroups in the form of denominations, sects, churches, schools, and the like; these may be local or global. Thus, a person may speak of their religious affiliation in terms of the Central Baptist Church located at the corner of First and Main, or of the True

Buddha School, which has thousands of students worshipping in temples around the world.

When a nurse begins her or his practice within a particular faith community, the uniqueness of that community may be easily recognized. It must be noted, however, that this uniqueness flows partly from the beliefs, values, and customs of the group's religion, and partly from the local community's distinct adaptation of the faith traditions within that religion. As the nurse becomes more familiar with these distinctions, she or he will benefit from further reflection on the following questions: What types of subgroups for shared reflection exist in this faith community? What topics of learning or reflection are being addressed here? Which aspects of the faith community's experience are not being talked about? How does the community celebrate meaningful events? How are new members welcomed into the faith community's special traditions and celebrations? What is the impact on members of the types of ritual or worship service performed by the group? By addressing these questions, the nurse will become familiar with the faith filters used by the group in their sharing of faith, spirituality, theology, and religion.

From the point of view of nurturing reverence (*religio*), nurses within faith communities can help cultivate respect for the whole person—body, mind, and spirit—by emphasizing the relationship between faith and health. Likewise, a nurse can foster repetition (*relegere*) and provide connection (*religare*) by serving as a health educator, health counselor, and referral agent within a faith community. Finally, the nurse can enable deepening levels of commitment (*re-eligere*) as members of a particular faith community experience practical opportunities for serving others in coordinated support groups and volunteer activities that not only express care, but also foster health and well-being. In this way, traditional world religions can be well served through the activities of faith community nurses, who contribute to a broader understanding of religion as a community within which to share reflection and celebration around experiences of being in relationship.

✍ Summary

This chapter has provided the reader with a general introduction to the concepts of *faith, spirituality, theology,* and *religion* as we are using them in this text. It also provided broad-based descriptions of each term constructed with reference to information and insights derived not only from nursing literature, but also from theology, philosophy, anthropology, and sociology. As each concept was introduced and developed, it took its place in an expanding approach to meaning regarding characteristics of faith communities. Accordingly, the descriptions discussed in this chapter can be summarized in Figure 2.1.

These descriptions can aid professional nurses as they observe and assess the wide variety of relationships and activities occurring within faith communities. When a nurse concentrates on the relational core at the heart of all faith, then the distinguishing elements outlined in this chapter can flow together and become parts related to a whole.

Faith	Spirituality	Theology	Religion
Being in relationship with...	Experiences of being in relationship with...	Reflection & celebration around experiences of being in relationship with...	Community contexts within which to share reflection & celebration around experiences of being in relationship with....

Figure 2.1. Characteristics of Faith Communities

Notes
_____

1. For more on the topic of *spirit*, please refer to Lane (1987), Newman (1989), and Starck (1992). On *spiritual*, see the following sources: Brittain and Boozer (1987), Burkhardt and Nagai-Jacobson (1985), Burnard (1987), Carson (1989), Chandler, Holden, and Kolander (1992), Conrad (1985), Ellison (1983), Fehring, Brennan, and Keller (1987), Goddard (1995a, 1995b), Haase, Britt, Coward, Leidy, and Penn (1992), Heliker (1992), Highfield and Cason (1983), Labun (1988), Morris (1996), Oldnall (1996), Piles (1990), Ross (1995), Shelly and Fish (1988), Soeken (1987), Stepnick and Perry (1992), Stiles (1990), Wald and Bailey (1990), and Walton (1996). With reference to *spirituality*, see the following: Barnum (1996), Belcher, Dettmore, and Holzmer (1989), Boutell and Bozett (1990), Burkhardt (1989), Clark, Cross, Deane, and Lowry (1991), Groer,

O'Connor, and Droppleman (1996), Leetun (1996), Ley and Corless (1988), Nagai-Jacobson and Burkhardt (1989), Oldnall (1995), Peri (1995), Roach (1997), and Stuart, Deckro, and Mandle (1989).

2. Two articles that consider the concept of *religion* are Emblen (1992) and Mickley, Carson, and Soeken (1995). For a discussion of *religiosity*, see Astedt-Kurki (1995), and for a discussion of *religious* factors in patient care, see Sampson (1982).

3. Regarding how to connect with the sacred in self and others, see Nagai-Jacobson & Burkhardt (1989). On how to provide spiritual care, see Clark, Cross, Deane, and Lowry (1991), Piles (1990), and Sardana (1990). For a discussion of how to identify and assess the spiritual dimension of persons, see Burkhardt (1989), Carpenito (1989), Goddard (1995a, 1995b), McSherry (1983), and Stoll (1979). For the importance of recognizing and responding to a person's spiritual needs, see Carson (1980), Emblen and Halstead (1993), and Highfield and Cason (1983). Finally, for an exploration of the concepts of spiritual distress and spiritual well-being, see Ellison (1983), Ellison and Smith (1991), Hungelmann, Kenkel-Rossi, Klassen, and Stollenwerk (1985), Shaffer (1991), and Stepnick and Perry (1992).

4. References related to various approaches to *faith* include the following: for considerations of faith as a noun or a verb, see Stokes (1989); as a disposition or an intuition, see Bowker (1997, p. 334) and James (1961, p. 201); as personal or inspired knowledge, see McBrien (1981); as given or developed, see Carson (1989, p. 28), Ford (1988), Fowler (1991), and Westerhoff (1976); and as religious or human, see Dulles (1994) and Panikkar (1971).

5. References discussing *spirituality* include the following: on its capacity for motivating a person "to choose meaningful relationships and pursuits," see Carson (1989, p. 6); with the "whole of life," see Nagai-Jacobson and Burkhardt (1989, p. 21); and on connecting one with the "inner resources" needed to find answers to questions about the meaning of life, see Belcher, Dettmore, and Holzemer (1989, p. 18). We also recommend, for a discussion of *spirituality*, that you read Highfield and Cason (1983, pp. 188-189) on the experiences of detachment; Ellison (1983, pp. 331-332) and Stuart, Deckro, and Mandle (1989, pp. 36-37) on well-being; and Haase, Britt, Coward, Leidy, and Penn (1992, pp. 142-143) on interconnectedness.

3 ~

Health, Healing, Wholeness, and Health Promotion

Joanne K. Olson

When invited to speak to local congregations interested in the concept of faith community nursing, I often begin with a three-part quiz, asking first that participants write the names of five health care agencies in their community, and then share these verbally with the larger group. Agencies commonly identified include the nearest hospital, a dental office, a physician's office, or a neighborhood walk-in clinic. The next questions to the group are, "Did you include your local congregation on the list?" and, "Why or why not?" Though there are no right or wrong answers to the quiz, the discussions that follow the questions are informative. They reveal much about how the group views health, and highlight which community agencies provide health care according to the participants' definitions of health. Ultimately, we arrive at a discussion about what health is and why a faith community might be considered a partner in providing community health care.

A similar exercise is used to begin classroom discussion for nurses preparing to become faith community nurses. There is much overlap in the words used by both congregations and nurses when discussing their goals and purposes. Words such as *health, healing, wholeness,* and *health promotion* surface in conversations with both groups. At times, additional words such as *disease, illness,* and *cure* also enter the conversation. But what do we mean by these frequently used words and phrases? Are there some common health goals toward which both faith communities and the nursing profession strive? It is only when we wrestle with the deeper meanings of these concepts that nursing services within a faith community context can be fully understood.

The purpose of this chapter is to challenge the reader to think about the following questions: What is *health*? What is *healing*? What is *wholeness*? What is *health promotion*? Where in our communities do health-related activities take place? This chapter emphasizes the discussion of the term *health* to highlight the complexity of the concept, and to stress the importance of knowing exactly what we mean when we use the term. Furthermore, this discussion helps to identify the definition of health that is foundational to nursing practice as we view it occurring within faith communities.

Before we talk about health, perhaps it is fitting to define several other terms, including *disease, illness,* and *cure.* In a presentation about the theological framework for parish nursing, Michael Nel (1998), drawing on the work of Kleinman (1980), differentiated between disease and illness. From the perspective of medical anthropology, disease is "a malfunctioning of biological and/or psychological processes"; illness, on the other hand, is "the psychosocial experiences and meaning of perceived disease" (Kleinman, 1980, p. 72). Such a distinction suggests that someone with a disease may not necessarily feel ill, and that someone without a disease could feel quite ill. Moreover, a cure is "a method or course of remedial treatment, as for disease" (*American College Dictionary*, 1970), and so is not explicitly linked with illness.

∽ What Is Health?

The word *health* comes from the Anglo-Saxon word *hal*, which means "sound" or "whole" (*Webster's*, 1991; see also Smith, 1990; Vine, 1966). Health is the central concept of nursing, and is often considered the goal of all nursing efforts (Meleis, 1990). Likewise, faith communities claim to be involved in health and health care (Droege, 1995; Evans,

1995; Westberg, 1984). Nel (1998) sees health as the opposite of illness, and as a condition in which all cultural, biological, relational, and spiritual factors that relate to illness are brought into balance. In a number of sacred texts, including Hebrew and Christian scriptures, health is seen as wholeness, *shalom*, and a total sense of well-being. As a word, it is linked with safety, salvation, fullness, completeness, and peace (Gold, 1989; Vine, 1966). From this point of view, the goal of disease treatment is a cure, but the goal of treating an illness is to find healing and restore health.

The mission statements of many faith communities include intentions to carry out a health or healing ministry. Yet when asked to name health care institutions in their communities, I find, as did Droege (1995) and Westberg (1984), that most congregational members think of health as the absence of disease, and so proceed to identify institutions known for treating disease. Although initial responses reflect this definition of health only as the absence of disease, further discussions reveal that congregational members know from experience that there is much more to health. Labonte (1993) notes that in open-ended health surveys, few responses concern disease. Rather, personal experiences of feeling energized, loved, in control, fit, happy, creative, spiritually content, and whole were synonymous with health. Furthermore, experiences of community—a sense of connectedness, shared values, discipline, activity, sharing, caring, belonging, and being respected—also contributed to an experience of health.

Of course, there are as many ways to define health as there are cultures and individuals. One's ideas about health are shaped by both personal and cultural worldviews. Authors such as Labonte (1993), Meleis (1990), and Pietroni (1987), however, have combined similar types of health definitions into categories to aid us in seeing the similarities. Meleis (1990) suggests that "the quest for a single definition of health is not appropriate, possible, or useful" (p. 109). She further argues that a diversity of ideas about health, along with an examination of what it is about health that we can all agree on, is necessary. Meleis further suggests that clinicians should understand and be able to speak clearly about many different meanings of health, and that there are appropriate times for the use of each meaning (see also Pietroni, 1987).

Absence of Disease

One way to view health is to see it as an absence of disease: If someone is not diagnosed as being "diseased," then they are healthy

(Smith, 1982). Health, disease, and illness are part of the same continuum, and depending on the amount of disease present, a person is more or less healthy. Once medical tests indicate the presence of disease, achieving higher levels of health involves removing the cause, decreasing the symptoms, or removing and/or replacing the diseased body part (Pietroni, 1987).

Some nursing models define health in a similar fashion, relying heavily on medical knowledge as they consider internal homeostasis (Johnson, 1980) or internal and external adaptation (Roy, 1984) to signify health. Some nursing definitions of health have moved away from this way of thinking, because seeing health and illness as a continuum renders nursing mainly a disease-oriented discipline (Allen, 1981). There is also a trend in the public to view health more as "experiences of capacity and connectedness than about . . . experiences of disease or disability" (Labonte, 1993, p. 16). It is interesting to note, meanwhile, that our health care systems seem to continue to operate largely on the assumption that health equates with an absence of disease.

Viewing health and disease or illness as discrete events becomes more difficult when we think of people living with disease, disability, unhealthy lifestyles, or terminal illness, yet who experience themselves as being quite healthy. Factors other than one's state of disease or nondisease must be at play here. Labonte (1993) suggests that these experiences of health seem inherently social or spiritual. In another vein, Jensen and Allen (1993) discuss one's state of wellness or illness as a human experience of perceived function or dysfunction. They view one's perception of their state of health or illness as affected by an interplay of numerous factors, including extrapersonal (sociopolitical and economic), interpersonal (social supports and relationships), and intrapersonal (personality, past experiences, and emotional state) considerations; health- and disease-related elements (health promotion, functional status, visibility of one's disease or health state, and severity of prognosis); and cognitive-affective factors.

Behavioral Health Definitions

A paper developed by Canadian health policy specialists, and named in honor of Marc Lalonde, the federal health minister in the mid-1970s, is credited with moving the thinking about health away from a purely medical or physiological definition to include more of a behavioral or lifestyle approach (Labonte, 1993). From this perspective, the definition of health moved beyond disease prevention to incorporate ideas about the promotion of well-being. In a similar fashion, some models of nursing view health as the ability to function in societal roles (Smith, 1982) or to carry out self-care (Orem, 1980).

Health as a Socioenvironmental Matter

These ways of viewing health have something in common with each other: In them, health is largely viewed as an individual matter. An individual is responsible for his or her own health, with lesser responsibility falling to families, communities, and society (Meleis, 1990). The article "Health: A Personal Commitment" (Parse, 1990a) exemplifies this view. More recent views of health have expanded to incorporate a sociological and ecological way of thinking. Labonte suggests that this shift occurred for several reasons: First, our view of health has changed because overall levels of education and socioeconomic status have improved in recent years (Labonte, 1993). Second, we have come to recognize the social and environmental contexts in which personal behaviors are embedded (Labonte & Penfold, 1981).

More recent conceptions of health see it as encompassing the whole person and incorporating the relationship between that person and his or her environment (Reynolds, 1988). This expanded approach to the definition of health is reflected by the Ottawa Charter for Health Promotion (World Health Organization, 1986), in which the prerequisites for health are expanded from strictly medical and behavioral health determinants, such as disease prevention and lifestyle, to include such psychological, social, environmental, and political elements as "peace, shelter, education, food, income, a stable ecosystem, social justice, and equity" (p. 1). The most important component of the Ottawa Charter, though, is a shift from treatment and prevention methods of health care to health promotion strategies that feature empowerment. Labonte (1993) defines empowerment as the process "that describes the means through which internal feelings of powerlessness are transformed, and group actions initiated to change the physical and social living conditions that create or reinforce inequalities in power" (p. 101), while capacity building is the ability to individually or collectively take action on health-related concerns.

Health as Lifestyle

Unwilling to settle for a narrow definition of health characterized only by negations, Pender has focused her career on defining health so that the many factors known to have an impact on it can be considered.

She views health as the primary life experience, with illness as a secondary process that may become superimposed on health (Pender, 1987). Furthermore, health and illness exist in a dialectic relationship; this means that health can exist without illness, but illness cannot exist without health as its context. Pender (1990) describes a system for classifying health using five dimensions of human health expressions and fifteen subcategories; in this system, she proposes that "each of the dimensions of health expression—*affect, attitudes, activity, aspirations,* and *accomplishments* [italics added]—should be assessed in terms of daily fluctuations as well as evolving patterns over time" (Pender, 1990, p. 118).

The dimension of *affect*, according to Pender, includes subjectively experienced emotions and feelings. Emotions frequently identified with high levels of health include serenity, harmony (feelings of relatedness to God and/or the universe, or being at peace with nature and fellow humans), vitality, and sensitivity (intense knowing of self and others). The second dimension of health expression—*attitudes*—structures the way people see their world. Subcategories include optimism (seeing possibilities for growth even in difficulty), which "is enhanced by reverence for life and trust in God or the orderliness of the universe" (Pender, 1990, p. 119); relevancy (grasping one's place in the world with an appreciation for unique, personal contributions); and competency (personal clarity about actual and potential capabilities, and a belief in the power to channel capabilities into meaningful patterns of work and play). "Optimism is enhanced by reverence for life and trust in God or the orderliness of the universe" (Pender, 1990, p. 119).

The *activity* dimension of health expression includes positive life patterns or lifestyle, meaningful work, and invigorating play. Suggesting that human beings are inherently purposeful, Pender (1990) describes self-actualization and social contribution as subcategories under the fourth dimension, *aspirations*. Finally, enjoyment, creativity, and transcendence characterize the dimension of *accomplishment*. Pender's work clearly demonstrates the complexity of a term such as health. Furthermore, her work indicates that health is largely a subjective and private experience that can only partially be observed by others. She urges all health professionals to work toward a view of health that is positive, comprehensive, unifying, and humanistic.

Health as a Way of Living and Behaving

Moyra Allen (1981) views health as a social and behavioral phenomenon, a way of living and behaving. In her view, people demonstrate a pattern of behavior, a way of thinking and acting, that is their way of coping with problems and of attaining goals. Allen urges health professionals to move beyond seeing health as an individual state reached only when certain health habits and disease prevention strategies, such as good nutrition, enough exercise, and no smoking, are implemented. In Allen's view, there are no external measurements of good health or bad health: Health is more about what works for the person or family. Furthermore, this view does not see health as part of a continuum with illness or disease, but rather sees them as two separate dimensions. A person could have a disease and still be living in a healthy fashion; conversely, a person could have no disease and be quite unhealthy. Health, here, is viewed as a process, a way of living and behaving that includes elements of developing or becoming. While disease is an attribute of the individual, health is a phenomenon of families and groups: Ways of being healthy are learned within a family and a community; therefore, individual health should be considered a social phenomenon, with family and community as the primary context.

Nurses using the McGill Model in their practice strive to promote environments in which individuals, families, or groups can learn ways of living that are healthful for them. When nurses involve individuals, families, and groups in learning about healthy living by focusing on the issues that are most pressing for them, people are more likely to feel in control over factors that affect their health. In addition, they acquire new skills and are more responsive to new situations in the long term.

The McGill Model view of health is consistent with what nurses, working in faith communities, are trying to accomplish in their nursing practice. It allows for health and illness to coexist, yet be viewed as distinct and separate ideas, thus emphasizing the social context in which health is learned and continues to develop. This view focuses on the strengths of individuals, families, and groups, and, rather than positioning the health professional as the main actor, as the one *doing* things *for* the person, this model enables the person to seek a more healthful way of life. Furthermore, the model focuses on growth and learning, allowing for the many dimensions of health: physical, psychological, social, and spiritual. It is also consistent with the five principles of primary healthcare (Reutter & Harrison, 1996) that emerged from the Alma Ata Declaration (World Health Organization, 1978): (a) health promotion, (b) public participation, (c) intersectoral and interdisciplinary collaboration, (d) accessibility, and (e) appropriate technology. To be in tune with international colleagues, Meleis (1990) warns that we must recognize that primary healthcare is the means to attaining health. Strategies consistent with primary healthcare include community participation, consciousness raising, and ensuring appropriate local resources, access, options, and empowerment.

✎ What Is Healing?

Many faith communities have, within their mandate, some reference to a healing ministry. Likewise, nurses use the term healing when describing some of the activities they undertake in working with people. What, then, *is* healing? Are faith communities and nurses talking about the same thing when they refer to healing? How does healing relate to health?

From a faith community perspective, healing has been referred to as a process that deals with restoring a person or community to health (Nel, 1998). Droege (1995), writing from a Christian perspective, says that "health and healing are the mission of the church" (p. 119). He believes that most Christian denominations would consider health and healing a part of their mission. Some give great emphasis to activities related to healing. These healing activities grow out of a belief that healing, health, and wholeness are related to the theological idea of salvation, which is an ongoing restoration process. It involves individuals and communities in their search for completeness or wholeness now and in the future. Although the language used here is of Christian origin, other faith traditions have parallel terms for healing as a soundness and harmony of body, mind, and spirit.

The word *healing* comes from the Anglo-Saxon word *hale*, meaning to care for or attend to the whole person (*Webster's*, 1991; see also Rew, 1996; Vine, 1966). Healing is an integration or balance of the physical, mental, emotional, and spiritual dimensions of oneself that leads toward personal growth and development. It is something that cannot be "given to" or "done to" another person: Healing must be personal and come from within; others can only facilitate the healing process. Nurses carry out the role of healer when they create environments and circumstances that promote self-healing or wholeness in others (Rew, 1996; Wells-Federman, 1996). Most literature on healing emphasizes the importance of beginning with self-healing or self-care. Since the nurse-patient relationship is often described as a therapeutic or healing relationship, some nurse theorists have focused specifically on the development of nursing models that see the interaction between nurses and patients as the essence of nursing (see, for example, King, 1981; Orlando, 1961, 1972; Patterson & Zderad, 1976; Travelbee, 1971; Wiedenbach, 1963).

✑ What Is Wholeness?

We alluded to wholeness in the context of faith communities earlier in this chapter. Geertje Boschma (1994), writing about the historical development of holistic ideas in nursing, indicates that the use of the terms *holism* or *wholism* in nursing is quite recent. The first use of the term *wholeness* occurred in 1969, in the title of an article by Myra Levine (1969). Two years later, Levine wrote an article that used the word *holism* (Levine, 1971). Blattner (1981) traces the term *holism* back to the Anglo-Saxon word *hal,* meaning "whole," "to heal," "sound," or "happy." In this regard, nursing and faith community meanings of wholeness are quite congruent. It is important to note not only that both health and wholeness share the same etymological roots, but that, when used by people to describe personal experience, such as feeling energized, loved, in control, fit, happy, creative, and spiritually content, *wholeness* and *health* share similar meanings (Labonte, 1993).

✑ What Is Health Promotion?

There are many definitions of health promotion and many perspectives on the nature of health promotion activities. After reviewing these definitions and views, we have selected Labonte's (1993) definition and view of health promotion as most congruent with the purposes of this text. Labonte defines *health promotion* as "any activity or program designed to improve social and environmental living conditions such that people's experience of well-being is increased" (p. 99). The Ottawa Charter, likewise, characterizes health promotion as "the process of enabling people to increase control over, and improve, their health" (World Health Organization, 1986, p. 1). Labonte describes this charter as marking the significant move from strictly medical and behavioral health determinants to more psychological, social, environmental, and political ones. This view of health promotion also introduces the idea of empowering or enabling people as a way of promoting health.

Health promotion is often confused with the concept of disease prevention, which is "any activity or program designed to prevent disease, disease being some deviation from physio-chemical normality upon which there is some professional medical consensus" (Labonte, 1993, p. 99). Disease prevention is often discussed in terms of primary, secondary, and tertiary prevention. Primary prevention is an action or program designed to help people grow up with or maintain healthy behaviors. Secondary prevention aims to help people change unhealthy behaviors and strives for early detection of disease. Tertiary prevention is treatment that prevents a person from becoming more ill or dying from a disease (Labonte, 1993). Health promotion, then, is not the same as disease control or disease prevention: Disease prevention is problem-oriented, with an emphasis on slowing, changing, or eliminating disease processes, whereas health promotion is more a matter of personal integration with one's world (Parse, 1990b). It is action taken to enhance the quality of life, and it encompasses the whole person (Smith, 1990).

ဆ Where Do Health-Related Activities Take Place?

Let us return to the original question: Where do health-related activities take place in our communities? By now we could ask the questions in a way that employs the meaning of all the words discussed: Where do *hal* or *wholeness* promotion activities take place within our community? Some activities will occur in the institutions that first come to mind when congregational members are asked this question: the hospital, the doctor's office, and the walk-in clinic. But Westberg (1984) is one of many who would suggest that what these institutions really offer is illness care. He suggests that at least five other institutions in our communities contribute to maintaining good health: homes, schools, places of worship, work places, and public health agencies. Looking specifically at local faith communities, health-promoting services of all kinds are being offered: worship experiences that instill hope and faith, social support networks, education, counseling, social experiences, family activities, and volunteer opportunities (Westberg, 1984). Acknowledging that not all churches are health-giving, with some actually having doctrines that could impede people's movement toward health, Westberg believes that every faith community has the potential to become more of a "wellness center" (on this idea of the church as a place of health and healing, see also Droege, 1995, and Evans, 1995).

◢ Summary

In this chapter, the reader has been invited to consider the meanings of the words basic to faith community nursing practice: *health, healing, wholeness,* and *health promotion.* We have discovered that all of these words have a similar origin, and all involve movement toward becoming more complete, balanced, or whole in the context of a community. We have proposed that faith communities might logically be considered community healthcare institutions. Nurses who work in faith communities are in a position to give attention to both faith and health. Drawing on the concepts of faith, spirituality, theology, and religion introduced in Chapter 2, together with the concepts of health, healing, wholeness, and health promotion discussed in this chapter, the nurse can bridge the two realms; this is to say, nurses, as they serve on ministry teams within faith community settings, may be in a position to build connections between the health sciences and the healing traditions of diverse faith groups. Thus, by participating in a dialogue and acting with respect, nurses can contribute to people's sense of harmony and balance, which healthcare circles call *health* and faith communities call *wholeness, peace, shalom,* and *salvation.*

4

Local Faith Communities as Places of Seeking

Margaret B. Clark

We are question-raising creatures. Think for a moment of all the questions that have come to your mind today. Think, too, of all the meetings you have attended, the people you have met, the television shows you have watched, or the computer time you have spent, and then consider the role that questions and curiosity have played in those activities. Inquiry is a part of our spiritual life, too. A number of years ago, I decided to look up the first question in the Bible, since this is the text that has been the most important source of religious heritage for me. What I found was the question, "Where are you?" (Gen. 3:9 NRSV). It is a question about *place*. Ever since I made that discovery, I have continued to ponder not only the phenomenon of questioning, but also the relationship between questions and place.

This chapter explores faith communities as *places* and as *places of seeking*. The ideas of faith seeking and health seeking, we recall from

Chapter 1, have been associated with exploration and discovery. In our current chapter, "seeking" will also be associated with the groundswell of spiritual hunger and searching evident in our world today. When faith community nurses enter local congregations, they meet questioning individuals, families, and groups, and they bring their own questions to that setting. In addition, nurses encounter the faith community as a place where spiritual hungers may arise and where many forms of searching may occur. Faith community nurses must therefore understand clearly how they can best support people moving through deepening cycles of spiritual question raising, hunger, searching, and discovery.

Our belief is that local faith communities are strategically situated to be what we call *places of seeking.* That is, when questions and spiritual hungers arise, local faith communities are uniquely positioned to assess these questions and hungers as indicators of spiritual health. Rather than being discouraged or defensive about decreased attendance at structured religious activities, faith communities need to wonder anew about the question of *place.* That is, they need both to reassess their position within the larger community and to think about how they might better be settings where intentional faith renewal and health promotion occur. Indeed, during our current times of global change, local faith communities will benefit by counting the number of ways they can respond to the biblical question, "Where are you?" with the reply, "We are here." We are here in many forms, many places, and with many names. We are small and large, simple and complex, local and global. We are here as communities within which people can share experiences of reflection and celebration around being in relationship with the divine, self, and others. Furthermore, we are here as community health resources. In this chapter, we invite faith group leaders and nurses of all religious traditions to envision their local faith communities as community health centers where faith seeking and health seeking are encouraged and wholeness is fostered.

✑ Questions Arising As Nurses Enter Local Faith Communities

Faith community nursing is an important emerging nursing specialty. In this section of the chapter, we look at nurses entering local faith communities as agents of health promotion. First, we touch briefly on the rise of parish nursing. Then we explore some of the questions that faith community nurses might ask themselves as they enter local faith group settings in a variety of religious traditions. Our interest continues to be the local faith community as a place of seeking.

In the late 1960s, a group of doctors, nurses, and clergy in the United States began to experiment with the idea of developing holistic health centers within faith communities (Westberg, 1990a). They discovered, as their work evolved through pilot projects and evaluation studies, that *nurses* in each of the holistic health centers bound together the three professions—doctors, nurses, and clergy—in a common appreciation for the healing talents of each (Tubesing, 1977; Westberg, 1990a). Nurses were seen to function as "translators" (Westberg, 1990a, p. 27), speaking the two languages of healthcare and religion. They played an important role in fostering interdisciplinary dialogue about matters of faith and health. Likewise, they were uniquely resourceful in facilitating a "whole person" approach to healthcare (Westberg, 1990a). The special contributions of nurses working within church-based holistic health centers has evolved over the past two decades into what we call *parish nursing.*

Parish nurses are agents of health promotion and disease prevention whose role is based on the care of whole persons within faith communities (Solari-Twadell & McDermott, 1999). According to one author, parish nurses work alongside other ministry professionals "to integrate the theological, psychological, sociological, and physiological perspectives of health and healing into the word, sacrament, and service of the congregation" (Ryan, 1990, p. 51). There are currently seven activities associated with parish nursing: Nurses act as (a) integrators of faith and health, (b) health educators, (c) personal health counselors, (d) referral agents and liaisons with congregational and community resources, (e) trainers of volunteers, (f) developers of support groups, and (g) health advocates (Holstrom, 1999).

In a manner of speaking, parish nursing is a type of nursing specialty where a unique pluriformity of function is integrated to the uniqueness of role. That is, terms such as *parish nurse* and *parish nursing* are more than descriptive phrases; they also serve as foundational concepts holding explicit meanings that need to be understood and preserved. Without this specificity, the unique role and functions carried forward by professional registered nurses within faith communities are at risk of diffusion and confusion (Solari-Twadell & McDermott, 1999). Building on our understanding of the vision and conceptual foundations integral to parish nursing, we see the need for an expanded multifaith and multicultural dialogue around the uniqueness of this role. We encourage both sharing with faith traditions around the globe about the idea of having registered professional nurses placed within their faith group settings, and exploring how these nurses might carry forward intentional health promotion activities within the unique contexts of traditions and structures represented by each religious grouping. In time, we believe such dialogue will occur.

As nurses enter faith communities of multicultural and multifaith origin, the need to raise questions will arise. We suggest that a first consideration is to ask, What is this place called? An earlier chapter mentioned the words *church, parish, synagogue, mosque,* and *temple* as ways of naming faith community settings. Words to be added to this list could include *stake, gurdwara, lodge, circle,* and many others. Respectful inquiry into the names local faith communities use to describe themselves can teach nurses valuable lessons. Take the word *temple,* for example. How would a Jewish person speak of its meaning as distinct from a Muslim or a Sikh? In another vein, if a nurse were to ask an Aboriginal elder direct questions about the meaning of a *lodge,* there might be indirect and nonverbal responses until the nurse has learned about the protocol of respect that needs to precede question-asking in that culture. With this kind of learning, faith community nurses expand their ability to serve as translators of not only verbal, but also the nonverbal, ritual, and symbolic languages of health and faith.

The second area of consideration for nurses entering local faith communities is to ask, What kinds of meaning are associated with the names given to the place? For example, according to Bowker, the building used by some Sikh communities for their worship is called a *gurdwara,* a Punjabi word that means "gateway of the Guru" (Bowker, 1997). With such an initial understanding, we are invited to wonder what some of the deeper meanings of this word are, as well as what place the stories of its development play in the history of the Sikh faith. Likewise, we may also be curious about the origins and meaning of the Christian *parish.*

Indeed, the etymology of *parish* leads one back, through the Middle English *parisshe,* the Middle French *parroche,* and the Latin *parochia,* to the Greek root *paroikia* (*Webster's,* 1991). This word is a composite of *para* ("beside") and *oikeo* ("to dwell"), and means "to dwell along-side others." It is a concept akin to the Hebrew *ger* and Arabic *jar*, both of which mean "protected stranger" (Milgrom, 5750/1990) or "neighbor," in the sense of a noncitizen who sojourns without official status (Kittel & Friedrich, 1967). Exploring the root meaning of *parish*, one thus finds that it describes a way of being in relationship with God. In addition to its etymology, *parish* has rich historical meanings. The words *paroikia* and *parochia* have been used to describe religious learning centers, communal settings, the territory of a bishop, churches with baptismal fonts, rural faith centers, and parcels of land claimed as property by a ruler, nation, or state (Boyd, 1952; Cross & Livingstone, 1974; Latourette, 1953; Poulet, 1934). Since we are not skilled in the historic or linguistic methods needed to pursue word meanings and historical development further, we simply draw attention to a basic principle of inquiry for nurses who enter local faith community settings; that is, names can be points of entry for learning about both the meaning and history of a place.

A final question that we urge nurses entering local faith communities to ask is, What kinds of relational systems and structures operate in this place? For example, does the faith community draw on a large, mid-sized, or small geographic base? Likewise, what is the population base? Do people have to travel long distances in order to gather for worship? Within this faith community, are decisions made by single persons, groups, committees, or some other entity? Who are the formal and informal leaders? What connections, if any, does the local congregation have with regional, national, or international faith group structures? What kind of access does the faith community nurse have to persons in leadership, or to policy-making and decision-making vehicles? In another vein, where does the faith community nurse's ministry plan fit into the overall vision of the faith community? Is the nurse's position integrated within congregational structures to such a degree that it can sustain changes in designated faith group leadership, or is the faith community nurse likely to lose her or his job with a change of rabbis, priests, imams, or pastors? Exploring these questions can provide the faith community nurse with important information related to place. That is, faith communities are organized social systems (Richardson, 1996), and a faith community nurse will want to know her or his place in that system.

✑ Understanding "Place" as a Dimension of Faith Communities

The question of place evokes many levels of response. In replying to the question "Where are you?" for example, one will hear literal answers, such as "I'm in Florida," or "I'm with the children in the kitchen." There are also emotional and metaphoric responses: "I'm feeling totally lost," or "I'm in the pits." Seen in this light, the notion of place within local faith communities needs to be approached as multidimensional, and faith community nurses will benefit from knowing how to listen for and recognize these various dimensions.

Thomas Groome, in *Sharing Faith* (1991), describes three important facets of place. First, he says, "our 'place' is always our first source of life and well-being" (p. 101). Think, for a moment of the place of an infant when held tenderly by its parents. It is essentially safe, secure, and the focus of loving tenderness. These are primary values associated with one's place. In another vein, can you remember a time when you felt truly alive, centered, and whole? What or who held you in that place, and how do you speak about it in terms of life and well-being? Finally, how does one, as a faith community nurse or faith group leader, go about encouraging others to speak about such places of safety, vitality, and wholeness?

A second point Groome makes is that place conditions one's "being" and "knowing." In other words, where we are has an impact on who we are and what we know. This point came home to me about ten years ago when I stood in a village in Botswana, Africa, looking into the night sky, and someone asked the question, "I wonder if we can see the Southern Cross?" Being from North America, I had never known what it was like to look among the constellations of stars for the Southern Cross. Conversely, the villagers with whom I stood in Botswana had never known what it was like to search the skies for the Big Dipper or North Star. Ever since that experience, I have noticed countless other ways in which place affects knowledge and being. Indeed, the location of one's birth and upbringing has an impact on the sights, sounds, smells, tastes, and textures we come to associate with the living of our lives.

Finally, Groome suggests that a deep sharing of faith requires one to give attention to the whole sociocultural context in which one lives. In other words, we are never mere "observers" of our place. Rather, "We take on as our own its patterns of meaning and role models, its attitudes and values, as constitutive of our identity" (Groome, 1991, p. 100). Seen in this light, our sociocultural location not only conditions our being and knowing, it also shapes who we are. In the language of the behavioral sciences, this formative dimension to place is called socialization or enculturation (Berger & Luckmann, 1966; Friedman, 1985; Westerhoff, 1976). As a helping professional, for example, how many times have you observed parents teaching values to their children? Think of the mother who encourages her daughter to "say 'thank you,'" or the father who comforts his son with "It's okay to cry." By contrast, think of the socializing impact on one's sense of self when one is referred to as "rich" or "poor," "smart" or "stupid," "pretty" or "ugly," or "popular" or "unpopular." Experiences of place related with these attitudes, roles, and values can have a lasting effect on a person's sense of well-being.

Applying these insights from Groome to faith community nursing, we suggest that nurses entering local faith communities ask at least three questions related with the multidimensional nature of place. First, what are the sources of life and well-being here? Second, how does this local faith community context condition the being and knowing of its members? Third, in what ways is this a formative setting? From these lines of questioning, additional observations and inquiries can be made. For example, in considering the faith community as a formative place, the nurse may seek to learn more about the role models, patterns of meaning, attitudes, and values that are in evidence. How are these indicative of faith sharing and health sharing?

Before leaving this section, we draw attention to one more point. The maturing of individuals, families, and groups occurs contextually; that is, maturation is a dimension of place. The condition of a musical instrument, for example, can affect a musician's ability to develop certain skills. Likewise, the presence or absence of supportive friends and mentors can affect one's ability to complete certain developmental tasks. Where we are influences what and who we have available to us in our various types of human development. On this matter, Groome (1991) points to a connection between development and learning. He asks, "What is the relationship between socialization and education—should education promote a dialectic between people and their 'place,' or should it simply be an intentional agency of socialization?" (p. 101).[1] This question suggests that it is possible to step back from a position of total immersion in one's place in order to reflect on it and converse with it. We need to be aware, therefore, that some methods of education support one's stepping back into a stance of reflection, but other educational methods simply reinforce social immersion. In this regard, it is our belief that methods of education and learning that promote inquiry contribute not only to reflection, but also to empowerment (Gros & Ezer, 1997).

Nurses entering local faith communities usually have their first experience of place by means of carrying out an assessment process. They observe, listen, ask questions, and gather findings. When the evaluation is carried forward by the use of inquiry methods, such as those found in the McGill model of nursing (see Chapter 6), a nurse's sense of place can be deepened and broadened. In other words, with the skills that promote inquiry, faith community nurses can both stand back in reflection and participate in conversations of exploration and discovery with individuals, families, and groups in the local faith community. More will be said about this in other parts of our book. For the present, we want to focus on the value of questioning as a tool for faith community nurses to use as they explore the multidimensional quality of place that exists in local faith group settings.

✍ Understanding "Seeking" in Local Faith Communities

Spiritual hunger is in evidence throughout our world. According to Reginald Bibby, increasing numbers of believers are experiencing disenchantment and disillusionment with both known and unknown gods (Bibby, 1993, 1995). They feel caught in an emotionally complex longing for something better than what they have already experienced within social structures and organized religions. They seem to live like aliens, dwelling alongside others but not yet knowing what it is like to be at home in our world. This ache of longing and this alienation are a serious problem of connection—versus disconnection (Bellingham, Cohen, Jones, & Spaniol, 1989). The phrases *spiritual need* and *spiritual distress* are used frequently in the literature (Clark & Brink, 1996; Clinebell, 1992; Ellison, 1983; Emblen & Halstead, 1993; Highfield & Cason, 1983).

In this section of the chapter, we will look briefly at insights found on the topic of seeking as they appear in *The Choice Is Always Ours* (Phillips, Howes, & Nixon, 1948/1975). The authors of this anthology speak broadly about a fundamental and universal human longing for meaning, joy, and creativity. For some people, they say, "this longing becomes so heightened that they penetrate to a perception of the way to its achievement" (Phillips et al., 1948/1975, p. 23). With this statement, the authors draw attention to the possibility that spiritual longings and hungers may help one to move beyond one's existing awareness to new levels of perception. Sometimes this phenomenon is referred to as transcendence (Underhill, 1911/1961).

Although nursing assessment usually approaches the spirit as a dimension of our humanity, it is important for faith community nurses to be aware of the transcendent potential within the spirit (Cobb & Robshaw, 1998; Emblen, 1992; Goddard, 1995a; Macrae, 1995). Nurses working in local congregations will encounter evidence of spiritual hunger, longing, and alienation among those they serve. A basic principle worth considering at such times of encounter is whether or not these longings and hungers could be spiritual health indicators. Not all aches and pains need fixing. Some aches, and even some episodes of illness, can be signs of growth. Seen in this light, not only skilled compassion, but also appropriate referral within various faith traditions to recognized spiritual directors, leaders, elders, guides, teachers, masters, or advanced meditation practitioners may need to occur. Attentiveness to whole-person health involves careful attunement to the interrelationship of body, mind, and spirit in the seeking of wholeness.

The chapter "The Searching and the Finding" in Phillips et al. (1948/1975), provides a catalog of eleven phrases used to describe motives for searching. The list draws not only from religious literature, but from other types of literature as well, in an attempt to highlight the universal nature of human seeking. Rather than try to describe each motive, we will simply list them, and allow the linguistic imagery to stimulate further reading and reflection. Searching, then, emanates in relationship with

- A great cry
- A surging purpose
- A desire for orientation
- The intent of nature
- The quest of consciousness
- A mystical aspiration
- An intricate longing for unity
- The desire for intentional living

- The desire for oneness with the universe

- The sense of being sought by "another"

- The fountain of spirit

There is a rich legacy of classic, period specific, and contemporary literature available in most faith traditions on topics in the spiritual life; we encourage readers to explore resources in their own and other traditions to add deeper understanding as well as meaning to the descriptive phrases listed here.[2]

Faith community nurses, meeting people in their local congregations who manifest spiritual hunger and who seem to be searching for intangible but meaningful spiritual capacities, can respond through collaborative learning interactions and referrals. Again, we must remember that seeking may be an indicator of spiritual health, one that orients an individual, family, or group toward the holistic integration of faith and health. The unique perspectives available through faith community nurses, especially their attentiveness to whole-person health, will benefit not only the search, but also discovery.

We supplement the summary list of motives for seeking by sketching where the search can lead, what Phillips, Howes, and Nixon (1948/1975) call "the finding of the way" (p. 38). We believe many faith traditions will be able to resonate with one or several of the descriptive phrases listed earlier, as they are ways of articulating the positive potential within spiritual hunger and searching. Again, the reader is encouraged to explore the wealth of resources in this area. "Finding the way" can be seen as

- A turning

- A hidden treasure

- "Steps" to real simplicity

- A voluntary change of will

- Total responsiveness to the best in each situation

- Commitment

- Purity of heart

- A denial of self-will

- Conscious fidelity to "inner vocation"

- An openness to the "new creation"
- The "voice of the beloved"
- The actualization of innate and individual wholeness

In keeping with our suggestion regarding the role of faith community nurses encountering spiritual hunger, we suggest that nurses respond to spiritual discovery with collaborative learning, skilled compassion, and appropriate referrals. Such a response is of optimum benefit to local congregations. The activities of seeking are multifaceted and richly diverse, and faith community nurses as well as faith group leaders can help those who are the focus of their ministry by promoting inquiry, engaging in collaborative learning, and simply offering an attentive presence.

໒ఄ *Local Faith Communities as "Places of Seeking"*

The previous two sections of this chapter have considered place and seeking as distinct entities; it is now time to bring these concepts together. We recall again the question, "Where are you?" and the potential for today's faith communities to say, "We are here." We firmly believe that local faith communities are strategically situated to be places of seeking. Faith communities have been fashioned in a multitude of forms and places all throughout history, which has enabled them to adjust the manner in which they responded to and related with members as well as potential members. Religious traditions around the globe give evidence of how they have drawn on geography, social structure, cultural symbols, and significant events to be able to say, "We are here."

A key factor in the adaptiveness of religious groups has been their ability to raise questions. In order to remain present *to* others, faith communities have needed to ask *of* others, "Where are you?" A function of local faith communities, therefore, is their outreach, or seeking to know the location of their members so they can proceed to be in meaningful relationship with them. In times past, this has meant traveling along trade routes, becoming familiar with both rural and urban population bases, crossing huge ocean waters, pioneering uncharted frontiers, and becoming established in a multitude of local and global settings. Today, we are living in times of change and transition, where terms such as *globalization, multinational, cyberspace,* and *the Internet* are in common usage. In such a context, how are local faith communities asking the age-old question, "Where are you?" in order to persevere in their ability to be with others? We believe faith community nurses and faith group leaders, as agents of this question, will find their congregational members in *dispersed places*. In today's world, local faith communities need structures of response that not only gather, but also go out to meet, sojourn with, and accompany their members.

It needs to be said, in this regard, that the organizational structures that support ministry activities seeking to find people in their dispersed places are products of value systems that may or may not be enduring. By this we mean to say that we are emerging from a historical period that has specialized in differentiation. Knowing how to draw attention to minute distinctions in matters of body, mind, and spirit has been a hallmark of the twentieth century. Because of our progress, we are heavily invested in the values of distinctiveness, multiplicity, and even disconnection. Some have referred to this as a process of "numbing" oneself in relationship to others (Herman, 1992; May, 1950/1977; Noer, 1993). Furthermore, our sociocultural structures and physical surroundings reflect back to us that we are a burgeoning global population of individuals, families, and groups who inhabit a planet whose resources are slowly but surely being depleted. With this eventuality in mind, we need to be aware that the values about place that have formed our surrounding physical and attitudinal structures are in a process of shifting. To quote a phrase from Christian scriptures, "the old order of things" is passing away (Rev. 21:3 NRSV). It is important, therefore, that faith communities position themselves to listen closely for indicators from within both their ancient traditions and contemporary cultures that may be giving rise to a new sense of place.

In addition to asking "Where are you?" in the light of our contemporary transitions, local faith communities and their ministering leaders have another significant task as *places of seeking*. It is the task of probing religious traditions for the enduring and unifying spiritual resources that will foster wholeness for today and for the future. Spiritual resources emanating from deeply rooted religious values are a strength that faith communities have to offer in times of transition. In this regard, we believe today's faith communities will be able to say,

"We are here," when they arrive at the points of connection where people are not only awakening to experiences of being in relationship with others, but are also reflecting on these experiences of spiritual awakening.

One crucial and significant point of connection where ministry professionals will find people awakening spiritually is in the domain of health. As we will discuss in the next chapter, healing and health-care have been linked historically with faith traditions. We therefore invite leaders and members within diverse faith communities to consider their potential as resources for health, healing, and wholeness. That is, we ask them to consider what, among the enduring and unifying values in religious traditions, are the healing arts and healing practices that connect with faith seeking and spiritual awakening?

Many faith traditions already know the value of combining outward oriented ministries with facility-based hospitality, education, and social support. Christianity, for example, has been noted for combining evangelism with proclamation, and religious instruction with works of charity. As they look to the future, local faith communities need to ask themselves how they can situate themselves more intentionally to connect healing arts and health practices with current expressions of spiritual awakening. What if local congregations begin to see themselves functioning as community health centers, where faith seeking and health seeking are encouraged, and wholeness is fostered? Likewise, what if the broader society begins to recognize faith community nurses as a unique resource within local congregations dedicated to the promotion of health and faith integration? We believe that such a combination of events would lead to a new sense of place for local faith communities.

Faith community nursing is a relatively new ministry specialty arising out of our changing times. Its historical roots in the values of faith and health integration are rich and varied, and much will be learned from them. (More will be said of this in our next chapter.) However, at the same time that it is historically rooted, faith community nursing is also new. It is being formed out of, and will embody, the values of today that hold a future promise for the integration of health and faith. We suggest, therefore, that faith community nursing is a unique health resource that can be made available through local faith communities to the larger society. Furthermore, it is a resource with the potential to mediate the enduring and unifying health values found in diverse religious traditions. For example, as the parish nurse functions as referral agent and liaison with congregational and community resources (Holstrom, 1999), she or he is in a position to reach out from the local congregation to connect with broader community health resources. At the same time, she or he is in a position to invite those in the broader society to reach into the local faith community for spiritual health resources. It is a pivotal location. As a ministry professional who works in collaboration with other faith group leaders, the faith community nurse is free to go out from the local congregation to meet, sojourn with, and accompany those awakening to health issues that are also faith issues. As a health professional, the nurse is also free to bring into the local faith community health resources that can also foster spiritual growth.

To speak of faith communities as places of seeking, therefore, is to see them as question-raising and explorative. In their outward reaching capacity, they seek spiritual sojourners in a multitude of dispersed places, providing an attentive and supportive presence. As *empowering places*, local faith communities welcome seekers into settings of safe and sacred space. Indeed, those who serve local congregations as faith group leaders and faith community nurses are in a unique position to foster enduring and unifying faith and health values. Envisioned as a form of community health center, local faith communities can say, "We are here" as agents of faith and health integration, of wholeness, both now and into the future.

ᴄ⃝ Summary

In this chapter, we explored local faith communities as places of seeking. We delved into questions that can be raised by registered professional nurses entering local faith communities to carry forward an intentional health promotion ministry. We also considered place as an entity related with one's physical, emotional, intellectual, social, and spiritual well-being. Furthermore, we considered questions that nurses may want to raise as they explore the multidimensional nature of place within local faith communities.

In addition to place, this chapter looked at the notion of seeking as an expression of both spiritual hunger and spiritual health. It highlighted the benefits of ministering to seekers by promoting inquiry, collaborative learning, skilled compassion, and appropriate referrals. Finally, the chapter attempted to draw the notions of both place and seeking together by considering faith communities as spiritual health centers. In this regard, faith community nursing is viewed as a unique ministry within local congregations that mediates faith seeking and health seeking through a collaboration with faith group leaders and community health resources. More will be said about these ideas in later chapters of the book.

Notes

1. The word *dialectic* means "to speak across." It comes from two Greek words, *dia* ("across") and *legein* ("to speak"). It is akin to *dialect*, and is essentially conversational, insofar as it reflects on ways of speaking across differences. It implies diversity, and can involve polarity, conflict, and struggle. For many hundreds of years, the word dialectic has been used by philosophers and theoreticians not only to describe a type of argumentation, but also to explore developmental processes.

2. Each faith tradition is the keeper of its own wealth of resources. Likewise, within each tradition, a person can find not only major themes of the spiritual life, but also significant subthemes pertinent to particular historical periods. *The Oxford Dictionary of World Religions,* by John Bowker (1997), has been a helpful starting point for me in discovering the spiritual and religious diversities that exist. In addition, faith community nurses may want to talk with one or several local faith group leaders regarding the spiritual literature that is available.

5 ❧

The History of the Relationship Between Nursing and Faith Traditions

Pauline Paul

This chapter provides an overview of the history of nursing, and illustrates how nursing has intersected with faith traditions. It is important to recognize that, to date, there has been little research related to this topic. This is not surprising, considering that the systematic study of the history of nursing is a relatively recent phenomenon. Likewise, it is only during the latter portion of the twentieth century that the study of women and women's activities has been increasingly recognized as a legitimate field of historical investigation. It is possible, however, to provide an overview of some aspects of this history based on general historical accounts and through the examination of selected nursing literature.

Essential to our discussion is the tenet that the history of nursing cannot be studied without taking into account the context in which nursing developed. As proposed in other sections of this book, the links among faith traditions, health, and healing seem universal in nature (Sullivan, 1989). Throughout history, human beings have also carried out activities that, today, we would consider to be within the realm of modern nursing. From a historical point of view, we can also affirm that the dominant views of any given society influence all forms of human activities; we can, therefore, state that the development of nursing is influenced by the views espoused by the society in which it develops.

To facilitate reading, this chapter is organized chronologically. First, I explore nursing in ancient times, defined here as before the common era (B.C.E.). This is followed by a more in-depth account of European nursing's place in the Christian faith tradition from the beginning of Christianity to the early 1800s. Emphasis is then given to the development of organized nursing in North America between 1639 and the late 1800s. I follow this with an overview of the history of modern nursing, with emphasis given to the American and Canadian contexts. Finally, I give an account of the birth and development of parish nursing in the United States, and briefly address its more recent migration to Canada and other countries.

It is important to acknowledge that the content of this chapter is colored by the availability of relevant literature in the English and French languages, by the fact that we, the authors of this book, are the products of Canadian and American societies, and that our Christian heritage also influences the way in which we view and understand the world. Those who write about history must be particularly cognizant of this reality, and they must acknowledge that those who wrote in the past were also the products of a given environment.

✍ Nursing in Ancient Times

Nutting and Dock (1907) were among the first to systematically document the history of nursing from ancient times to the modern era. Their work is frequently cited, especially in respect to the early history of nursing. These two authors, who are considered to belong to a select group of founders of modern nursing in North America, deemed it important to provide nurses with knowledge about the history of nursing from the beginning of time. Their writings are particularly important, because they acknowledged that although modern nursing was a new phenomenon, nursing itself certainly was not. They wrote, "The art of nursing, at once the oldest of the occupations of women and the youngest branch of medical science, must have been co-existent with the first mother who performed for her little ones all those services which made it possible for them to live and thrive" (p. 3).

Nutting and Dock (1907) described the healing arts in the ancient cultures of India, Ceylon, Egypt, Babylon, Assyria, Greece, Rome, and Judea. Included in this description is information about how religious beliefs colored activities related to healthy living and healing practices. In most of these cultures there is little evidence to indicate that nursing was an entity separate from medicine, yet it is very likely that activities similar to some of those found in modern nursing were being conducted. For example, Deloughery (1995) proposed that "much of the ancient Greek physician's craft falls under what modern nurses would claim as their practice" (p. 3). Although it is difficult to determine the extent to which the healing arts were performed by women, we do know that modern nursing is predominantly carried out by women.

The development of early nursing in India is unique. In contrast with other cultures, compelling evidence shows that nursing had an existence of its own, and that it was seen as an appropriate occupation for women. In the sacred text of Ayurveda (1500 B.C.E.), nursing is considered to be "one of the four legs on which therapeutic stands. The physicians, the drugs, the attendant [the nurse] and the patient constitute the four basic factors of treatment" (Ghai & Ghai, 1997, p. 131). There is also evidence that hospitals already existed in India in the third century B.C.E., that Buddhist monks had developed advanced surgical techniques, and that nurses cared for the patients treated by these surgeons. Excerpts from the text of Kasyapa Samhita published in Ghai and Ghai (1997) indicate that, to be good nurses, women had to "possess considerable intelligence, good education, healthy physique, good manners, an even temper, a sympathetic temperament and deft hands" (p. 132). The "good nurse" also had to be "knowledgeable, devoted to helping patients, clever and pure in body and mind" (p. 133). This description is remarkably similar to those written in the early twentieth century. The inclusion of the notion of purity, which has often been associated with the popular image of the nurse as an "Angel of Mercy," is particularly striking. The images of nursing throughout history are further discussed in Chapter 8.

❧ Nursing in Europe From Early Christianity to the Early 1800s

Hebrew and Christian scriptures espouse a holistic vision of human beings (Brittain, 1986). The Christian New Testament includes "more than forty stories of physical healings . . . which, with the discussion surrounding them, account for almost one-fifth of the whole text" (Catholic Health Association of Canada, 1996, p. 17). Carson (1989) and Wylie (1990) have noted that the authors of the four gospels show that Christ put great emphasis on healing and on psychological, spiritual, and physical health. This holistic healing mission has been continued by his followers, and particularly by members of nursing religious orders.

There is evidence that as early as the first century of Christianity, lay women of good social standing were appointed by bishops to visit the sick. Named deaconesses, these women performed functions similar to some of those of the modern community health nurse. One of the most famous of these deaconesses was Phoebe, a Greek women who delivered St. Paul's epistle to the Romans (Deloughery, 1995). According to Amundsen and Ferngren (1986), Christian concern, particularly for those in need, led to the establishment of the first Christian hospitals in the fourth century. One of the most well-known of these hospitals, the Basileias, was established around 372 by Basil the Great, Bishop of Caesarea in Cappadocia. This hospital had nurses, and it "provided a model for many others that spread throughout the eastern Roman Empire and from there into the West in the fifth century" (Amundsen & Ferngren, 1986, p. 49).[1]

The gradual appearance of religious orders devoted to the care of the sick, the wounded, and the poor was a result of these beliefs, and these orders largely contributed to the rise of nursing as an occupation primarily devoted to the care of human beings (Donahue, 1985). In the early Middle Ages, the role of the deaconess expanded in the Church of Rome. Famous deaconesses, such as Marcella, Helena, and Fabiola, devoted their lives to the care of the sick and the poor (Carson 1989; Donahue, 1985; Nutting & Dock, 1907). The simultaneous spread of the Roman Empire and of Christianity in Western Europe saw more women involved in the establishment of hospitals and monasteries, where nursing continued to flourish. For example, St. Brigid (425–523) established a monastery in Ireland (Dolan, Fitzpatrick, & Hermann,

1983), and Hildegard of Bingen (1098?–1179), who has been considered to be a physician, a nurse, and a scholar, did the same in Germany (Nutting & Dock, 1907). It is recognized that military nursing was also a development of the early Middle Ages, insofar as the Crusades gave rise to nursing orders devoted to the care of the wounded.[2]

The Renaissance, which began in the early 1400s, brought important changes to the Christian world.[3] Evidence suggests that the Reformation,[4] which was one of these important changes, had a profound impact on the development of nursing. The Reformation resulted in a division of the Western Church, and gave birth to new expressions of the Christian faith tradition; groups such as Lutherans, Mennonites, Presbyterians, and Anglicans, to name only a few, emerged as a result of this division. This historical event greatly affected the delivery of nursing care. In countries like France, where Roman Catholicism remained the primary religion, religious nursing orders continued their healing missions in ancient hospitals such as the Hôtel-Dieu of Paris (established in 650) and the Hôtel-Dieu of Lyon (established in 542). In fact, the Counter-Reformation, which occurred in France in response to the Reformation, gave a renewed strength to the Roman Catholic Church and its institutions.

The rise of Protestantism in other countries, however, generally brought the suppression of nursing religious orders and, with it, the disappearance of a large number of hospitals and organized nursing. England has been seen as the prime example of a nation where nursing entered a very dark period, lasting from the 1550s to the 1850s. In that country, the Reformation officially began when Henry VIII, in 1534, established the supremacy of the Crown over the church, rejected the Roman Catholic pope, and by doing so gave birth to the Church of England (Booty, 1986). By 1539, Henry had dissolved the monasteries, resulting in the elimination of nursing religious orders and of most of their hospitals. In practical terms, the nursing workforce was decimated, and the only means left to serve the sick and the poor, which some English citizens still believed needed to be done, was to hire women willing to replace the sisters. Since few volunteered, convicted women and others with limited options began to staff the few institutions that had survived. The image of Sairey Gamp, a character created by Charles Dickens, is a well-known symbol of what went wrong in British nursing during that era.

What were the cultural and social factors that led to this dark age of nursing? Among the many, two key factors need to be addressed in our discussion.[5] First, nursing in that era could be seen as a life-threatening occupation. The absence of vaccines, antibiotics, and other means for controlling the spread of infectious diseases meant that those who treated the ill often themselves became ill, a fact that played a significant role in making nursing seem unattractive. We can postulate that although women who entered religious orders faced the same dangers, their faith in God and their sense of vocation gave them the courage and fortitude to devote their lives to the care of the sick. Specific examples of this will be provided when I address early nursing in North America.

Second, members of Protestant groups became increasingly ambivalent toward the poor and the sick, a sentiment that corresponds to the values that accompanied the rise of capitalism in these countries. Donahue (1985) describes this ambivalence:

> The seeming ambivalence of Protestant countries toward the sick and the poor was the result of two conflicting influences: the desire to make money, to be rich and powerful, and the desire to be chosen of God by doing works that would provide a state of "grace." Laws and customs discouraged the humane care of the downtrodden and the weak, yet tremendous efforts were made to raise money to provide the necessities of life. (p. 193)

It must be mentioned that German Lutherans saw a rebirth of nursing's mission of healing through the work of two important leaders. In 1823, Amalie Sieveking from Hamburg began developing a sisterhood akin to the Roman Catholic Sisters of Charity, and 10 years later she organized a women's society devoted to the care of the sick and the poor. Inspired by her work, Lutheran pastor Theodore Fliedner gave a new life to the deaconess movement by establishing the first motherhouse at Kaiserwerth in 1836 (Lindberg, 1986).[6] An innovator, he began training salaried nurses. In 1851, Florence Nightingale spent a few months at Kaiserwerth, and this experience played a role in shaping her views about the need to educate nurses.

In summary, the early days of Christianity saw the rise of groups of women whose function was to minister to the sick. The orders of sisters and deaconesses of Europe, which arose over centuries as expressions of the varied Christian faith traditions, contributed to the development of organized nursing. The events of the English and French Reformation and Counter-Reformation illustrate the extent to which nursing was linked to faith traditions. The development of nursing in Canada and the United States further exemplifies this link.

∽ *The Development of Organized Nursing in Canada and the United States*

Nursing in the French and British colonies, established in the 1600s in areas of current Canada and the United States, reflected the systems and traditions that existed in their motherlands. It should, therefore, be evident from previous discussion that the provision of nursing services in the French colonies was very different from that offered in the British colonies. The fact that the French monarchy was supportive of the services offered by Roman Catholic nursing orders explains, in part, why organized nursing and hospitals almost immediately appeared in New France. Conversely, the fact that the British crown had eliminated these orders contributed to the much slower development of nursing and hospitals in the 13 colonies of New England. In their history of nursing in Canada, Gibbon and Mathewson (1947) write,

> If the settlements along the St. Lawrence River had been colonized in the seventeenth century by the English instead of by the French, the history of nursing in Canada might have been very different. Fate, however, decided in favor of the French, and that was fortunate for both the Huron and Algonquin Indians and for the white pioneers, since in the wake of the fur traders and *coureurs de bois*, came the Augustinian Hospitallers or Nursing Sisters of Dieppe to Quebec and the St. Joseph Hospitallers of La Fléche to Montreal on their missions of healing and of mercy—missions which had no counterpart in the colonizing efforts of the Protestant English in North America. (p. 1)

Hospitals appeared very rapidly in New France. Founded in 1608, Quebec City had its first hospital by 1639. In 1642, Jeanne Mance, a lay nurse and the cofounder of Montreal, immediately worked to construct a hospital in that community. This clearly shows that providing nursing services was considered a priority in New France.

Like other monastic orders, the Hospitallers of the Hôtel-Dieu of Quebec kept a detailed diary of their life in New France. *Les annales de l'Hôtel-Dieu de Québec, 1636–1716,* provides a rich account of the activities of the sisters and the faith that motivated them to help other human beings. The writings of Mother Marie-Andrée Regnard Duplessis de Sainte-Hélène, in 1648, are particularly interesting, because they show that the sisters were preoccupied with what we would today call health promotion activities:

> Every year, new French people came with their families to settle in this country; we helped them in many things and did not wait until they became sick to offer assistance. They found in our house the relief or at least the support which they needed and considered the Hôtel-Dieu to be their refuge. Also we were pleased to house them, feed them, and teach them about the customs of Canada, while they were building their own house. (Juchereau de Sainte-Ignace & Duplessis, 1939/1989, p. 71)[7]

In 1738, Marie Marguerite d'Youville founded the Sisters of Charity of Montreal, better known as the Grey Nuns. This was one of the greatest developments in New France nursing, because d'Youville created a noncloistered nursing order, which meant that her sisters could bring nursing services into the homes of those who were ill. For this reason, d'Youville is considered the mother of community health nursing in Canada, and during the nineteenth century, her Grey Nuns developed an unequalled tradition of nursing in the most remote areas of Western and Northern Canada.

Margaret Allemang (1985),[8] who has been instrumental in the development of the Canadian Association for the History of Nursing, summarizes the delivery of nursing care in New France as follows:

> The period dramatically illustrates a comprehensive type of community service in a precarious environment, conducted by women motivated by strong beliefs in Christian charity. This early model of community nursing developed at a time when two alien cultures met, medical science and technology were unknown, and trained nurses did not exist. Intuitive concepts of community nursing can be recognized in the relationships between the persons giving and receiving care, in the attention given to people without community supports, and in the stark political and financial problems that had to be confronted. . . . Their care was unconditional and beyond distinctions based on race, creed, culture, or nationality. (pp. 4-5)

As stated earlier, organized nursing care did not develop immediately in the British colonies. Nursing was left in the hands of a few individuals who did not have any particular training, but who were willing to assist those in need. "The English settlers," according to Donahue (1985), "lacked the organized service of the convent or the mission, the experience of nuns and priests. Consequently hospitals developed slowly in the original thirteen colonies. Social welfare was considered to be the responsibility of the individual, the family, or the neighborhood" (p. 269). Hospitals did not develop rapidly in the colonial United States. Donahue identified only five hospitals in existence before the American Revolution (1776–1784).

In the first half of the 1800s, Roman Catholic nursing orders devoted to the care of the sick began to spread in the United States. In 1809, Elizabeth Seton founded the Sisters of Charity of Emmitsburg, Maryland. In the years to follow, many orders began to offer services to the growing population. According to Doyle (1929a), between 1840 and 1871, 70 new hospitals either were established by or began their operation under the direction of Roman Catholic sisters. In 1849, the first Lutheran deaconesses arrived to take charge of the Philadelphia Infirmary, and they were soon followed by other deaconess nursing orders of the Lutheran Church and by sisterhoods of the Episcopal Church (Doyle, 1929b, 1929c).

One trend emerges when one examines the growth of nursing orders in the United States in the 1800s: Immigration played an important role in the establishment of orders devoted to the care of the sick. Immigrants coming from nations where nursing religious orders were present likely wanted to see the development of nursing services similar to those found in their motherland. To a large extent, one can follow the history of these nursing orders in the United States by examining immigration patterns; once a group reached a critical mass, an order of the religious denomination of that group became involved in the provision of nursing services. This trend can readily be seen, for example, with the establishment of Roman Catholic orders and hospitals in the Northeast once a critical number of Irish immigrants had settled in that area. Likewise, the rise of Norwegian Lutheran hospitals in the Midwest, where Norwegian immigrants settled, can be linked to these population movements. The nursing sisters and deaconesses offered important services to the population, and it is relevant to note that for immigrant populations the fact that these nurses shared their faith and could speak their mother tongue must have been comforting. That alone likely gave a holistic flavor to the services being offered. Similar patterns continued to be found during the modern era of nursing; the rise of Mormon nursing in Utah between 1890 and 1920 supports this hypothesis very well. As stated by E. Shaw Sorensen (1998), the birth of professional nursing in Utah emerged from women working in the context of their faith and culture.

✍ Modern Nursing: From the 1850s to the 1990s

Florence Nightingale (1820–1910) is considered by most to be the mother of modern nursing. As stated earlier, Nightingale was influenced by the work of Fliedner and the deaconesses. We know that she also sought instructions from Roman Catholic sisters who were well versed in nursing care. To a large extent, Nightingale adapted and refined methods she had learned in other parts of Europe; her talent resided in her political and organizational abilities, which led to the spread of her ideas and to a degree of fame achieved by very few other nurses. Of relevance to this chapter is the role she played in the development of nursing education.

In 1860, Nightingale opened the first official school of nursing in association with London's St. Thomas Hospital (Wake, 1998; Woodham-Smith, 1950). Nursing schools soon began to open throughout the Western world, and thus increased the opportunities for lay women to become nurses. This development was very significant, considering that until that time, and especially in countries where religious sisters were numerous, it had been difficult for lay women to choose nursing as an occupation; the creation of the Nightingale school was among the factors that contributed to removing the negative stigma previously associated with nursing. The fact that Nightingale developed her school at a time when Britain and other European countries were still significantly involved in colonial activities also led to the spread of Western nursing practices throughout other parts of the world; an important fact, if one considers that Western nursing, which had its roots in Christianity, was thus brought to countries where other faiths were predominant.[9]

Although schools of nursing rapidly spread through the Western world, a large number did not have financial independence from the hospital with which they were affiliated (Donahue, 1985; Ross Kerr, 1996a). This was an important departure from the Nightingale model, and it significantly contributed to the use of nursing students as the main hospital nursing workforce for decades to follow. The consequences of what Estelle Brown (1948) calls this "historical accident"[10] were important, and numerous contemporary writers in the field of nursing history have examined the long-term effects it had on the development of nursing and nursing education in North America. Authors such as Reverby (1982), Petitat (1989), McPherson (1996), and Ross Kerr (1998), to name only a few, have shown the negative impact that this error had, leading as it did to the exploitation of nursing students, contributing to the precarious conditions of employment in the field, and hindering the development of the discipline of nursing. To a degree, this situation contributed to the notion that the role of nurses was to serve in a totally altruistic way.

It is essential to mention here that the rise of the modern hospital also played a significant role in the development of modern nursing. Although it is beyond the scope of this chapter to examine the development of the modern hospital,[11] it is critical to note that the hospital became the workshop of medicine, and that gradually the poor and the rich became dependent on this institution for the delivery of curative medical and nursing services. From a relatively marginal institution, which in most parts of North America had predominantly offered services to the needy, the hospital became the key feature of the twentieth-century health care system. This growth meant, among other things, that nursing sisters and deaconesses increasingly had to rely on a lay nursing workforce, and that networks of hospitals not affiliated with religious denominations also developed at an unprecedented level.

We can hypothesize that these developments gradually altered the nature of the long association that had existed between nursing and Christian faith traditions; indeed, the evolution of nursing in French Quebec supports this theory. In that province, until the 1960s, health and social services, including nursing education, were almost entirely under the auspices of Roman Catholic sisterhoods. Nursing truly was seen as a vocation. This makes more visible than elsewhere the modification of the link between nursing and the Christian faith. As proposed by Petitat (1989), in that Canadian province during the 1900s, nursing evolved from a vocation to a profession.

> The mutation of nursing reflects a mutation of the internal logic of the profession: actions no longer have the same meaning, neither in terms of relationship to the self, nor in terms of the relationship to the patient.... The moral logic or the religious logic is replaced by the scientific logic; the logic of giving to others first is replaced by the logic of collective bargaining. (p. 16)[12]

These words echo those of Barnum (1996), who writes about the changes that took place in the United States. She states that nursing students were once taught to care for the body, mind, and spirit of their patients; later, after adopting the scientific ideology, they were taught to care for the biopsychosocial being.

Barnum (1996) notes that during the biopsychosocial era, from the late 1950s to the 1980s, students learned little about the spirit. They were taught about special diets and rituals of religious practice; they also learned from one another not to venture into what was seen as the territory of the chaplain or clergy. Articles published in the *Canadian Nurse* and the *American Journal of Nursing*, the nursing journals with the greatest circulation in each country, reflected these trends.[13] However, a few articles showed that important questions were being asked. For example, Schumacher (1964), a nursing leader in Alberta, proposed that it was not sufficient to phone and invite a pastor to visit or to report that someone wanted to take communion; nurses themselves needed to pay attention to spiritual issues. Acknowledging that scientific medicine had brought important gains, she also wrote,

> There is a growing uneasiness that in the process something was lost—a genuine concern for the true worth and dignity of every person. We have erred in fragmenting man. The ill have spiritual needs equally important with their physical and emotional needs. Recognizing this, we are attempting to see them as a whole human being, realizing that a man's spirit may affect his body, that his interior strength (or lack of it) may be a real factor in recovery. This is not a new idea; rather it is the re-discovery of an old one. (p. 774)

Ashbrook (1955), an American clergyperson, echoed Schumacher's call, stating, "We acknowledge the nurse's obligation to meet her patient's physical and emotional needs, but what of his spiritual and religious needs?" (p. 164).

Meanwhile, Wallace (1967), a Canadian chaplain, stated that chaplains were not an excuse for nurses to avoid personal involvement with patients in the dimension of the spirit. Sister Dickinson (1975), an American nurse, wrote that referring patients to chaplains was insufficient, stating that "to redefine spiritual care, we do not need a watered-down version of past religious practices but a broader grasp of man's present search for meaning and a practical way of integrating spiritual care in every day nursing" (p. 1789). Ellis (1980), a Canadian nurse, wondered why it had almost become taboo to discuss spiritual matters and religion with patients, writing,

> Did not nursing historically develop in a religious milieu in which love of God and mankind was expressed through care, compassion and charity to the sick, the poor, the orphans and the outcasts? . . . The spiritual dimension is not a separate department of an individual's life but an integrated and integrating force of the total person. (p. 42)

Early in this chapter, I stated that the history of nursing could not be examined without taking into account contextual factors. North American authors writing about current trends and issues in the nursing profession have shown that these factors play a role in the life of the profession.[14] They have, for example, documented the roles played by the changes in the status of women, the dramatic growth of university education after World War II, changes in healthcare systems, and economic factors that affect the supply and demand for healthcare professionals. It is likely that some of these factors, by having an impact on nursing, have helped to alter the link between nursing and the Christian faith tradition. Other factors, such as the sexual revolution of the 1960s, the rejection of authority characteristic of our era, Vatican II, and the secularization of North America, were also probably instrumental in reshaping this link. It is difficult, however, to make a definitive statement about the recent history of the relationship between nursing and faith traditions, because we are still too immersed in this period of time. The historian of the future will be in a better position to examine the recent and current nature of this link, and to establish which factors were the most determinant.

Changes made for numerous reasons, not necessarily related to the link between nursing and faith traditions, may also have affected this relationship. For example, between the 1960s and the 1980s, nursing education rejected many of the rituals that had marked the life of generations of nursing students. In particular, capping ceremonies and the use of nursing caps were abandoned. The capping ceremony of the past, we should note, was intertwined with symbols linked to the Christian tradition, and to a sense of hierarchy and authority. Older nurses certainly recall the white candles, the kneeling, and the admonitions to service that marked these ceremonies. The degree of connection between a school and a specific Christian faith group also shaped the extent to which these events included a component reflecting that particular faith.[15] We cannot say if this movement away from rituals related to an alteration of the relationship between nursing and faith traditions, if it played even a small role in changing this relationship, or if the change was primarily related to other societal factors. However, it remains that the reduction of ritual in nursing occurred during the period when nursing and the Christian faith tradition seemed to be growing apart.

As I stated earlier, some nurses in the 1960s and 1970s were asking questions about spiritual matters in nursing and about the apparent shift that had taken place in the previous decades. Nurses were not the only individuals wondering about the spiritual dimension or about its role in the health and life of Americans and Canadians. For Barnum (1996), societal manifestations of this new quest of the 1980s were represented by the growth of self-help groups, increased questioning within the Christian faith tradition, and emerging New Age ideologies. Barnum also proposes that the rise of parish nursing is an effect of this resurgence in spiritual seeking among both nursing groups and the general population.

✍ The Birth and Development of Parish Nursing

Parish nursing has its roots in the work of Granger Westberg (1913–1999), who in the late 1960s and 1970s worked with physicians, nurses, pastoral counselors, and congregations to establish Holistic Health Centers (Westberg, 1990a). Although these centers showed that they could contribute to the provision of holistic care, it was soon realized that they were too expensive to sustain. However, Westberg had observed that the nurse's role in these centers seemed to provide the "glue" connecting the faith community with the medical community. Evaluators of the program from nonreligious backgrounds noted that

> most of the nurses employed in these clinics could speak two languages: the language of science and the language of religion. The

nurses were translators. They helped the doctor and the minister communicate in ways that were helpful to a "whole person" approach to health care. (Westberg, 1990a, p. 28)[16]

In 1984, Westberg approached the Lutheran General Hospital in Park Ridge, Illinois, and asked them to become involved in a pilot project that would link their institution with six local congregations who would each have a parish nurse (Djupe, Olson, & Ryan, 1994). The functions of parish nurses are discussed in other chapters of this book; however, it is relevant to state that parish nursing seems to be reclaiming aspects of nursing that were cherished earlier in the profession's history. Parish nurses are concerned with caring for people as more than biopsychosocial beings. Like nurses from past eras, they consider the spiritual dimension to be important to human health. They also provide services directly to the community, and, like the first nurses of North America who came to New France in 1639, they do not wait until people are sick to assist them. They are health promoters, and this makes them very much in touch with the 1990s.

The first parish nurses in the Westberg project must have brought something important to the members of faith communities, because the number of parish nurses exploded during the next decade. By 1994, there were 2,500 parish nurses in the Midwestern United States alone (Djupe et al., 1994). Recently, Olson, Clark, and Simington (1999) have documented the development of parish nursing in Canada; likewise, Australian parish nursing developments have been described by Van Loon (1999).

◡ꙅ *Summary*

We have seen in this chapter that nursing existed in ancient civilizations, but that it emerged as a distinct entity with the birth of Christianity. We also examined how generations of nursing sisters and deaconesses were the main providers of nursing care in the West. To them, nursing was a form of ministry, and by helping others who were healthy, sick, or in need, they were emulating the work of Christ. We saw how contextual factors played a role in the development of nursing in Europe and North America. Addressing the birth of nursing in Canada and the United States showed that the early nurses of our countries were the product of the dominant faith traditions and cultures of their European homelands. We examined the role played by Florence Nightingale, looking in particular at her experiences with deaconesses and nursing sisters. We have seen that modern nursing evolved in a society where values, beliefs, and authority were increasingly questioned, noting that during this period the link between nursing and faith traditions became blurred. However, as we enter a new millennium, nursing may be recapturing some of its roots, and parish nursing is a concrete manifestation of this phenomenon. It may well be that the roots of nursing, which grew from generations of nurses, are talking to us, and letting us know that the role of the nurse is, was, and will be to assist human beings in holistic ways, and that faith traditions can be important in achieving this goal.

Notes

1. It is necessary at this point to refer to the Great Schism, which divided Christianity into the eastern church (the Eastern Orthodox Church, also known as the Byzantine Church), which emerged in Byzantium, the eastern part of the Roman Empire, and the western church (Roman Catholicism), which emerged in the western part of the empire, what is roughly western Europe. This division took place over a long period, spanning from the ninth to the thirteenth centuries, and was caused by cultural, political, liturgical, and doctrinal factors (see Harakas, 1986). In this chapter, we primarily focus on nursing in the West, and thus on the Western faith traditions.

2. Major armed conflicts are not positive events. However, they have played important roles in the development of nursing and medicine. For example, the Crimean War of the 1800s was instrumental in the refinement of Nightingale's views about nursing, and significant advances were made in the field of surgery during World War II.

3. The Reformation and the travels of Europeans to the Americas are two examples illustrating aspects of the rebirth (the meaning of the word *renaissance*) that was taking place in the old continent.

4. The Reformation of the sixteenth century was initiated by Martin Luther (1483–1586), and gave birth to the Protestant churches of Europe.

5. Some of the other factors not discussed here are the place of women in society and the belief that poverty and illness were the result of laziness and bad behavior.

6. Fliedner was also influenced by the English Quaker Elizabeth Fry and the Mennonite deaconess movement of Holland (Lindberg, 1986).

7. The original text in seventeenth-century French reads as follows:

Le païs se peuploit tous les ans par de nouveaux François qui amenoient leurs familles pour s'y établir; nous les aidions en bien des choses, et nous n'attendions pas qu'ils fussent malades pour les secourir. Ils trouvoient dans nôtre maison le soulagement ou du moins la consolation dont ils avoient besoin, et regardoient l'Hôtel Dieu comme leur azile. Aussy nous faisions nous un plaisir de les loger, de les nourrir et de les instruire des usages de Canada, pendant qu'ils préparoient leur demeure. (Juchereau de Sainte-Ignace & Duplessis, 1989, p. 71)

8. Dr. Margaret Allemang is professor emerita of nursing from the University of Toronto. She has been instrumental in the development of the Canadian Association for the History of Nursing.

9. Bringing western nursing practices to these countries was not without difficulties. Hermani (1996) writes about the early years of western nursing in India and Pakistan, stating,

Admissions to nursing were exclusively reserved for Anglo-Indian and Europeans, . . . thus both Hindus and Muslims were prevented from enrolling in nursing programs. A primary reason for this policy was prohibition by their own culture. The caste prohibitions among Hindus, especially Brahmins, the upper religious class, promoted the belief that touching or coming in contact with any physical thing was not hygienic and forbidden for them.

Current issues related to the appropriateness of being a nurse in some Muslim groups have been well documented. See, for example, El-Sanabary (1993) and Mura and Mura (1995).

10. This term was used by Estelle Lucille Brown, an important nursing leader in the United States. See Brown, E.L. (1948). *Nursing for the future*. New York: Russell Sage Foundation.

11. For an in-depth analysis of the development of the modern hospital, see Rosenberg (1987) and Rosner (1982).

12. The original citation in French reads as follows:

Cette mutation de la médiation infirmière recèle une mutation de la logique interne de la profession: les actes n'ont plus la même signification, ni par rapport à soi, ni par rapport au patient. . . . La logique morale ou religieuse s'efface devant la logique scientifique; la logique du renoncement fait place à celle des syndicats. (Petitat, 1989, p. 16)

13. A systematic review of these two journals revealed that, between 1945 and 1980, articles related to religion spirituality mainly addressed these topics.

14. For more information, see Deloughery (1995) and Ross Kerr and MacPhail (1996).

15. Popular histories of schools of nursing usually offer detailed descriptions of these ceremonies.

16. These words are particularly striking to me because they evoked the words of Emile Legal (1916), a Roman Catholic bishop, who stated that nursing sisters were to take care of body and soul; they were to be competent to assist physicians and priests.

6

The McGill Model of Nursing

Joanne K. Olson

In this text, as we have said, a faith community nurse is defined as a registered professional nurse hired or recognized by a faith community to carry forward an intentional health promotion ministry. As a ministry team member, the nurse works with others who have been prepared in various disciplines, such as theology, education, the behavioral sciences, and the fine arts. Each professional brings to the team a perspective unique to that individual's discipline. It is out of this diversity that the beauty and challenge of team ministry is born. As a professional registered nurse, the faith community nurse carries out a professional role using a set of assumptions, values, and ideas that form an explicit or implicit nursing conceptual model. Simply stated, conceptual models are the road maps that guide a professional's practice on a day-to-day basis, and they flow out of the worldview the professional holds regarding the concepts central to a particular discipline. In this chapter, we will discuss what it means to operate out of a nursing frame of reference, and examine the concepts considered central to all nursing professionals: *health, person, nursing,* and *environment*. We will consider various ways that these terms can be viewed (i.e., the ways in which they are worldviews), as well as how a faith community nurse might think about these important concepts.

Although there are a number of nursing models used by parish nurse practitioners (Bergquist & King, 1994; Bunkers, 1998, 1999), we focus on the McGill model of nursing. The McGill approach has been valued in Canada for over two decades, and we believe it has tremendous relevance for broad-based application to faith community nursing. To encourage additional investigation into this model's assumptions and core concepts, this chapter will be devoted to discussion of the McGill model of nursing (Gottlieb & Ezer, 1997). Later chapters will draw on these foundations in applying theory to faith community and parish nursing practice.

✍ Nursing Conceptual Models and Worldviews

All nurses have private images of their nursing practice. These private images influence how individual nurses interpret information, make decisions, and act in relationship to the people to whom they give care (Reilly, 1975). These images could be referred to as the nurse's personal conceptual model of nursing. When nurse leaders make formal presentations of or publish their private images of nursing, these conceptualizations become one of the many models of nursing. These published conceptual models facilitate discussion and communication among nurses, and provide a systematic approach to nursing practice, education, and research (Fawcett, 1995).

What are the concepts that are central to the nursing discipline and about which nurses need to communicate? Fawcett (1995) describes four generally accepted concepts of interest to nursing: *health, person, nursing,* and *environment*. Together, these four concepts form nursing's "metaparadigm," or the phenomena of central interest to the nursing discipline (Fawcett, 1993). Each nursing conceptual model involves a unique definition of these terms, as well as a description of how these terms relate to one another in the practice of professional nursing from that model's perspective. In most of nursing's conceptual models, *health* is the goal of nursing care, the reason for nursing action. (See

Chapter 3 for various definitions of health.) Each model identifies how a *person* is viewed, and whether individuals, families, communities, or other types of groups are considered recipients of nursing care. In describing *nursing,* a model usually defines the actions taken by nurses either on behalf of or in conjunction with the *person,* the desired goals or outcomes of nursing actions, and how nursing action is carried out within that particular nursing model. Finally, each nursing model defines *environment* as the context within which persons move toward health.

A worldview can be described as a particular way of viewing the phenomenon of concern within a discipline. Our worldview filters what we see, hear, and experience about the people for whom we care. Parse (1987), for example, identifies two main ways of viewing the phenomena of concern to nursing: the totality paradigm, and the simultaneity paradigm. Fawcett (1995), on the other hand, presents three different worldviews: the reaction worldview, the reciprocal interaction worldview, and the simultaneous action worldview. When comparing these various paradigms, we can sense a tension between mechanistic and relational understandings of how people achieve and maintain health. The paragraphs that follow describe these worldviews further. We suggest that, in reading the descriptions of these worldviews, you consider how a nurse with such views, working within a faith community, might view health, persons, environment, and nursing.

If a nurse sees people and the world through what Parse (1987) identifies as the *totality paradigm,* persons are not only complete, total persons, but also a sum of their parts, the combination of biological, psychological, social, and spiritual features. Furthermore, in this worldview, the environment is seen as both internal and external to the person, consisting of stimuli with which the person interacts, and to which he or she adapts to maintain balance while striving toward health, a state of well-being. The nurse in this worldview is the prime decision maker, with limited involvement from the person being cared for. Parse (1987) credits nursing's emergence as a natural science alongside medicine as the main reason that the rather mechanistic views of the totality paradigm have dominated nursing's thinking for quite some time. She argues that the nursing models developed by Roy (1976, 1984), Orem (1985), and King (1981) fall within this worldview.

In contrast, Parse places her own work (Parse, 1981) and that of Martha Rogers (1970) in the *simultaneity worldview*. In this paradigm, persons are viewed as more than and different from the sum of their parts. People are open, free beings who can make their own choices while living in a mutual rhythmical interchange with their environment. Health in this view is seen as a process of becoming, something that can only be experienced and described by the individual. There is no optimal level of health; health is how one experiences personal living. The goal of nursing includes a focus on quality of life from the person's perspective. The prime decision maker in this paradigm is the person rather than the nurse.

Fawcett (1995) uses three categories to label various nursing worldviews, but the similarities with Parse's two categories can easily be seen. Sometimes referred to as a mechanistic worldview, the *reaction worldview* addresses the needs of a compartmentalized human being. The person responds in a reactive manner to environmental stimuli. Stability rather than growth is valued, with change occurring only for survival purposes. In the *reciprocal interaction worldview*, humans are seen as holistic, yet also made up of parts. They are active and in reciprocal interaction with their environments, although here, too, change occurs in individuals mainly for the purpose of survival. In the *simultaneous action worldview*, persons are seen as more than and different from the sum of their parts. There is mutual, rhythmic, and constant change in both the person and the environment. In this view, growth and change are seen as positive, and health is considered a process rather than a state.

How would a nurse practicing in a faith community view the concepts *health, person, nursing*, and the *environment*? I ask this of nurses preparing to be faith community nurses because, articulated or not, they all have ideas about the nature of these terms. Classroom discussions reveal that most faith community nurses believe that health is very different from "no disease." They know well from experience that people living with disease can be quite healthy, and that those with no diagnosed disease can be quite unhealthy. They see change and health challenges as possible opportunities for growth in people, families, and communities. Furthermore, students in my classes view persons as biological, psychological, social, and spiritual beings. Faith community nurses give great emphasis to seeing people as spiritual beings in constant relationship with others and with a divine being. They see life as a sacred gift in trust from God, however God or the divine being is defined.

Finally, most faith community nurses, no matter what their personal faith beliefs are, want to function from a nursing model that views people broadly enough to include all faith traditions and perspectives. In their view, the role of the nurse is to help people grow and change, using all available resources. The nursing assessments and interventions used by these nurses include those that are physical, psychological, social, and spiritual in nature. These nurses know that spiritual distress, if left unattended, may later surface in psychological pain or physical illness. They know, too, that people's overall health would be enhanced if they could be taught to reach deep within for the resources that result from spiritual growth and development; moreover, these nurses see themselves only as facilitators of health and healing, believing that all true healing comes from a higher source. Faith community nurses generally define environment as both internal and external surroundings, with the important difference that these surroundings include the faith community environment. People who are members of a faith group share common beliefs and values, gather together regularly to outwardly express their inner beliefs through worship, and provide social support to one another on a regular basis.

Our next challenge is to review existing nursing models to see which ones are compatible with the views of faith community nurses. If nursing models were placed on a continuum, we would find the more mechanistic models of Roy (1976, 1984), Orem (1985), and King (1981) at one end, and more relational models, such as the McGill model or the views of Rogers (1970) and Parse (1981, 1987) at the other end. From the description of the worldviews of faith community nurses, it is clear that there is a leaning away from mechanistic ways of viewing nursing, and a gravitation toward more relational nursing models. As mentioned earlier, models such as those of Parse (Bunkers, 1998, 1999) are being used to guide nursing practice in some faith communities. In this book, we have selected the McGill model of nursing for several reasons. First, it focuses on health promotion. It also has an emphasis on strengths and potentials; it features the process of inquiry; it focuses on the relationship that develops during shared learning; and, finally, it is compatible with and understood by other professionals who minister within a faith community setting.

✎ Development of the McGill Model of Nursing

The McGill model of nursing was developed by Moyra Allen and other faculty at the McGill School of Nursing, McGill University, Montreal, Quebec, Canada. Beginning in the early 1970s, the principles of the model have guided nursing education in Quebec and other parts of Canada for over two decades. Moreover, the model has changed nursing care practices in many health care agencies in Canada, the United States, and even Asia (Gottlieb & Ezer, 1997). Impetus for the model's development largely grew out of changes in Canada's healthcare system in the early 1960s, when healthcare services became universally available to all Canadians. With the thought that nursing would play a major role in the restructured healthcare system, many debated what the nursing role would encompass. Many nurse leaders encouraged the development of nurse practitioners to extend physician services within Canada. Moyra Allen (1979), however, argued that a new way of practicing nursing was needed:

> The major shortcoming of our present health insurance plan is that, although it has undoubtedly improved the organization and delivery of health care, it is providing the same type of health care as in the past, mainly diagnostic and curative with some prevention. This type of health care has been viewed as satisfactory by health care planners to the extent that it is available, accessible, and universally distributed. To this end, we have seen a resurgence of ideas relative to health care planning—availability of services at the local or community level, health professionals working together in teams, and a rational distribution of the tasks of health professionals. Herein lies the basic fallacy: the assumption that we need more of the same type of health care, and that the real problems are ones of organization and delivery of health care services. (p. 56)

Later, Dr. Allen (1981) spoke about the real health problems that face society:

> It is said that cancer and cardiovascular disease are the two major health problems in our society. However, the real populations at risk are families. We are burdened with unhealthy families whose development in living leads not to better health, but to disruption, divorce, loss of job, juvenile delinquency, battering, mental illness, crime, and on it goes. In spite of our enviable health manpower situation in Can-

ada, the greatest portion of sickness and death relates to the consequences of destructive lifestyles and health practices. (p. 153)

Rather than expanding the nurse's role into the medical domain,
Allen (1977) envisioned nurses functioning in a "complemental role."
She firmly believed that nurses possess knowledge and skills different
from and complementary to physicians and other professionals. Furthermore, their range of knowledge and skills were being wasted if
they were merely doing more of what was already being done in
healthcare. Moyra Allen envisioned a healthier society brought about
through the health promotion activities of nurses collaborating with
individuals and families. The model she developed, then, addressed a
gap that existed in Canadian healthcare services. Allen (1997b) said
that "this gap is demonstrated in the lack of community resources
whose primary goal is directed toward the healthy development of
families throughout their lifespan" (p. 165). Long before the health
reform sweeping North America in the 1990s, Moyra Allen saw the
importance of moving healthcare into the mainstream of community
settings.

✍ *Assumptions and Concepts Basic to the McGill Model of Nursing*

Congruent with the definition of health promotion in the Ottawa Charter (World Health Organization, 1986), the McGill model of nursing
enables people to increase control over and improve their health. It is
unique in its emphasis on the family as client and on the empowerment
approach to the process of health promotion. We will now examine the
assumptions that underlie the McGill model, and consider each of
nursing's metaparadigm concepts as described in this model. While
reading about these assumptions and concepts, continue to think about
the potential fit between the McGill model and faith community nursing practice.

Assumptions

In a conceptual model, any basic belief of the theorist accepted
without empirical testing is called an assumption (Kravitz & Frey,
1989; Stevens, 1979). Central to the McGill model is the underlying
belief that the health of a nation is its most valuable resource (Gottlieb

& Rowat, 1987; Kravitz & Frey, 1989). The similarity between Allen's beliefs and those published in health minister Marc Lalonde's *A New Perspective on the Health of Canadians* (1974) can easily be seen. As Lalonde himself articulated it, "Good health is the bedrock on which social progress is built. A nation of healthy people can do those things that make life worthwhile . . . and good physical and mental health are necessary for the quality of life to which everyone aspires" (Lalonde, 1974, p. 5).

Following also from the Lalonde report, the second assumption of the model is that individuals, families, and communities aspire to, are motivated toward, and strive for better health. In other words, the potential to develop and achieve better health resides in people themselves (Gottlieb & Rowat, 1987; Kravitz & Frey, 1989). The belief that this "better health" is best learned through active involvement and personal discovery is the third assumption of the model. Additional assumptions include a belief that health is a phenomenon of the family, and that nursing is a primary health resource for families and communities (Gottlieb & Rowat, 1987; Kravitz & Frey, 1989). Following from these assumptions is a belief that nurses have the necessary broad knowledge and skills to be a primary health resource through a variety of nursing roles in society (Gottleib & Rowat, 1987).

Core Concepts

Health. We considered, in a previous chapter, how the essential elements of health as discussed in the McGill model contrast with other possible ways of viewing health. We will now expand on that introduction. Moyra Allen (1997b) said, "The quality upon which the nurse focuses is health . . . [the nurse] is oriented to the health aspect of the patient/client situation across settings—hospital, home, or other community facility" (Allen, 1997b, pp. 166-167). For Allen, the phrase "health aspect" meant "the patient/client/family's accommodation to, dealing with, or coping with events of daily living including both customary and unusual or crisis situations" (p. 167). Health is not a state, but a developmental process, the intentional work of achieving life's goals (Warner, 1981). Health, then, becomes something that can be learned; disease, however, is more a phenomenon of the individual. Health is an attribute learned in the context of the family or group to which a person belongs.

Most critical to the McGill model definition of health is the idea that health is not part of a health-illness continuum, and it is not a state or an end point. Rather, health and illness are viewed as very separate entities that can coexist, but that are not on the same continuum (see Figure 6.1).

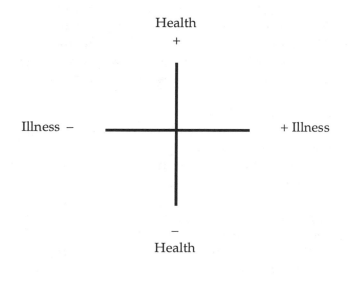

Health

+

Illness –   + Illness

–

Health

Figure 6.1. The Relationship Between Health and Illness

Source: This figure originally appeared in "The Health Dimension in Nursing Practice: Notes on Nursing in Primary Health Care," by M. Allen, 1981, *Journal of Advanced Nursing, 6,* p. 154. Copyright 1981 by Blackwell Science, Ltd. Reprinted with permission.

The most desirable situation is when there is much health and no illness. Less satisfactory states include times when there is no illness, but feelings of health are low, or when there is illness, but also a high level of health. The least desirable state is when there is illness and also little health (Kravitz & Frey, 1989). Subsumed under the definition of health are two processes: the process of coping and the process of development (Gottlieb & Rowat, 1987). Coping refers to efforts made specifically to deal with a problem. Development, in contrast, is not problem oriented; it refers to recognizing, mobilizing, maintaining, and regulating resources that reside within the individual, family, and the larger social context (Gottlieb & Rowat, 1987). The focus of nursing, then, is on the health aspects of people's situations: The nurse looks for potential and strength, rather than for areas of weakness (Kravitz & Frey, 1989).

It should be noted that, in this model, *learning* is viewed as a bridging concept, because it relates to several of the metaparadigm concepts, especially health. First, this model holds that persons—individuals, families, and communities—have the capacity to learn. Second, health itself is viewed as a learning process. The environment, then, is seen as the context for learning. Finally, knowing how people learn is considered knowledge basic to effective nursing care (Kravitz & Frey, 1989).

We should remember that when a nurse focuses on health rather than illness, illness is not being ignored. Rather, it is subsumed by the focus on how the individual, family, or community copes with and manages the impact of illness (Kravitz & Frey, 1989). Furthermore, as Feeley and Gerez-Lirette write, "Illness and the related issues are viewed as only one aspect of a family's health concerns" (Feeley & Gerez-Lirette, 1997, p. 300). The overall health of the individual and family is the nurse's primary concern (Allen, 1997b). Speaking as a nurse using the model in a hospital ambulatory setting, Tyler (1997) says, "The nurse does not abandon helping the family to understand and follow treatment and medication schedules prescribed, but fits this in an overall context of health that allows the exploration of other issues which are important to the family" (p. 328).

Person. In the McGill model, the "person" or unit of concern is the family, because the individual's health needs to be considered within the context of the family. Furthermore, health is seen to be learned in a family context (Gottlieb & Rowat, 1987). Much as individuals can be understood through cultural and faith "filters" (Burley-Allen, 1995; Jones, 1989, 1992), individuals need to be seen through a family filter (Allen, 1997b). The McGill model broadly defines the family as any natural living group in which learning takes place (Allen, 1982a). Families are viewed as subsystems within such larger systems as communities. From a systems perspective, nurses need to see families as having shared history, emotional and instrumental needs, developmental stages and tasks, boundaries, subsystems, roles, rules, and myths (Wright & Leahy, 1984).

Individuals and families are viewed as being on a life journey, where change and challenges are inevitable. At the same time, the individual and the family are seen as active problem solvers capable of learning new ways to cope with situations and problematic events. Each experience is thought to serve an educational function, where the family learns something in the process. Underlying the model is the belief that the solutions to problems or situations exist within the family and individual, and do not come from the nurse. The individual and family, then, are active participants in seeking healthier living, and the nurse collaborates with the family in achieving the goals they have set for themselves (Gottlieb & Rowat, 1987). This model operates from an empowering position, where the individual and family are seen to possess strengths, resources, and the energy needed to work on their own health issues. The nurse "coaches" the individual and family, using knowledge of the principles of health promotion and strategies based on knowing how people learn.

Nursing. In the McGill model, health is the primary focus of nursing (Attridge, Ezer, & Macdonald, 1981), and health promotion is nursing's primary goal (Gottlieb & Rowat, 1987). Within this broad view of nursing, there are few limits to what legitimately falls into the nurse's role (Attridge et al., 1981).

Rather than function as an expert, directing the care of individuals or families, nurses using the McGill model work collaboratively with individuals and families, functioning in the following roles: awareness raiser, coach, coordinator or liaison, resource, focuser, integrator, listener, negotiator, provider of care, reinforcer, supporter, role model, and stimulator. What, then, is the act of nursing in this conceptual model? Kravitz and Frey (1989) suggest that

> nursing is . . . a professional response to the person's natural search for healthful living. Nursing engages the client-family in the search for healthy being. The nurse structures and tailors appropriate learning situations wherein clients have access to pertinent health information, opportunities to discuss and share, and are able to test appropriate action plans. (p. 314)

As described, then, "this nursing role of health promotion is complementary to the medical role of preventing or treating illness" (Murphy, 1997, p. 288). The nurse possesses knowledge and skills different from and complementary to those of the physician (Feeley & Gerez-Lirette,

1997). For example, in an ambulatory care setting, nurses demonstrated their knowledge of the impact of chronic illness on individuals and families, as well as their expertise in areas such as nutrition, growth and development, the family life cycle, community resources, and strategies for pain relief. Nurses are able to provide long-term support to families, playing a key role in helping them learn to cope with or anticipate health-related situations. When carrying out these roles, the nurse works in partnership with the family, because each has their own areas of expertise. The family is expert in knowledge of themselves as a family, but the nurse brings skills in helping families to identify, prioritize, and plan strategies to achieve their goals for health (Feeley & Gerez-Lirette, 1997).

In any nursing model, the nursing process usually consists of assessment, planning, intervention, and evaluation phases. The process of nursing in the McGill model is a situation-responsive approach that emphasizes the family as client, and seeks to work with families over a period of time (Laforet-Fliesser & Ford-Gilboe, 1997); it places the nurse-client relationship at the center by focusing on the health aspects of their situation, and, throughout the relationship, emphasizes the client's concerns, strengths, and potentials. Collaboration between the nurse and the client or family is the key to each phase of the nursing process. The data collection and assessment phases of the nursing process are open, exploratory, and ongoing. The McGill plan focuses on the strengths, resources, and positive forces in the family (Attridge et al., 1981).

Warner (1997) describes using the McGill model as a knowledge-seeking way of nursing, a type of nursing that depends largely on a process of inquiry. She divides the nursing process into three phases: the *exploratory phase,* the *working phase,* and the *discovery phase,* which correspond to Allen's (1997b) *assessment, practice mode,* and *evaluation* stages. If we think about health as something that is learned, it makes sense that the nursing process would begin with an exploratory phase (Warner, 1997). This is the time when a nurse becomes initially acquainted with a family and their health-related issues, and begins to involve the family in actively working on the issues and learning to be healthy. A working phase follows, in which the nurse collaborates with the family in developing a plan for the steps that will be taken to deal with the health-related issues facing them. The nurse gives the family space and time to begin testing out their own ideas so that they get satisfaction from their efforts without much interference from the nurse. In the discovery phase, the nurse and the family review the previous two phases to discover which actions can be linked with which consequences.

The *assessment* or exploratory phase is marked by attempts to obtain an overall profile of the client or family, and of the health issues with which they are living. The nurse seeks answers to the following questions, sometimes referred to as the "questions to guide inquiry": What is the client or family working on or dealing with? What does the family want, or what is the family working toward? How is the family going about it? What is the family's potential to develop and find healthier ways of living? What resources are the family using, and what others could be mobilized? What aspects of the broader context of family life might explain the family's present health behavior or situation? (Allen, 1986, 1997b; Warner, 1997). While seeking answers to these questions, the nurse is already including the family in information-gathering activities, thereby fully involving them in work on their own health-related issues. At the same time, the nurse is searching for family strengths that can later be used as the basis for future health promotion activities. This phase ends with the nurse and family negotiating a way to continue working together, with roles and expectations of the relationship being clearly defined.

In the *practice mode*, also called the working phase, nursing practice becomes more focused (Warner, 1997). It begins with a summary of the outcomes of the first phase. The nurse states health-related issues in terms of the goals of the family, what they want to accomplish during the nurse-family relationship. The nurse next leads sessions that focus on strategic planning with the family. A plan of action is drawn up after the family brainstorms about ways of dealing with the health issues on which they are working; the strategies are then considered in light of existing resources, as well as additional resources that the nurse can bring to bear on the situation. Next, the nurse allows the family time to try out the plan that they themselves have established with coaching from the nurse.

In the final phase of the nursing process, the *evaluation* or discovery phase, the nurse and the family reflect back, evaluating their relationship and how the plans have worked in moving the family closer to their health goals. The nurse includes herself or himself in the reflection process, because each nursing situation is an opportunity for the nurse to learn alongside the family.

Environment. Drawing on social learning theory, environment is defined as those social contexts in which healthy living is learned: the home, school, workplace, community group, hospital, or clinic (Gottlieb & Rowat, 1987; Kravitz & Frey, 1989). People and their environments, in the McGill model, are not viewed as separate entities, but are seen to be in constant interaction with each other. Nursing is capable of structuring environments that assist individuals and families in learning new ways of dealing with situations, thereby achieving healthy ways of functioning (Gottlieb & Rowat, 1987).

✍ *Relevance of the McGill Nursing Model to Faith Community Nursing*

It is significant to note that, in working with professionals in pastoral care ministry, the congruence between the conceptual models from which ministry personnel function and the McGill nursing model are pronounced. At least three similarities surface immediately in discussions of how both disciplines approach interactions with people. First, life is viewed as a journey; in the case of faith community leaders, life is viewed most often in terms of a faith journey. Second, both groups are familiar with the process of inquiry; such a questioning approach is the basis of the McGill model of nursing, and in a pastoral care ministry, it is natural to use a process of inquiry in learning about the faith tradition of another. Finally, in models of pastoral care ministry, the focus is on emphasizing and building on people's strengths, and on seeking answers and resources from within the person. The consistency between the ideas of health promotion and faith development will be expanded further in future chapters of this text.

7

The Nurse and
Theological Reflection

Margaret B. Clark

In an earlier chapter, we described *theology* as *reflection and celebration around experiences of being in relationship*. This description situates theology at the service of *spirituality*, in the same way that reflection is at the service of experience (Hellwig, 1992). Both individuals and groups have experiences of being in relationship with the self and others, including transcendent or divine others. These experiences constitute a person or group's spirituality; they also form the foundation for a person or group's theology. Thus, we can speak of marital or family spiritualities, as well as of theologies of marriage and the family. Perhaps one day soon, we will also be speaking about spiritualities and theologies of faith community nursing. Moving from experiences of being in relationship with the self and others to an exploration of one's theology is the work of theological reflection (Shea, 1997).

In this chapter, we will look at the definition of theological reflection provided by Patricia O'Connell Killen and John deBeer in their book *The Art of Theological Reflection* (1994). We will then explore the implications of this definition for faith community nursing by developing four approaches to theological reflection: theological reflection as a way to self-knowledge, as learning about others, as discovering the collective story of a faith community, and as doing social analysis. In order to promote and benefit from a more in-depth exploration of each of these approaches, we then look at some of the tools for theological reflection that are available to nurses working in faith communities. Finally, we will present a conceptual framework for theological reflection that draws all four approaches together in one diagram. The diagram is intended to serve as a resource for nurses who enter faith communities to carry out the unique functions of parish nursing (Holstrom, 1999). It is also meant to assist nurses facing complex relational experiences within their various faith group settings in choosing which of the four approaches to investigate more deeply as they make theological reflection an integral dimension of their work.

✍ What Is Theological Reflection?

According to Killen and deBeer (1994), theological reflection is, first, "the discipline of exploring individual and corporate experience in conversation with the wisdom of a religious heritage" (p. 51). Second, in theological reflection, "the conversation is a genuine dialogue that seeks to hear from our own beliefs, actions, and perspectives, as well as those of the tradition. It respects the integrity of both" (p. 51). Third, theological reflection may "confirm, challenge, clarify, and expand how we understand our own experience and how we understand the religious tradition" (p. 51). Finally, the outcome of theological reflection is "new truth and meaning for living" (p. 51).

Looking at this complex definition, we can abstract its key elements. First, theological reflection is a discipline; and it is in particular a discipline of exploring individual and corporate experience. *To explore,* according to the dictionary, means "to cry out" (*Webster's,* 1991). It involves investigation, study, and analysis. The focus of exploration is experience, and this emphasis on experience is in keeping with what previous chapters of our book have been saying about faith and spirituality as preconditions for theology. When individuals and groups are able to "cry out" from within the uniqueness of their experience, they further the work of theology.

Second, exploring involves conversation. The conversation being proposed here is a *dialogue*, which means "to speak across" (*Webster's*, 1991). Dialogue is also what Paul VI (1964) called "the art of spiritual communication" (p. 36), characterized by clarity, meekness, trust, and prudence. In Killen and deBeer's definition, there are two main dialogue partners: The first is a person's "beliefs, actions and perspectives," and the second is the "wisdom of a religious heritage" (Killen & deBeer, 1994, p. 51). Both individual and communal points of view are integral to the conversation of theological reflection; if one of the partners dominates the other, dialogue is impeded. Both the person and the tradition need to coexist in a relationship of mutuality in order for theology to flourish.

Third, successful dialogue requires that both partners in the discourse be viewed with respect. Respect derives from the ability to see another as distinct and separate from oneself. The Latin root *respicere* means to "look at," in the sense of looking back on or reexamining. The implication is that the dialogue process is one of continual review and repeated encounter with the other until it is seen for what it is—or they are seen for who they really are. As a relational activity, respect requires that a person think, reason, question, and wonder until they get below the surface of the obvious, and perceive the deeper issues. In this sense, we may say that respect is a way of seeing another into visibility. Thus, as a person becomes visible to the tradition, and as the tradition becomes visible to an individual, there can be a rich exchange of not only deductive, reason-based principles, but also inductive, experience-based narratives.

Fourth, theological reflection will have an impact on how experience is understood. As an individual or group and a religious heritage get to know one another through exploration, dialogue, and respect, changes begin to occur in the ways they experience both themselves and one another. Seeing, hearing, touching, tasting, inquiring, and imagining give way to the discovery of meaning. This is what one theologian refers to as understanding (Lonergan, 1957, 1972). Likewise, with one's understanding "confirmed, challenged, clarified and expanded," there is a possibility for individuals or groups to weigh the evidence of increased awareness, and to discern "new truth and meaning for living" (Killen & deBeer, 1994, p. 51). Thus, experience flows into understanding, and understanding provides insight for evaluating, choosing, and implementing what one has understood.

We believe Killen and deBeer (1994) provide a definition of theological reflection that is broad enough to be used by a number of faith traditions and cultures: It recognizes both individual and communal experiences; it proposes an environment of exploration, dialogue, and respect; and it anticipates change occurring through the four activities of confirmation, challenge, clarification, and expansion. Furthermore, with the inclusion of ongoing change, theological reflection becomes an ongoing process; that is, reflection changes us, change proceeds to new experiences, and these new experiences invite further reflection in a perpetual cyclic process. Finally, the definition used by Killen and deBeer communicates a sense of hopefulness about the outcomes of theological reflection. As new truth and meaning are generated, living is fostered. Since in our book we are interested in nursing within a faith community as a ministry of health promotion among those who are living in times of transition, we believe that new truth and meaning for living is not only an outcome of theological reflection, but also a sign of hope and health.

✐ Four Approaches to Theological Reflection

Theological reflection needs to be appreciated as a multifaceted activity. To begin with, it fosters self-knowledge in the nurse who seeks to function as a spiritual caregiver within a faith community. In the unique functions of parish nursing (Holstrom, 1999), for example, nurses come to know themselves in new ways. Experiences of changing self-awareness awaken questions about meaning and purpose in the nurse. At such times it is important for a nurse to reflect theologically on her or his personal and professional identity, to ask the following questions: What does it mean to call myself a parish nurse or a faith community nurse? How do I experience myself being a spiritual caregiver? How do I understand my nursing as a foundation for ministry? If I were to observe myself doing faith community nursing, what would I see? Each question is an entry point to theological reflection as an activity of self-discovery.

Another facet of theological reflection has to do with learning about others. While working in faith community settings, nurses will get to know many types of people. These may include individuals during all phases of the life span, families in various aspects of their development, groups or aggregates of people with differing needs or interests, and large assemblies gathered to worship around many types of events. In keeping with the whole-person approach characteristic of the nursing profession, it is important for faith community nurses to develop spiritual assessment skills that are well grounded and comfortably integrated into their nursing practice. Furthermore, it is important for them to see spiritual assessment as something distinct from, but also related to, theological reflection. That is to say, spiritual assessment is a way of listening to other persons as they relate with themselves, their social networks, cultural heritages, faith traditions, life events, and transforming experiences. While attending to the spiritual may mean identifying spiritual distress (Kim, McFarland, & McLane, 1989) or recognizing a human dimension that transcends one's biological and psychosocial nature (Reed, 1998), it can also mean listening to a person speak about divine beings, experiences of evil, a sense of vocation, memories of previous incarnations, and mystical approaches to self-transcendence.

Theological reflection as an activity of learning about others may lead the nurse to entertain some of the following questions: What is the person's story? What relationships are uplifting for the person? What relationships are troubling to the person? Are there beliefs, symbols, or rituals that figure prominently in the person's experience? How do faith, spirituality, theology, and religion play a part in the person's current circumstances? How is the person's spiritual health or distress related to other dimensions of the person's total health or distress? Information gathered through questions like these are a form of spiritual assessment that parallels theological reflection as an activity of learning about others. The complementarity of both activities working together can help the nurse know how to respond with spiritual caregiving.

In addition to self-knowledge and learning about others, theological reflection has to do with discovering the collective story of a faith community. Each faith group is situated within a network of beliefs, values, and assumptions. Some of these derive from religious tradition; others are rooted in geographical, sociopolitical, or cultural perspectives. One of the tasks of a nurse beginning to work within a faith community is to gain an appreciation for that community's uniqueness. What are the faith filters that guide the community to think, choose, and act the way it does? Who are the storytellers in the faith community? What types of experiences do they include in their history, and what do they leave out? Who are the heroes and heroines of the faith community? Who are the troublemakers and villains? What faith traditions are referred to? Would this community, in light of its religious heritage, be considered conservative, moderate, liberal, radical, or some other such term? Questions like these will enable the nurse to learn about the community's unique qualities, and to discover its collective faith story.

Finally, theological reflection has to do with social analysis. Each faith community exists within a broader sociocultural context. This may include local neighborhoods, businesses, and resources; it may also broaden to include society at large as a complex, high-tech, multicultural, and multifaith global civilization. In some instances, a faith community's vision may even include an awareness of itself in relationship with Mother Earth, seeing our tiny planet, situated within a solar system that is located among millions of other solar systems, spin both mysteriously and scientifically in an incomprehensibly far-reaching universe (Swimme, 1984). The possibilities are many. It is not enough, therefore, for a nurse to reflect theologically in isolation; rather, she or he will benefit from reflective processes that dialogue with a world where structures of globalization have an ever increasing effect on the ways in which we communicate, purchase goods, invest resources, and experience health.

Nurses who are able to draw on a variety of tools for theological reflection will be better equipped in their role of linking faith with health. This requires some familiarity with theological studies; it also requires awareness and appreciation of the complex fields represented by both behavioral and health sciences. Issues of increased self-awareness, spiritual consciousness, social justice, global harmony, and universal well-being do not need to be split off from practical nursing interventions. Nor do these issues need to become central to all forms of nursing care; rather, with the support of skills developed in the area of theological reflection as social analysis, nurses can think globally and act locally. Questions similar to the following may foster this type of holistic approach: How broadly does the faith community think beyond itself? How is the faith community perceived by those in the local neighborhood? How aware is the faith community of educational and health resources in the area? In what ways does the faith community reach out to those whom society considers "different," "strangers," "unimportant," or "a threat"? How does the faith community draw on its religious heritage to inform itself in matters of involvement with other faith groups, cultural practices, and sociopolitical issues?

Together, the four approaches of self-knowledge, learning about others, discovering the collective story of a faith community, and social analysis constitute the rich subject matter for theological reflection by faith community nurses. In order to facilitate a more in-depth exploration into each of these approaches, we will now look at some of the tools for theological reflection that are available to nurses working in faith communities.

✐ Tools for Theological Reflection

The tools presented here are nothing more or less than conceptual frameworks through which theological reflection can be carried forward. They assume faith (understood here to mean being in relationship with) and spirituality (understood as experiences of being in relationship with). Each tool seeks to promote reflection on one's experience. Each tool can be used by anyone, though our focus is on nurses working within faith community settings, whom we believe will enjoy these tools and benefit from their use in accomplishing the unique functions of parish nursing (Holstrom, 1999). We believe, furthermore, that faith community nurses will increasingly enjoy and benefit from their use of these reflective tools if they also seek to gain familiarity with the language and study of theology.

Every academic discipline and, likewise, every profession has its own terminology or jargon. Thus, when nurses use the term "BP," we know they are talking about blood pressure and not British Petroleum. Likewise, when theologically educated faith leaders use terms like "Practical" or "Systematic," we know they are speaking about fields of study within theology, and not about a need to be more organized. In the field of faith community nursing, we have members of one profession entering professional working relationships with members of another profession. Thus, faith community nurses and theologically educated pastoral leaders need to learn from one another about the academic disciplines and professional languages that inform their respective work.

There are definite background and language differences that need to be taken into account. One way to conceptualize these differences is by means of the following comparison: For the past fifteen years I have worked as a hospital chaplain, which situates me in an environment where the predominant language derives from medicine and other health care disciplines. By contrast, the language of my profession derives from theology and the behavioral sciences. In order to communicate effectively within the hospital context, I have needed to study basic medical terminology and to understand a number of fundamental healthcare concepts. With this additional learning, I am better able to bring my theological background and faith-based perspective to the healthcare setting. In a similar fashion, the nurse who seeks to practice within a faith community enters an environment where the predominant language derives from religious or faith traditions and theology. In order to communicate effectively within this context, faith community nurses need to study basic theological terminology and to understand a number of fundamental concepts related to religious heritage. With this additional learning, the nurse will be better able to bring her or his nursing background and health-based perspective to the congregational setting.

Professionally prepared nurses working within faith community settings do not seek to replace other ministry professionals or to duplicate the functions of other faith group leaders; rather, the unique role of the faith community nurse is to carry forward an intentional health promotion ministry. This requires education in the fields of both nursing and theology to foster familiarity with the two languages of health and faith. In this way, faith community nurses can become the kind of translators Granger Westberg (1990a) envisioned them to be, and a greater depth of communication in matters of faith and health will be fostered.

Theological Reflection Tools for Self-Knowledge

Reference has already been made to Killen and deBeer's *The Art of Theological Reflection* (1994). It is an excellent resource for nurses working within faith community settings in two ways: First, it can help nurses gain knowledge about themselves as theologically reflective persons, and, second, it is a resource that nurses can use in helping members of their faith communities grow in self-knowledge through theological reflection. A basic assumption of the book is that, if we look honestly at our life, it will lead us to the tradition; and if we openly enter the tradition, it leads us to our lives. This is a circular thought well worth pondering.

According to Killen and deBeer (1994), if we slow down our "habitual processes of interpreting our lives," we will arrive at a better understanding of the "frameworks for interpretation" we are using (p. x). A first step in slowing down is to catch ourselves in one or another of three "standpoints" named in the book. First, there is the standpoint of *certitude.* This is when we "see the unfamiliar only in terms of what we already believe" (Killen & deBeer, 1994, p. 4). In this stance, predetermined categories filter our new experiences and constrain their meaning. There is a danger that this filtering process, when exclusive of other points of view, can result in our "entering the tradition" in ways that fail to lead us to life. The danger with this stance is that we can come to exclude other points of view, that we become advocates of the philosophy that it is "either our way or the wrong way." Such thinking is self-limiting.

The second standpoint is that of *self-assurance.* This is when we look honestly at our life, but do so in such a way that it fails to lead us to the tradition. We think, when we are in this stance, that what we think and feel, right here and right now, is all that matters. The risk in this is that "we do not notice distortions or inaccuracies in our perspectives on life" (Killen & deBeer, 1994, p. 11). We can become isolated and rigid.

The third standpoint provides us with greater balance. It is the standpoint of *exploration.* From this standpoint, a circle of communication and discovery can be created between personal experience and the wisdom of religious heritage. It is a place of "paying careful attention to where we are" (Killen & deBeer, 1994, p. 16), and then moving onward from that point with curiosity and a desire to learn. Killen and deBeer (1994) encourage us to seek the standpoint of exploration.

When we open ourselves in exploration, we experience our human "drive for meaning," and awaken a reflective "movement toward insight" (Killen & deBeer, 1994, p. 20). This movement toward insight, according to Killen and deBeer (1994), is both the "human process of coming to wisdom" (p. 20), and the threshold of theological reflection (p. 46).[1] What they develop is a five-part process of making meaning that involves the following steps: (a) entering into experience, (b) encountering feelings, (c) working through these feelings with the images that arise from them, (d) recognizing insight as the fruit of working with images, and (e) putting insight into action. We move from human reflection into theological reflection when we connect the human process of coming to wisdom with the collective wisdom of a faith tradition—the sacred texts, stories, teachings, and popular lore of a religious heritage.

The major part of Killen and deBeer's *The Art of Theological Reflection* (1994) develops a framework through which exploration can occur in a four-part dialogue. The four points of entry to dialogue are through an individual or group's (a) positions—convictions, beliefs, and opinions; (b) culture—ideas and artifacts, social structures, the physical environment, and so forth; (c) lived narratives—stories and events that make up our day-to-day living; and (d) the faith tradition. In Killen and deBeer's approach, the process of discovering how to engage in theological reflection is so gentle and natural that, before one knows it, one is thinking theologically. In the rich blend of down-to-earth stories and exercises provided in the book, nurses within faith community settings will be able to integrate skills and insights as they also come to know themselves in new ways. They will then be in a position to facilitate use of this process of making meaning among those with whom they work.

In addition to the tools provided in *The Art of Theological Reflection* (Killen & deBeer, 1994), faith community nurses may want to access a variety of other tools for personal growth and continuing education. These could include workshops on a number of topics related with self-discovery and self-care, personal journal writing, an independent or guided reading program, vision quests, dream awareness groups, personal therapy, and book or journal article study clubs. Faith community nurses might also enroll in college or university courses in the fields of practical, pastoral, or spiritual theology, or in clinical pastoral education (CPE), where their work in faith community nursing is the focus of personal and supervisory learning. Finally, nurses will benefit from annual retreat experiences with other nurses working in faith community settings, as well as with parish nurse interest groups established by their provincial or state nursing associations. The important thing is for the nurse to continue learning and growing holistically. Such ongoing development among faith community nurses is a necessary element for the therapeutic use of self in one's nursing profession.

Theological Reflection Tools for Learning About Others

Although spiritual assessment and theological reflection are distinct activities, we believe spiritual assessment is one way of engaging in theological reflection. Spiritual assessment seeks to learn about others in a particular dimension of their experience, the *spiritual* dimension; it rests, however, on an assessment of the whole person. Currently, a number of spiritual assessment tools exist, and additional instruments are being developed all the time. These instruments need to be examined carefully to ensure that they include not only human and religious approaches to spiritual health, but also the broad spectrum of a person's experiences of being in relationship with self and others (including divine and/or transcendent others).

An author from within the pastoral care field who has done some clarifying and innovative work in this area is George Fitchett. In his role as Director of Research and Spiritual Assessment in the Department of Religion, Health and Human Values at Rush-Presbyterian–St. Luke's Medical Center in Chicago, Illinois, he has worked closely with nurses and other health professionals. His first book, *Spiritual Assessment in Pastoral Care: A Guide to Selected Resources* (1993b), provides not only a summary of the literature studied by Fitchett, but also a process through which future searches of the literature on spiritual assessment can be conducted. Fitchett evaluated models of spiritual assessment according to six criteria: (a) applicable contexts, (b) concept of spirituality, (c) relation to other disciplines, (d) norms against which the client or parishioner is being assessed, (e) connection to the ministry process, and (f) user friendliness. He then went on to organize those various models of spiritual assessment into ten types:

- Overviews of spiritual assessment
- Historical models
- Models based on the work of Paul Pruyser (1976)
- Models based on the work of Edgar Draper (1965)
- Models based on the work of James Fowler (1981)
- Models designed for the hospital context
- Models designed for the outpatient context
- Models designed for the hospice context

- Nursing models

- Research models

What George Fitchett found was that, in all the models he studied, no model existed that was both functional and multidimensional. As a result, he wrote a second book, *Assessing spiritual needs: A guide for caregivers* (1993a). This book was initially directed at pastoral care providers whose methods of spiritual assessment Fitchett had observed in his role as a clinical pastoral education supervisor. What he found in that role was that the focus of education in pastoral care has been in four areas: (a) the sharing of relevant knowledge from the behavioral sciences, particularly psychology; (b) the attainment of counseling skills; (c) the integration or correlation of psychology, counseling, and the behavioral sciences with theology; and (d) the development of the self and of the identity of the pastoral caregiver (Fitchett, 1993a).

He goes on to say, however, that "in none of these areas has assessment been a major focus" (Fitchett, 1993a, p. 15). Thus, the introductory section of his book emphasizes the importance of spiritual assessment as a foundation for action, communication, relational or social contracting, evaluation, personal accountability, quality assurance, research, and as the touchstone of a profession's identity. Fitchett concludes this section with a statement that, we believe, affirms the point we made earlier about spiritual assessment being one way of doing theological reflection:

> Emphasis on the importance of assessment is rooted in the conviction that revelation about the divine nature and foundation of existence is continuing and that it proceeds through persons. . . . Attentive listening to another is attentive listening to God. . . . In assessment we are concerned to know how God is at work, in ourselves or in another, and to consider what implications that knowledge has for our lives. (Fitchett, 1993a, p. 23)

The remainder of *Assessing Spiritual Needs* introduces Fitchett's own spiritual assessment model. He calls it the "7 × 7 Model" (Fitchett, 1993a, p. 39). It begins with an assessment of seven holistic dimensions of the person, which is followed by a seven-part exploration of spirituality. Fitchett (1993a) believes that our "spiritual lives in general and our spiritual needs and resources at any particular moment are strongly influenced by what is happening in the rest of our life. . . . Our spirits are not separate from our bodies, our emotions, and our thoughts. . . . [E]ach of us is one whole person" (p. 42). Holistic assessment explores a person's (a) physical dimension, (b) psychological dimension, (c) psychosocial dimension, (d) family systems dimension, (e) ethnic and cultural dimension, and (f) societal issues dimension. Based on the foundation created by these first six dimensions, holistic assessment then goes on to explore (g) the spiritual dimension of the person. This spiritual dimension is, in turn, assessed through the seven approaches of

- Beliefs and meaning
- Vocation and consequences
- Experience and emotion
- Courage and growth
- Ritual and practice
- Community
- Authority and guidance

Together, Fitchett's *Spiritual Assessment in Pastoral Care* (1993b) and *Assessing Spiritual Needs* (1993a) provide excellent resources for accessing tools of spiritual assessment. They also reinforce the idea that spiritual assessment is one way of doing theological reflection. Finally, they provide a means through which the nurse working within a faith community can gain a great deal of information in learning about others.

Theological Reflection in Discovering the Story of a Faith Community

The nurse entering a faith community is keenly aware that this community does not exist in isolation from its religious tradition or the surrounding culture. In fact, the community's experience of itself is shaped in part by these aspects of interconnectedness. In order to discover the collective story of a faith community, a nurse will need to familiarize herself or himself with both the tradition and culture of that community. A helpful resource in this endeavor is *Method in Ministry*, by James D. Whitehead and Evelyn Eaton Whitehead (1995). Although their book has a Christian emphasis, we believe the principles they address can be reflected on by a number of faith traditions.

According to the Whiteheads (1995), theological reflection in ministry is the process by which "a community of faith engages the religious information" gained from tradition, experience, and culture "in pursuit of insight that will illumine and shape pastoral response" (p. x). The reader will notice the compatibility between this definition and that of Killen and deBeer (1994). There is, however, also a notable difference; in the Whiteheads' approach, it is "a community of faith"—and not the individual alone—that enters into theological reflection, and this reflection is in pursuit of "pastoral response."

In a manner similar to Killen and deBeer, the Whiteheads (1995) see the central activity in theological reflection being conversation. They believe that participating in a conversation reminds us that "pastoral reflection is meant to be a communal exercise, not a monologue nor a lecture" (p. 4). Furthermore, such a "community dialogue is a habit, both pleasurable and painful, in which our faith is tested and matures" (p. 4). From these starting points, the Whiteheads go on to develop both a *model* and a *method* for doing theological reflection in ministry settings. In their words, the *model* "points to the participants in the conversation, helping us recognize the different voices and alerting us to their authority" (p. 4). Participants identified by this model are the religious tradition, the surrounding culture, and the experiences of a believing community. The *method* "shows us how the conversation proceeds—how the different participants in the dialogue present their case, engage one another, and move toward a practical response" (p. 4). Elements of the conversational process include attending, assertion, and pastoral response.

The model of theological reflection proposed by the Whiteheads (1995) looks at religious tradition in two ways. First, the model sees religious tradition as pluriform, which is to say that it assumes there will be a variety of expressions of belief and practice within a faith tradition. Second, religious tradition is ambiguous; in order to arrive at clarity or certainty, a faith group will usually need to travel a path of obscurity, doubt, and confusion. Indeed, the core beliefs of most religious traditions include assertions that appear both profound and inconceivable. Sorting through these ambiguities is one task of theological reflection.

The Whitehead model also views surrounding culture in two ways. First, as with the religious tradition, the surrounding culture is seen to be pluriform. There are many cultures and subcultures in every faith community; some commonly understood variables of culture are nationality, age, gender, race, religious heritage, office or role, access to information or privilege, and life circumstances. Second, in addition to being pluriform, the surrounding culture is also ubiquitous, meaning "existing or being everywhere at the same time" (*Webster's*, 1991). We have all had experiences of noticing something new, and then seeing it everywhere. This type of personal experience has a cultural parallel, sometimes referred to as a *paradigm shift* (Barker, 1992; Kuhn, 1970). Within the twentieth century, for example, we have seen the introduction of electronics and computer technologies. Over a period of less than four decades, we have come to see computers everywhere; that is, they are ubiquitous. Understanding the importance of these sorts of cultural shifts, and discerning their relationship to the core teachings of a faith tradition, is another important task of theological reflection.

The Whiteheads' use of the word *experience* in their model reinforces insights in Killen and deBeer (1994) that we discussed earlier. One point worth noting, however, is the Whiteheads' emphasis on communal, as well as personal, experience, which complements our own emphasis on discovering the collective story of a faith community.

In addition to the model, there is a three-stage method of theological reflection put forward by the Whiteheads (1995). Their method "suggests a process by which we pursue this communal discernment" (p. 13). The first stage in the Whiteheads' model is *attending*. To attend, according to the Whiteheads, means "to listen critically while suspending judgment" (p. 14). The second stage in the method is *assertion;* assertive engagement, according to the Whiteheads, is a style of behavior that "acknowledges the value of one's own needs and convictions in a manner that respects the needs and convictions of others" (p. 15). The final stage is one of *pastoral response,* which involves "moving from discussion and insight to decision and action" (p. 13). It requires planning, acting, and evaluating.

The majority of *Method in Ministry* (1995) discusses theological reflection at work in a variety of pastoral settings. It includes a chapter contributed by Peter Buttitta (1995) on "Theological Reflection in Health Ministry: A Strategy for Parish Nurses," which introduces parish nurses to a way of theological thinking that seeks to discover the collective story of a faith community. With the aid of this book and the tools it provides, the nurse will be better able to become familiar with the body of religious teachings, practice, and polity held by the faith group; and this familiarity will both shape the relationship being formed between the nurse and faith community, and contribute to the effectiveness of the faith community nurse's ministry of spiritual caregiving.

Theological Reflection in Doing Social Analysis

The final approach to theological reflection we will discuss in this chapter is that of social analysis. This term assumes that a faith community exists in connection with expanding spheres of relationship. For example, if a parish nurse were to study church bulletins and information boards within the faith community, she or he would discover a rich network of individuals, businesses, church organizations, and global concerns. As humans, we exist in relationships, not in isolation. In order for the parish nurse to be an "integrator of faith and health" (Holstrom, 1999), she or he must be able to recognize linkages between local, civic, state or provincial, national, and global faith and health communities. The metaphor of a pebble being dropped into a tranquil body of water is often used to demonstrate this point: From the central point at which the pebble enters the water, a ripple occurs that reaches far beyond the point of entry. In a similar way, beliefs, values, assumptions, and activities within a faith community can have far-reaching implications.

In the mid-1980s, at approximately the same time parish nursing was gaining popular recognition, Joe Holland and Peter Henriot wrote *Social Analysis: Linking Faith and Justice* (1986). Their work evolves from two important premises: First, they point to culture as a key to the ongoing creative transformation of human civilizations; second, they see the task of theological reflection to be that of linking "faith energies with energies of justice and peace" (p. xiv) in the service of a divine-human creative transformation. "Our path back to healing," they say, "is via the human, but through the human to the divine. . . . The human is not safeguarded without its foundation in the divine, and the divine is not accessible except through the human" (p. xviii). They propose social analysis as a tool connecting human and divine energies, and as a vehicle for channeling these energies into pastoral action.

According to Holland and Henriot (1986), social analysis is "the effort to obtain a more complete picture of a social situation by exploring its historical and structural relationships" (p. 14). Their book suggests we analyze the following dimensions to social situations: distinct issues such as unemployment or hunger; the policies that address these issues, such as job training or food aid programs; the structures of economic, political, social, and cultural institutions out of which such issues arise and to which such policies are addressed; and the systems on which the economic, political, social, and cultural structures are based, such as ideologies, organizations, or behavior patterns, and so forth. In order to conduct a social analysis, Holland and Henriot say that it is important to explore a number of societal elements, including the historical dimensions of a situation, structural elements of the situation or society, the various divisions of a society, and multiple levels of the issues involved. What this approach does is foster the art of observation. It is like standing in the basket of a hot air balloon as the balloon begins to lift above the surface: As it rises higher and higher into the air, the observer is able to take a broader look at structures, patterns, and unique features in the geography below. In relationship with theological reflection, social analysis looks out at a faith community setting and identifies the broad historical, social, economic, political, and religious concerns that are operative.

A nurse who is familiar with community health nursing will recognize the affinity between social analysis and community assessment. At the conclusion of Holland and Henriot (1986), the reader will find two questionnaires: "Beginning Social Analysis" and "Evaluating Social Action Responses" (pp. 106-112). As the faith community nurse reads through the questions provided in these questionnaires, as well as in a number of other sections of the book, she or he will find helpful ways to reflect theologically on the links between local and global communities, faith and justice, and faith and health.

∽ Drawing the Four Approaches Together

Figure 7.1 provides a conceptual framework for theological reflection that draws together the four approaches addressed throughout this chapter. It is a conglomerate composed of the sphere of experience depicted by Killen and deBeer (1994, p. 60), the triangular model of James and Evelyn Whitehead (1995, p. 6), and the pastoral circle of Holland and Henriot (1986, p. 8). We believe it can assist the nurse who is working within a faith community to make theological reflection a more integral dimension of her or his ministry.

Conceptual Framework for Theological Reflection

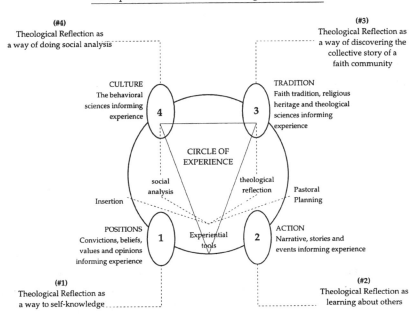

Figure 7.1. Four Approaches to Theological Reflection

Source: This conceptual framework is based on graphics found in *Social Analysis: LinkingFaith and Justice,* by J. Holland and P. Henriot, 1986, p. 8 (Copyright 1986 by the Center for Concern. Reprinted with permission); *The Art of Theological Reflection,* by P. Killen and J. deBeer, 1994, p. 60 (Copyright 1994 by Kathleen O'Connell Sievers. Reprinted with permission); and *Method in Ministry: Theological Reflections and Christian Ministry,* edited by J. D. Whitehead and E. E. Whitehead, 1995, p. 6 (Copyright 1995 by Sheed & Ward. Reprinted with permission).

In the diagram, one sees a circle of experience. Near the circumference are four entry points into this circle. These are *positions, action, tradition,* and *culture.* Inside the circle is a triangle, which connects *culture* and *tradition* with *experiential tools. Experiential tools* are also linked by proximity with positions and action. The terms *insertion, pastoral planning, social analysis,* and *theological reflection* are also situated both inside and outside the circle, with a connection to experiential tools. Finally, there is a line drawn from *culture* to *social analysis,* and another line from *tradition* to *theological reflection.* Each of these concepts and terms are taken from the sources referred to previously (Holland & Henriot, 1986; Killen & deBeer, 1994; Whitehead & Whitehead, 1995).

When working in a faith community, a nurse will encounter a number of experiences inviting theological reflection. At times, the experience will originate from within the nurse, awakening questions of meaning and purpose. In terms of our diagram, at this point the nurse is standing at the entry point of *positions* (#1). The way into greater depth of awareness and understanding is through theological reflection, which fosters self-knowledge. Examining one's beliefs, values, convictions, and opinions will lead the nurse into relationship with action, tradition, and culture, but the weight of attention will be on the development of the nurse in her or his unique identity and on parish nursing functions.

At other times, the experience will originate within a parishioner, faith group leader, or community event. Here, the nurse is at the entry point of *action* (#2). Now it is important here to approach theological reflection as a way of learning about others. Drawing on holistic spiritual assessment tools will lead the nurse into relationship with tradition, culture, and self, but the weight of attention will be on respecting the story and the uniqueness of the other.

At still other times, and especially when first entering a new faith group setting, the focus of experience will be on the faith community in its uniqueness. Here, the nurse is at the entry point of *tradition* (#3), and it is important to approach theological reflection as a way of discovering the collective story of the faith community. Using tools that emphasize theological reflection as a faith community endeavor will put the nurse in touch with culture, self, and actions of others, but the weight of attention will be on various forms and ambiguities within the religious tradition.

Finally, there will be the times when societal issues are the focus of attention in the circle of experience. This is when the nurse is at the entry point of *culture* (#4), and will benefit from seeing theological reflection as a way of doing social analysis. Instruments that explore the links of faith and justice, combined with community assessment tools that explore connections between faith and health, will serve the nurse well as she or he attempts to discern how the local is global, the personal is political, and so forth. Again, social analysis will put the nurse in touch with self, others, and a faith tradition's rich heritage, but the weight of attention will be on the issues, policies, structures, and systems emanating from society as a whole.

In conclusion, we hope this conceptual framework, which brings theological reflection into the domains of self-knowledge, learning about others, discovering the collective story of a faith community, and social analysis, will foster nursing practice. We believe that in the ongoing process of experience and reflection many things occur, including personal growth, interdisciplinary professional learning, individual or family healing, and theology as reflection and celebration on experiences of being in relationship. The faith community nurse who is able to approach theological reflection holistically can serve as a unique resource in linking faith and health. Drawing on tools gained from a variety of approaches to theological reflection, a faith community nurse can facilitate exploration into the broad spectrum of relationships included in the concept of theology.

Note

1. For a more detailed discussion of the process of coming to wisdom, see Chapter 2 of Killen and deBeer's *The Art of Theological Reflection* (pp. 20-45). For more on theology as a form of reflection, see Chapter 3 of the same volume (pp. 46-75).

PART III

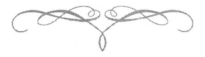

NURSE AS HEALTH PROMOTER

8

Images of Nursing

Joanne K. Olson

Many congregations express interest and enthusiasm about having a nurse on their ministry team. However, on closer examination of how this would be implemented, the question often arises: "Exactly what would a nurse *do* within our faith community?" At the heart of this question is public confusion about the educational preparation and scope of practice of professional registered nurses. If faith community nurses are to carry out their roles effectively, faith group leaders, congregational members, and nurses themselves need to view nurses as skilled professionals capable of both independent and collaborative practice within the faith community. In this chapter, we begin by considering the power of images, then proceed to an overview of how nurses have historically been viewed in society. Next, we consider how nurses view themselves, and how faith group leaders view nurses. Our focus then turns to presenting more accurate information about nursing as a profession. Finally, we propose an image of nursing that is consistent with the health-promoting roles of a faith community nurse.

◢ The Power of Images

An image is defined as a mental picture or representation, an idea or conception (*American College Dictionary*, 1970). In her book *Image as Insight* (1985), Margaret Miles reminds us that images are powerful, in that these representations of reality ultimately inform our emotional, spiritual, and intellectual lives. When congregational members and faith group leaders think about a nurse functioning on a faith community staff, personal images of nurses and nursing immediately come to their minds. What beliefs and ideas about nursing do these images carry? Although nursing's goal is to improve health and quality of life by meeting specific human needs, the misunderstandings about the nature and extent of nursing education and practice serve as major obstacles to achieving this goal. Public beliefs, attitudes, and interpretations of nursing are extremely powerful forces in determining where nursing fits into society and how effective the profession can be in achieving its goals (Kalisch & Kalisch, 1987).

◢ Public Images of Nursing

Historical Public Images of Nursing

Because many members of the general public do not have regular contact with nurses, they acquire much of their information about nursing from the mass media. Kalisch and Kalisch (1987) have spent several decades researching the public's image of nursing as it is expressed in novels, movies, and television. Believing that nurses today have both the willingness and ability to participate in expanded healthcare roles, they find nursing's potential being weakened by inaccurate and sometimes even negative societal images. Following a systematic analysis of the popular media of the time, Kalisch and Kalisch have categorized public nursing images into five time periods: the eras of the "Angel of Mercy," the "Girl Friday," the "Heroine," the "Mother," and the "Sex Object" (Kalisch & Kalisch, 1987, p. 8).

The "Angel of Mercy" era (1854–1919) included two phases. In the first phase, nurses were seen as poorly educated and doing mainly domestic duties in deplorable surroundings. Sairey Gamp, from Dickens's *Martin Chuzzlewit* (1843–1844), exemplifies this image. She had little or no education, worked in appalling surroundings, and was generally unreliable in her patient care. In the second phase, which began to emerge during the Crimean War (1853–1856), nursing's image moved from being disrespectable to becoming a more noble profession. Much of this positive movement has been credited to Florence Nightingale (Kalisch & Kalisch, 1987; Wicks, 1987). As uniformed nurses communicated human dignity and caring amidst the chaos and destruction of battle, they were seen as idealized symbols of moral integrity. Along with the angelic image, nursing was emerging as noble work to be practiced by respectable women (Kalisch & Kalisch, 1987).

After World War I, the "Angel of Mercy" image gave way to that of the "Girl Friday" (1920–1929). This image of nursing was largely antiprofessional. Nurses were seen as subordinate to physicians, and much more interested in romance and marriage than in nursing; they were viewed as reliable workers, but worked as nurses only until they married. Educational standards decreased, and students were exploited for the long hours of free service they could offer to hospitals. This was a decade marked by materialism, and one in which the image of nursing suffered a setback (Kalisch & Kalisch, 1987).

Between 1930 and 1945, in the "Heroine" era, nursing became recognized as a profession again. As with previous wars, when World War II broke out, women gained employment opportunities because of the vacuum created when men were sent to war. Viewed as educated, skillful professionals, nurses contributed during World War II, and were seen as heroines (Kalisch & Kalisch, 1987).

When World War II was over, and for some twenty years after, women concentrated their efforts on being at home to raise their "baby boom" children. With this societal change in women's roles came a new nursing image, the "Mother" (1946–1965). Nurses were seen as women with limited knowledge and skill, but deserving of such descriptions as "maternal, nurturing, sympathetic, passive, expressive, and domestic" (Kalisch & Kalisch, 1982, p. 15). A nurse was a "mother away from home" (Wicks, 1987, p. 244). Although positive in nature, the image of nursing held by the public was not one of an educated, competent professional.

From 1966 to the present, the "Sex Object" image of nursing has dominated the media. Kalisch and Kalisch (1982) describe this era as the most negative media image of nursing since Dickens's Sairey Gamp. The maternal image gave way to a nurse shown in movies and soap operas as "a sensual, romantic, hedonistic, frivolous, irresponsible, promiscuous individual" (Kalisch & Kalisch, 1982, p. 17). It was—and still is—common to find that movie and novel plots included nurses being sexually involved with male patients and with physicians. In relating to physicians, nurses were usually portrayed in demeaning ways as being subordinate (Kalisch & Kalisch, 1987).

Recent Public Images of Nursing

In the late 1980s and early 1990s, the public's image of nurses and nursing was researched using interviews and telephone survey methods. In 1988, such a study was conducted in Alberta, Canada (Payne, Cook, & Associates, 1990). Using a telephone survey method, people were asked to describe their perception of the nursing profession. Over 87% of the responses were positive. Descriptions of nurses included such adjectives as *caring, compassionate, knowledgeable, intelligent, helpful, devoted, dedicated, professional, responsible,* and *hardworking.* Although, according to the respondents, the media had influenced over 60% of the subjects' responses, some 80% had formed their opinions, at least in part, through personal contact with nurses or by hearing of others' experiences with nurses. It is worth noting that 79% of subjects did not see nursing as an autonomous profession: They believed nurses should always consult a physician before administering patient care; furthermore, 72% of the subjects thought that physicians had total authority over patient care. In another study (Reichelt, 1988), American adults were found to perceive nurses as demonstrating care and concern more than providing unique services or utilizing cognitive skills.

In a discussion of nursing images, MacPhail (1996) noted that both of these studies demonstrated that not all members of the public see the need for nurses to continue their education. When nurses with diploma or associate degree levels of nursing education return to universities to seek a baccalaureate degree, their family, friends, and patients often wonder why. MacPhail sees this questioning as a reflection of a misconception that a registered nurse never needs to pursue further education. This misconception seems to be based on a lack of knowledge about the pattern and nature of nursing education and practice.

Although Kalisch and Kalisch (1982, 1987) looked mainly at the entertainment media, and the Payne, Cook, and Associates (1990) and Reichelt (1988) studies used survey methods to uncover public opinion about nursing, a 1998 U.S. study by the University of Rochester School of Nursing took a different approach to determining how nursing is viewed in society. In this, the Woodhull Study, researchers reviewed 20,000 articles published during the month of September 1997 in newspapers, magazines, and trade publications, examining them for attitudes about nurses and the nursing profession, as reflected in news media (University of Rochester, School of Nursing, 1998). The major finding of the study was that the largest group of health professionals in North America is largely invisible in the articles reviewed. Although more than 2.5 million registered nurses practice in the United States (University of Rochester, School of Nursing, 1998) and over 270,000 practice in Canada, nurses were cited only four percent of the time in the over 20,000 health-related articles examined in sixteen news publications. In fact, nurses often would have been the appropriate health professional to seek in learning more about the issue being considered by a particular article. The researchers cited, for example, an article about the care of AIDS patients in the community. Rather than interviewing nurses, who currently provide most of the HIV/AIDS care and education in the community, others were sought. A physician, an HIV policy operations coordinator, and a pharmacy educator were cited when nurses would have been the more appropriate health professional to question (University of Rochester, School of Nursing, 1998).

The public's image of nurses as portrayed in popular media has gone through a number of phases, from angels of mercy to sex objects. Recent studies that directly surveyed the public about perceptions of nurses and nursing were quite positive in nature, but demonstrated limited public knowledge regarding nursing education and the scope of nursing practice, with one very recent study suggesting that nursing is nearly invisible in the media. How, then, do nurses become more visible? Is there a relationship between nursing's invisibility and the self-image of nurses?

✍ Nursing's Self-Image

In addition to nursing having a public or external image, MacPhail (1996) discusses the self-image or internal image of nursing. Insofar as one's self-image serves as a basis for the image one portrays to others,

MacPhail believes that assessing this representation is very important. Studies show that the interactions of nurses with the public were more influential than media depictions in creating nursing's public image (Payne, Cook, & Associates, 1990; Reichelt, 1988). Nurses have, as a group, sometimes been described as having low self-esteem (MacPhail, 1996).

It is important that nurses value themselves, what they know, and what they do, and that they take every opportunity to affect nursing's image positively through their daily interactions with clients, families, and other professionals. MacPhail (1996) suggests that nurses need to remain unified in these actions in order to make constructive and desirable changes in their group self-perceptions and in perceptions of nursing by the public. Nurses need to realize for themselves, and then communicate to the public, that "nursing is more complex than most people think. . . . Developing the knowledge, skills, attitudes, and values needed to practice nursing is a very complicated undertaking" (MacPhail, 1996, p. 61).

The self-image of nurses practicing in faith communities will affect how they carry out their role within faith communities and, conversely, the role that they see themselves carrying out will affect their self-image. In a previous chapter, the role of faith community nurses was summed up by nurses themselves as that of helping people grow and change in various life situations, using all resources available to them. Seeing nursing in this positive, health-promoting light emphasizes the importance of relational qualities, and the need for extensive and rigorous education as a foundation for these health promotion activities. Although nurses practicing in faith communities might have confidence in their knowledge and skills related to health promotion, and might therefore possess a good self-image, this image needs to be communicated to clergy, other faith group leaders, and congregational members. Is this happening?

∽ Clergy's Image of Nursing

Because faith community nurses work in partnership with clergy, other faith community leaders, and congregational members, it is important to consider the images of nurses from the perspectives of these people. To date, no studies have been done that have looked specifically at the image of nursing from the perspective of congregational leaders or members of various faith communities. In a recent study of the feasibility of faith community nursing within the Edmonton, Alberta, area, however, Christian clergy spoke about their images of nurses and the profession of nursing (Olson, Simington, & Douglass, 1995). It was encouraging to learn that clergy have quite a thorough and accurate understanding of nurses and nursing. Questions asked in the survey included the following:

> Does your denomination view its mission as including responsiveness to the health and healing needs of people?
>
> Do you as a representative of your denomination believe that the clergy play a role in meeting the health needs of people?
>
> Do you see value in adding another professional to the pastoral team to assist in meeting the total needs of congregational members?
>
> Do you believe that a nurse would be the appropriate professional to fill such a role?

In response to the last two questions, clergy replied that they saw value in having another professional on the ministry team to assist with meeting health-related needs in the congregation and beyond, and readily identified nurses as the appropriate professionals; this concurred with Westberg's (1990b) findings. The study by Olson et al. (1995) showed that nurses had demonstrated to clergy their ability to view people holistically, easily seeing the interconnectedness of all dimensions of people. Many clergy indicated that they already utilize the broad knowledge and expertise of nurses who are members of their congregations, and would very much like to be able to do so in a more formal way. Past experience had provided a basis for their comment that nurses and clergy "think alike." According to clergy, both professions work with people even when there is not a cure, helping people to move toward acceptance and personal growth despite life circumstances.

Clergy clearly indicated, in the Olson et al. (1995) study, a respect for the profession of nursing, and a full appreciation for the knowledge and skills that nurses embody. They saw nurses as professionals who can bridge the worlds of faith and health, skilled in understanding both the language of the church and of health care (Westberg, 1990a). The study of the feasibility of faith community nursing within Alberta (Olson, et al., 1995) led us to believe that clergy had a positive and accurate image of nursing; we saw further work needed only in the area of helping clergy to realize the full potential of a nursing role within a faith community.

✍ A Holistic Image of Nursing

The final report of the Woodhull Study on nursing and the media (University of Rochester, School of Nursing, 1998) offers a description of nursing as it is and should be seen in the media and in the minds of the general public. The description includes many of the same ideas that need to be conveyed to people within faith communities regarding the preparation of nurses and the scope of nursing practice. We have termed this a holistic image of nursing because it emphasizes the broad-based and holistic nature of nursing. The Woodhull Study report emphasizes that nurses need to be seen as capable of working toward creating a "life-enabling environment" and as focused on improving the quality of life across the life span (University of Rochester, School of Nursing, 1998, p. 37). Nursing, then, involves far more than working with people in times of illness. The public has seen a move from episodic treatment of illness to a more proactive approach to health and health promotion. Along with that change in society, the public needs to know that nursing has kept current by changing its methods of education. Although the twentieth-century nurse may have seemed more focused on manual tasks, the nurse of the twenty-first century will be knowledge-oriented, will be a critical thinker and a problem solver (University of Rochester, School of Nursing, 1998, p. 37). The public should know, too, that nursing education is broad based in nature, drawing from the sciences, the arts, and the humanities, as well as from the knowledge base that has been developed within the nursing discipline.

The public needs also to understand the differences between nurses and physicians. Though nurses today have a knowledge base similar to physicians, they also have a broad-based knowledge grounded in the humanities as well as the sciences. Furthermore, nurses use the knowledge they have in common with physicians differently than do physicians; although medical practice is largely focused on individual medical diagnoses and treatment with a goal of a cure, nursing practice focuses on health assessment in times of illness and health, and on interventions that affect whole persons, families, and society at large (University of Rochester, School of Nursing, 1998,

p. 37). These thoughts are in keeping with the insights of Moyra Allen, as she developed the McGill nursing model and proposed that nursing has a unique role to play in society.

The authors of the Woodhull Study report (University of Rochester, School of Nursing, 1998) want the public to realize that nurses work as members of an interdisciplinary team that requires much integration, both with clients and with other healthcare providers. In this team model, the nursing roles include resource liaison, communication facilitator, services coordinator, personnel manager, and hands-on care provider. Nurses often teach, assist, and guide patients, helping them to understand health issues and to share responsibility for their own care.

Nurses tend to develop a more intimate relationship with their patients than other health care providers, largely because they spend more time with clients and they address a broad range of topics. Nurses function as advocates for the rights and needs of clients. These nursing roles can flourish in the faith community setting.

The public often does not fully understand that nurses are both autonomous and collaborative in working with other professionals. Researchers in the Woodhull Study (University of Rochester, School of Nursing, 1998) want the public to know that nurses perform physical, psychological, social, and spiritual assessments, diagnose positive and negative states of health, plan care, implement interventions, and evaluate the outcomes. Nurses are also involved in scientifically designed research that helps to set standards of patient care.

As autonomous professionals, nurses undergo extensive professional education, and function under a code of ethics and standards of practice as determined by each state or province. Although some nurses hold diplomas in nursing from hospital schools of nursing, more and more nurses are receiving university level education. Following a baccalaureate degree in nursing, nurses may pursue further nursing education at the masters or doctoral level, as well as education in disciplines other than nursing. As members of a self-regulating profession, registered nurses must pass a licensing examination, and annually demonstrate their continuing competence for relicensure.

It is these facts about nurses and the nursing profession that people within faith communities need to know in order to envision the potential for a nursing role in this setting. What are the characteristics of a nurse who portrays this holistic, health-promoting, professional image of nursing?

∽ Health-Promoting Images of Nursing

As we move into the twenty-first century, nurses must become more visible and known for the unique contribution that they can make to society. Kalisch and Kalisch (1987) proposed an ideal nursing image, which they termed the "Careerist." In this image, nurses are viewed as "intelligent, logical, progressive, sophisticated, emphatic, and assertive women or men who are committed to attaining higher and higher standards of health care" (p. 184). Building on these qualities, we propose the "Confidant" as the ideal nursing image for the twenty-first century: the nurse as knowledgeable, professionally autonomous, collaborative, empowering, self-aware, emotionally and spiritually mature, relational, and trustworthy. The word *confidant* comes from the Latin *con* + *fide*, which means "with faith." Such a root meaning returns us to the concept of faith as being in relationship with, as described in an earlier chapter. The nurse as confidant is one who is in relationship with people where they live, work, play, learn, and worship. The nurse as confidant is also in relationship with herself or himself through healthy self-esteem and good self-care. Finally, the nurse as confidant is in relationship with the idea that life is transcendent. In this sense, the nurse actualizes her or his full nursing potential, reaching beyond the limits of healthcare and human knowledge to more holistic values and universal truths. The nurse sees herself or himself as only a part of a larger universe, much of which is beyond human comprehension.

The idea of nurse as confidant is one that, for me, has long described the ideal nurse, and the one that best describes the nursing image toward which I hope all professional nurses strive. Over my career in nursing, I have seen many nurses who live up to this ideal image of nurse as confidant. In particular, I remember a young nurse who exemplified nurse as confidant. Mary (this is not her actual name) was a staff nurse on the county public health nursing team for which I served as nursing supervisor. In a low-income area of a large Midwestern U.S. city, my team of six public health nurses carried a general caseload of clients and families requiring home care and health promotional nursing services. As I think back over the team I supervised, I remember that Mary was a young but emotionally and spiritually mature nurse. Her spiritual maturity was especially evident on a day-to-day basis. I sensed that her own clarity about who she was as a person, and who she was in relationship to others and to a higher power, affected how she approached her nursing practice and how she respected people no matter what their situation. Though we worked for a county public health institution and she said little about her personal beliefs, I sensed that Mary viewed her nursing work as a ministry. She was sincere about her work and caring in all of her interactions with clients, families, and coworkers. Above all, I sensed a confidence about Mary and a solidness in all that she did. She was probably one of the most effective members on my nursing team.

The characteristics of the nurse as confidant, as described earlier and exemplified in Mary, are in keeping with the characteristics required for parish nurses to function as described by Holstrom (1999): The nurse acts as integrator of faith and health, health educator, personal health counselor, referral agent and liaison with congregational and community resources, trainer of volunteers, developer of support groups, and health advocate. As the nurse as confidant begins to carry out these functions successfully, people will begin to see nurses as educated, competent, confident, and skilled in meeting the demands of this independent and collaborative nursing practice. How will this most likely happen?

Several recent studies have determined that the public's views of nurses and nursing were most influenced by personal contact with nurses or by the experiences of others (Giovannetti, 1990; Lippman & Ponton, 1989; Payne, Cook, & Associates, 1990). The images that clergy tend to hold of nurses and nursing described earlier in this chapter bear out these findings; it was mainly the clergy's personal experiences with nurses that had contributed to their positive and accurate views of nursing. Likewise, the view of nurses among the public within congregations will be changed most by parishioners' personal experiences with faith community nurses. As more and more faith community members experience nurses in health-promoting roles, nursing's image will change. In turn, nurses will then be more able to carry out fully their health-promoting roles within faith communities, because they will be viewed as knowledgeable and capable health-promoting professionals. It is possible that faith community nursing could be a vehicle through which nursing's full potential in society will become more visible.

9 ∽

Characteristics of Health-Promoting Faith Community Nurses

Joanne K. Olson
Margaret B. Clark

F aith community nurses strive to promote the health of a faith community by working with faith group leaders and other staff to integrate the spiritual, psychological, sociological, and physiological perspectives of health and healing into the activities of the congregation. They do this by working to promote health when such concerns as interpersonal relationships, grief, guilt, stress, lifestyle adjustments, and life changes emerge. Nurses are prepared to assess the needs of the whole person, facilitating positive change through health assessment, health counseling, self-help groups, health education, and referrals to other healthcare providers and community resources (Ryan, 1990). Being a faith community nurse is more than a job in a new location or another opportunity for employment. We believe, with others, that faith community nursing involves a call to ministry, and can be seen as a vocation (Evans, 1995; Striepe, 1993; Striepe, King, & Scott, 1993; Widerquist & Davidhizer, 1994).

Viewing faith community nursing as a ministry, the nurse collaborates with pastoral staff and congregational members to actively transform the faith community into a place of health and healing (Nel, 1998). Believing that all people are sacred and to be treated with respect and dignity, the faith community nurse empowers people to become active partners in the management of their own personal health resources. While understanding health to be a process that involves the spiritual, psychological, physical, and social dimensions of a person, faith community nurses also believe that spiritual health is central to well-being and orients the person toward wholeness (Solari-Twadell, McDermott, Ryan, & Djupe, 1994). As a ministry that focuses largely on spiritual care in facilitating holistic health promotion, faith community nursing involves much more than being a professional who is a "human doer"; the position requires the development of skills that draw out the "human being" part of the nurse's professional self.

In this chapter, we discuss the following questions: What does it mean to say that faith community nursing is a ministry? What are some of the behaviors, characteristics, and attitudes needed by nurses involved in the health-promoting ministry known as parish nursing or faith community nursing? What abilities are needed for working with the spiritual dimension of people? How do faith community nurses use the "human being" part of their professional self in a therapeutic rather than a nontherapeutic way? How do nurses, practicing nursing as a ministry, promote health by empowering others?

✍ Faith Community Nursing as a Ministry and Vocation

Faith community nursing has been described as a response to a call to ministry (Evans, 1995; Striepe, 1993; Striepe et al., 1993; Widerquist & Davidhizer, 1994) and as a vocation (Lane, 1987). In Chapter 1, we defined a ministry as an orientation to serve others that is both representative of and carried out in relationship with a faith community's reason for being. Furthermore, ministry is seen to be endowed with and accountable to a public trust. In this definition, there are three major components to ministry. First, a ministry is representative: The one who ministers reveals the human face of a faith community's mission or purpose. Second, a ministry is carried forward in direct relationship with a particular faith community. Ministering persons do not act in isolation, but rather as part of a larger whole; that is, they are part of the faith community's reason for being as it gives practical shape to values emanating from spiritual and religious traditions. Third, a ministry is endowed with the trust of those being served. The one who ministers, therefore, is accountable to that public trust; within the context of ministry, one is never mandated to carry forward a personal agenda (McBrien, 1987) or create a private venue (Drummond, 1996). On the contrary, one's ministry is always open to established standards for public scrutiny as well as theological reflection.

Most faith traditions are grounded in core human values out of which service to others emanates. Buddhism, for example, evolves from four noble truths and an eightfold noble path; values of right understanding, intention, speech, action, means of livelihood, effort, mindfulness, and concentration promote harmonious relationships between oneself, all beings, and the environment. The meaning of being Christian is a matter of responding to a call both to live as a follower of Jesus Christ in the world and to serve God by serving others in that world (Feucht, 1974). Hinduism promotes belief in the sacredness of all living things. The Sikh religion promotes a life of truth, contentment, compassion, patience, and service. Finally, many Aboriginal traditions are founded on a belief in the fundamental interconnectedness of all natural things and all forms of life, with primary importance being attached to the land as Mother Earth (Ontario Multifaith Council on Spiritual and Religious Care, 1995).

Faith community nurses describe a feeling of being called to this type of multidimensional work. They desire to serve both a divine or transcendent other and the people of the world by using their professional nursing knowledge and skills. This kind of work addresses a need many nurses have to experience meaning and purpose in what they are doing on a day-to-day basis. People need a reason and a goal for living, and nurses are no exception. To be truly meaningful, life invites expansion in both vertical and horizontal directions. In this regard, faith community nursing can be called a vocation, because there is a sense of call or summons to the work. This sense of call and purpose can also foster a sense of tremendous satisfaction and meaning.

Lane (1987) addresses the idea of vocation affecting the nurse's ability to care spiritually for people as a three-step process. First, the nurse feels called to nursing or to a particular kind of nursing. With this call, the nurse views the professional work as having deep personal meaning, either in terms of religious or humanitarian values. Second, seeing nursing as a vocation involves an awareness of the effect one can have on the spirit of others. To maintain this sensitivity, the nurse takes time for personal reflection, prayer, and other spirit-enhancing activities or disciplines. Finally, with a sense of call and spiritual awareness, the nurse is able to see more fully the health-promoting benefits of spiritually supportive resources for those to whom care is given. "Nursing becomes a partnership with the source of all healing" (Lane, 1987, p. 337). Healing in this context means to become whole or complete, as opposed to being relieved of a physical disease or condition.

✐ A Story About Helping

Close your eyes for a minute, and think about a time when you have been anxious, worried, upset, or fearful. Perhaps this was a time when you were dealing with a very difficult life situation, a time when you needed someone's caring and healing presence to calm you. Next, think of an occasion when someone took the time to listen or did other acts that made you feel less alone in your suffering. Can you remember what that person did or said, and how the person acted that made you feel better? What, specifically, did that person do to promote your well-being? Whether the person you thought about was a friend, a relative, a coworker, or a helping professional, there are certain behaviors and characteristics that all helpful or health-promoting people have in common.

In doing the above exercise with you, I (Joanne) thought of a friend who happens also to be a professional nurse and who, at the time of being helpful to me, was a coworker. Thinking back to a time when I needed someone to be there for me, she was there. This friend demonstrated her "being there" in so many ways, but above all, she was an excellent listener. I did not feel rushed, nor did I ever feel that she was going to start talking if I stopped talking. She was just there, listening with her whole being. Her body posture and her occasional verbal responses indicated that she was with me, hearing my story as I related it. When I got emotional, and cried too much to carry on talking, she still listened, now more to my emotions than to my words. What I remember the most, though, is that my crying did not make her feel uncomfortable; she did not seem to feel that she had to do something to make me stop crying. She just waited with me, allowing me to cry and express my feelings. When I was done crying, I talked some more, and she continued listening. There was no judgement in her voice, and she never offered any type of advice. She listened and let me think aloud, coming up with my own ideas as to what I needed and wanted to do next about the situation that was facing me.

The door to the room we were in was closed, and the telephone answering machine was on to decrease unwanted interruptions. It was comforting to realize that I had my friend's undivided attention, and that no interruptions would interfere. My friend in no way minimized my situation; she realized its importance to me. Occasionally, she helped me to put some of my feelings into words when I had trouble doing so. When I did express feelings, she would sometimes restate those feelings, verbally sharing with me the fact that she understood not only what I was feeling, but also the reasons I was attributing to those feelings. Finally, she offered to be there for me in the future; I felt welcome. I sensed, even though we did not talk about it specifically, that what I had shared with her was confidential. What an amazing gift this friend gave me at a time when I desperately needed someone's caring presence. At that time, the faith community nursing concept had not yet reached Canada. If it had, I might have sought out the professional services of a faith community nurse in my congregation. My friend was a wonderful substitute, and it is with fondness that I reflect on her excellent helping skills.

৬ Characteristics and Attitudes of Health-Promoting Helping Professionals

The literature on professional helping is filled with terms that describe characteristics of professional helpers. Some of the characteristics that have been identified include congruence, unconditional positive regard, empathic understanding and active listening, well-established self-worth, an awareness of one's own vulnerability, and a belief that other persons' answers lie within them (Carkhuff, 1983; Clinebell, 1984; Rogers, 1951, 1961). Each of these characteristics will now be considered in more depth.

Congruence

Congruence is the outward display of inner genuineness, integration, and openness. Skilled helpers who are at home with themselves can afford to be transparently real with the person being helped (Egan, 1982). Rogers (1951, 1961) refers to congruence as the correspondence or harmony between a helper's basic attitudes and behaviors. Sometimes words like *credibility* or *authenticity* are used to explain what congruence means. Effective helpers are genuine people. They work with others without masks or façades, allowing their feelings and attitudes to be easily available to them through highly developed self-awareness skills. Their work with others engages the uniqueness of the other with the uniqueness of the self. When people being helped feel this kind of genuineness modeled for them, they, too, can move toward a greater congruence between attitudes and behaviors (Brammer, 1979).

Unconditional Positive Regard

Unconditional positive regard is an attitude that expresses concern for another's situation, as well as respect for his or her individuality and worth as a person (Brammer, 1979). The phrase *unconditional positive regard* was developed by Carl Rogers (1951, 1961) to describe a combination of helper qualities, including warmth, caring acceptance, and an interest in and respect for the other. This combination of qualities in the helper gives those being helped permission to be who they are, knowing that they will be respected for it. Warmth is described by Gerrard, Boniface, and Love (1980) as communicating caring to a person; it means being friendly by smiling, greeting the person by name, and showing genuine interest in the other person.

To have respect means valuing another person because they are a human being. According to McDougall, Lasswell, and Chen (1980), respect is the core value of human rights. They define respect as an interrelationship among humans in which they reciprocally recognize and honor each others' freedom of choice, worthiness as humans, and opportunity for equality. Following a review of the literature, Browne (1993) proposed that respect is a nursing ethic that acknowledges the dignity, inherent worth, and uniqueness of humans, and the potential for self-determination. Respect is more than just saying that one values the other person; a value is only fully a value when it has been acted on and expressed behaviorally. It is through verbal and nonverbal expressions that the helper shows those being helped that they are respected (Egan, 1982).

Empathic Understanding and Active Listening

Empathic understanding is the quality that allows helpers to encounter another person in such a way that both deep feelings and the reasons for those feelings are shared by the person being helped and fully understood by the person doing the helping. It is a quality essential in all helping relationships. People naturally develop some level of understanding of others as they grow up; to be an effective professional helper, however, further understanding about the theory and skills of empathy are essential (Combs, Avila, & Purkey, 1971). When these skills are well developed in the nurse-client relationship, measurable differences in client outcomes have been shown (Olson, 1995; Olson & Hanchett, 1997). Helpers who have developed skills in empathy are able to achieve a deep understanding and appreciation of the persons with whom they work, giving clients a sense of reassurance and acceptance. Empathy has been described as a process whereby the helper is sensitive to another's feelings and reasons for those feelings and can communicate verbally that he or she understands the client, and the client feels understood by the helper (Bradley & Edinberg, 1982).

Closely related to the development of empathy is the development of active listening. According to Bolton (1979), it is helpful to make a distinction between hearing and listening. Hearing emphasizes physiological, sensory processes. Listening, on the other hand, refers to a "more complex psychological procedure involving interpreting and understanding the significance of the sensory experience" (Bolton, 1979, p. 32). This distinction between merely hearing and really listening is deeply embedded in our language. Bolton says that the word *listen* is derived from two Anglo-Saxon words: *hlystan,* meaning "hearing," and *hlosnian,* meaning "to wait in suspense" (p. 32). Helping professionals who can wait in suspense are not only listening with their ears, but also hearing what is not being said with words. By observing body language and nuances of emotion, one can listen to the whole message. Active listening means being silent most of the time so that the other person can talk (Brammer, 1979).

A Sense of Self-Worth

An effective helper is one with a strong sense of self-worth and a feeling of confidence in her or his work. Sometimes identified as the main factor in influencing our ability to communicate with others, self-worth is the positive value that we place on ourselves as individuals (Bradley & Edinberg, 1982; Satir, 1976, 1988). Often we look to others' opinions of us to determine our self-worth. Sometimes when we receive praise, blame, or critique, we allow our self-worth to be affected, although others are evaluating only our behavior, not us as whole persons. Self-worth need not be associated with performance of various tasks. Maintaining one's high self-worth is even known to be helpful in changing some of our undesirable behaviors. Becoming skilled at ongoing self-assessment can assist in linking our feelings of self-worth to other feelings and behaviors. It can be one way to grow personally, and to promote self-understanding that contributes to self-worth (Bradley & Edinberg, 1982). When people are cared for by a confident person who possesses positive self-worth, they feel safe and in competent hands.

Awareness of One's Own Vulnerability

Good helpers are aware of their own vulnerability. They realize that they have much in common with the one seeking help. The helper realizes and appreciates that she or he could as easily be experiencing the health issue being discussed. Having this attitude of vulnerability keeps the helping person grounded and less likely to offer false reassurance or simplistic answers. Being grounded in one's own vulnerability makes the helping person more human, and allows the healing and helping to proceed (Becker, 1985; Niklas, 1981; Tournier, 1987; Vaughan, 1987).

Belief That a Person's Answers Lie Within Them

Basic to an effective helper's work with others is a belief that each person is unique and that each person comes with strengths and resources, as well as issues and concerns. Such a helper supports the uniqueness of others in seeking to uncover their hidden coping abilities and strengths (Egan, 1982). In his classic text on caring, Mayeroff (1971) states this well when he says, "In helping the other grow I do not impose my own direction; rather, I allow the direction of the other's growth to guide what I do. . . . I appreciate the other as independent in its own right with needs that are to be respected" (p. 9).

✍️ Special Characteristics of Helpers Working in the Spiritual Dimension

In addition to the characteristics outlined previously, qualities of help-ers working in the spiritual dimension include an ability to access one's own spirituality, to respect the spirituality of others, and to recommend spiritual resources when these seem appropriate (Becker, 1985; Niklas, 1981; Tournier, 1987; Vaughan, 1987; Wicks, Parsons, & Capps, 1985). We now turn to a consideration of each of these qualities.

The Ability to Access One's Own Spirituality

In Lane's (1987) classic article about care of the human spirit, she emphasizes that the nurse giving spiritual care does not necessarily need to be knowledgeable in a particular set of religious beliefs and practices. Such care does, however, require that the nurse consider her-self or himself a "spirit in the world" (Lane, 1987, p. 332), who needs to participate in spiritual activities. Lane says, "the greater the awareness of the nurse in the work and activities of the spirit, within himself or herself, the greater the awareness of the work and activities of the spirit in the patient" (p. 335).

There are several steps to this increased spiritual self-awareness. First, the nurse must gain awareness of her or his gifts and limitations. Reflection and turning inward are the means by which to accomplish this. The need is to connect with not only inner joys, but also feelings of loneliness, doubt, anger, and guilt (Lane, 1987). Following reflection are the steps of surrender and commitment. Surrendering means let-ting go, and knowing that opportunity for gain comes with letting go. Commitment refers to the ability to attach or bond to another person, community, or ideal. These activities of the spirit result in hospitality, a gracious warmth, and a generosity that opens the self to others. This hospitality is a form of total presence for the person being helped. Finally, the nurse who is in touch with her or his own spirituality is comfortable with struggle. This involves dealing with one's own and with other's pain, fear, suffering, despair, and joy. It also means being able to articulate these feelings and respond to others with compassion rather than trying to avoid their pain (Lane, 1987).

There are many ways to grow spiritually. Many accomplish spiri-tual growth by attending retreats or workshops, or by reading about topics related to spiritual development. Others go further, seeking opportunities to work with a spiritual director, or to enroll in courses such as clinical pastoral education. These experiences strengthen the nurse's ability to focus on both their own spiritual aspects and the spiritual aspects of others in a clinical setting under the guidance of a knowledgeable director or certified supervisor. Of special note regarding clinical pastoral education is the strength of its action and reflection learning method. Using nursing practice in a faith community as the basis for reflection, students learn from interaction with peers, from individual conferences with the supervisor, and through written assignments, such as verbatim reports and theological case studies reflecting on clinical experience. Nurses in these courses also focus on the assessment of spiritual needs, learning from didactic presentations on a variety of topics, and growing through a written self-, peer, and supervisory evaluation process.[1]

The Ability to Respect the Spirituality of Others

True spiritual care applies to the care of every person, be they Aboriginal, Buddhist, Christian, Muslim, or atheist. According to Lane (1987), respecting the spirituality of others means seeing every human spirit as a "fragile vessel holding the essence of who we are" (p. 335). When nurses care for the spirit of another, they "must approach with a sense of awe and deep humility" (Lane, 1987, p. 335). This is sometimes referred to as standing on holy ground or in a sacred place.

Respecting and attending to the spirituality of others includes many activities. These may involve sitting quietly with someone so that they can reflect (Berggren-Thomas & Griggs, 1995), allowing the person to talk about their spiritual feelings, or using touch to connect with the other person.

The Ability to Offer Spiritual Resources

When working intentionally in the spiritual care of people, nurses will gain comfort in assessing spiritual needs (Clinebell, 1992; Fitchett, 1993a, 1993b; Kim et al., 1989), as well as recommending and using spiritual resources in providing care when appropriate. These spiritual resources may include prayer, sacred texts, devotional and spiritual writings, worship, sacraments, spiritual health counseling, healing services, or meditation. Spiritual resources are always offered with the needs and wishes of the other person in mind, and not from the perspective of what the nurse would view as helpful to the person (Clinebell, 1984).

✍ Therapeutic Use of Self

In addition to developing certain characteristics and attitudes, an effective and health-promoting professional develops very specific therapeutic or facilitative helping behaviors and skills. These assist in creating a therapeutic, empowering, and health-promoting relationship with those being helped. Specific therapeutic techniques are (a) broad opening statements and questions, (b) verbal encouragement, (c) reflective statements and verbal acknowledgement of feelings, (d) the appropriate giving of information, (e) the clarification of information received, and (f) appropriate self-disclosure. Although these approaches to a therapeutic use of self are defined and developed briefly in the paragraphs that follow, the faith community nurse who wishes to become skilled in the use of these techniques will need to consult other texts and seek opportunities for continued learning. Preferably, that learning will occur in situations where supervised practice and feedback from those skilled in helping can be provided.

When working with people in a therapeutic way, it is best to use *broad opening statements and questions* that allow the person being helped to set the direction of the conversation. An example of such a statement would be, "Tell me how that experience made you feel," or, "Give me some examples of times when you have felt like this before." In addition, using *verbal signs*, such as, "Uh-huh" and "Go on," can encourage the person being helped to continue talking by indicating interest and understanding in what he or she is saying. *Reflecting* all or part of the person's statement, or slightly rephrasing it, can indicate that you have understood what was said, and are encouraging the person to continue. For example, the nurse might say, "So you were quite relieved when the doctor was finally able to see your mother." *Acknowledging feelings* shows acceptance of and respect for the person's experience, and encourages continued expression of feelings with the assurance that judgment will not be placed on them: "The situation with your son is causing you to feel embarrassed?"

Giving information by answering questions and dispelling misconceptions, when appropriate, decreases anxiety and establishes trust. Faith community nurses can often give health-related information that will be helpful to families. For example the nurse, in talking to an anxious grandmother-to-be, might say, "You probably were in the hospital for four to five days when your daughter was born. Now it is common to release new mothers and babies from the hospital in less than 24 hours."

Clarifying is a helpful technique in which the helper makes a statement or asks questions that help to make meaning clearer: "Did you say that you have never had a mammogram and are wondering what is involved in the test?" *Summarizing* is often used at the end of an interaction to pull together several ideas or feelings in order to review a lengthy discussion. For example, the nurse, after a visit with a parishioner, might say, "We've discussed many things today, Mary. You have shared your concerns about your relationship with your mother. We looked for some of the positive areas in that relationship, and talked about ways you could relieve stress related to your relationship with your mother. Next time we meet, I'd like to hear which methods you tried and which ones worked best for you."

Helpful professionals also use *appropriate self-disclosure* in their interactions. While self-disclosure creates trust and a sense of a human-to-human interaction, it is best to remember that self-disclosure needs to be appropriate, with the helper sharing only the information about herself or himself that will be of assistance to the other person. If nothing about the helper is shared with the person being helped, that person may be reluctant to open up totally to the helper. An example of appropriate self-disclosure might be, "I have teenagers too. I know they can be hard to understand at times."

Beyond using helpful attitudes and verbal behaviors, another way to be helpful and health promoting with others is to be physically present when interacting with them. A useful acronym, SOLER, has been developed to assist helpers in remembering to be physically present to the person being helped (Egan, 1982). The *S* is a reminder that the helper should *squarely* face the person, thereby adopting a posture that indicates involvement and a desire to be with the person. The *O* of SOLER means *open* posture. This nondefensive posture, where arms and legs are not crossed, invites the person being helped to feel comfortable and willing to share with the helper. The *L* refers to *leaning* toward the person being helped. The leaning needs to be enough to indicate genuine interest in the person, yet not so much as to frighten the person. It is suggested that the body act as if it has a hinge at the waist with the upper body moving forward and backward depending on the stage of the particular interaction. In the beginning, the person being helped might need some distance from the helper; as the interaction progresses, the helper may be able to move in closer to the other person. The *E* represents maintaining good *eye contact*, and is the fourth critical physical helping behavior. This action also tells people that you want to be with them. Good eye contact needs to be culturally sensitive, and may fall somewhere between looking directly into another person's eyes and looking away from the person. In some cultures, for example, to look directly into another's eyes is perceived as disrespect and an invasion of personal space; in other cultures, looking away from the person too often can signal that you are not interested in what they are saying. Finally, the *R* in SOLER refers to being relatively *relaxed* when with the people being helped. This means not fidgeting nervously or using distracting facial expressions. These behaviors can make the other person anxious, wondering what is causing you to be so uncomfortable. Egan (1982) reminds us that these are not rules to be applied rigidly, but are to be used as a set of guidelines to assist us in remembering how to physically attend to the people with whom we are working.

∽ *Nontherapeutic Behaviors*

At the opposite end of the helping behaviors spectrum are nontherapeutic or blocking behaviors. These behaviors are obstacles to good communication between a helper and a person being helped. They are not health promoting or empowering, and need to be avoided in all helping encounters (Bolton, 1979; Gordon, 1970).

Reassuring cliches and stereotyped comments are unhelpful. Likewise, trite comments given automatically, such as "Everything will be fine," or "It's not that bad," tend to convey to the person being helped that the helper is disinterested or lacks understanding of the situation. Giving *advice* is tempting, but needs to be avoided. Advice takes away a person's decision-making power by imposing the helper's opinions or solutions, and fails to assist the person to explore and arrive at his or her own conclusions. Likewise, when a helper *approves or agrees*, making comments like "That was a good idea," or "That will be very good for you," the focus is shifted from the person's values to those of the helper; such comments impose on the free expression of the person being helped. *Requesting an explanation* for the feelings or actions of the person being helped involves "Why" questions, which need to be avoided. They can be intimidating to the person being helped, and may promote conformity on the part of that person as they seek the helper's approval. *Disapproving or disagreeing* means placing negative judgment on a person's actions, thoughts, or feelings, and again introducing the helper's own values into the situation. This can be intimidating for the person, again prompting conformity in seeking the helper's approval.

Belittling refers to indicating that a person's experiences are not unique or important, thus shifting the focus away from the person. An example might be a comment like, "What you are going through is nothing compared with so many other people with whom I have worked." *Changing the subject* is the introduction of new or unrelated topics. It takes the lead in a conversation away from the person being helped, and may block that person from further attempts to make their needs known. The person may feel cheated that they have not been fully heard. *Closed questions* are questions that require "yes" or "no" answers. They limit the person's responses, and suggest that the helper is searching for a specific, correct answer. This type of question is not helpful in allowing a person being helped to open up and share his or her own story. Closely related to closed questions are *leading questions*, which move a person toward a certain answer rather than leaving all options for answers open to the person being helped. Finally, *inappropriate self-disclosure* is a blocking behavior. Such disclosure may make the person being helped feel confused about the relationship; that is, the person may feel that he or she is being placed in a helping role if the helper shares so much that it burdens the person being helped (Iwasiw & Olson, 1995).

We often forget how healing and empowering we can be to another person when we give them the gift of our true presence. Indeed, true presence can be health promoting in and of itself. Likewise, knowing how to practice nursing in an empowering way is important for the nurse working within a faith community.

✍ Practicing Nursing in an Empowering Way

What does it mean to practice nursing in an empowering way? According to *Roget's Pocket Thesaurus* (1982), *empowering* can be equated with "to make possible," "commission," "permission," "enable," "authorize," "endow with power," and "allow capability as well as potentiality." In the context of a conceptual analysis, empowerment is described as "a helping process whereby groups and individuals are enabled to change a situation, given skills, resources, opportunities and authority to do so" (Rodwell, 1996, p. 309). It is also described as a partnership that respects both self and others, and aims to develop a positive belief about oneself in the future. Inherent in the previous statement is the belief that empowerment is about changing the distribution of power, and the implication that power originates from self-esteem. Empowerment involves mutual decision making and allowing people the freedom to make choices and accept responsibility (Rodwell, 1996). The definition attributed to empowerment in helping relationships is "the process of enabling people to choose to take control over and make decisions about their lives. It is also a process which values all those involved" (Rodwell, 1996, p. 309).

When working with people in an empowering, health-promoting way, nurses function more from an attitude of being responsible *to* others, than from an attitude of feeling responsible *for* others. This means that they approach people with the aims of listening, empathizing, encouraging, and coaching, rather than protecting, rescuing, and fixing. This frees the nurse to serve as helper and guide, rather than as one controlling the situation and making the person live up to the nurse's expectations. As a result, the person being helped is free to act on her or his own behalf, and the nurse is free to assist and support. Such freedom can affect nurses' self-esteem, because they are now in a position to observe the person learn and grow, rather than feeling anxious, fearful, or overwhelmed with a sense of responsibility for the other's life. It is a win-win situation!

Another characteristic of those working with people in an empowering way is that they work with the strengths of the person or family being helped. Every person and every situation has strengths and positive elements present. The empowering helper knows how to find these strengths, and how to use them in moving the person toward health. In doing so, the helper assists people being helped to see their own strengths while working to develop new ones.

∽ Summary

When faith community nursing is viewed as a ministry, every person is seen as a whole person to be respected and cared for with awe and reverence. Flowing from that basic belief will be the attitudes and behaviors that promote health in every encounter within and beyond the faith community. Thus, others will benefit and nurses will feel satisfied and fulfilled in their role.

Note

1. For more information on CPE courses, contact the Association for Clinical Pastoral Education (ACPE), 1549 Clairmont Road, Suite 103, Decatur, GA. 30033 (telephone, 1-404-320-1472; fax, 1-404-320-0849; Website <www.acpe.edu>) or the Canadian Association for Clinical Practice and Pastoral Education (CAPPE/ACPEP), at 47 Queen's Park Crescent East, Toronto, Ontario M5S 2C3 (telephone, 1-416-977-3700; fax, 1-416-978-7821; Website, <www.cappe.org>)

10 ఎ

Functions of the Nurse as Health Promoter in a Faith Community

Joanne K. Olson

What does a nurse do in a faith community? Looking at the typical job description for a parish nurse position, it is evident that the faith community nurse is considered an employee of the faith community and a member of the ministerial team. The position is designed for the purpose of bringing to members of a congregation health services that focus on the holistic integration of body, mind, and spirit. This is achieved by assessing, planning, and implementing nursing care that addresses the strengths and limitations of individuals, families, and groups in the congregation. Health promotion activities may extend beyond the congregation to aggregates or the community as a whole, if the congregation recognizes these as part of its ministry. The faith community nurse functions to facilitate health and promotes, whenever possible, the congregation's mission of healing.

Job descriptions tend to be rather global in nature. Let us now look more specifically at the functions of a faith community nurse. In the early years of parish nursing in the United States, Rev. Granger Westberg identified five health-promoting functions carried out by parish nurses: health educator, personal health counselor, coordinator of volunteers, one who helps people relate to the complex medical care system, and one who assists people to integrate faith and health (Westberg, 1990b). Since that time, the functions of parish nurses have been further developed to include acting as integrator of faith and health, health educator, personal health counselor, referral agent and liaison with congregational and community resources, trainer of volunteers, developer of support groups, and health advocate (Holstrom, 1999; Solari-Twadell & McDermott, 1999). Although we use the term *faith community nurse* rather than *parish nurse* in this text, we see the functions carried out as being identical. We will describe each of these functions in this chapter, offering examples of situations where faith community nurses serve in these various functions. For purposes of clarity, each function will be described individually. In faith community nursing ministry, however, there is much overlap among the various functions. In particular, we view the first function, acting as an integrator of faith and health, as one that regularly interfaces and overlaps with the other six functions.

∞ Integrator of Faith and Health

In earlier chapters, we described faith as being in relationship with, and health as both a social phenomenon and a way of living and behaving that includes elements of developing and becoming, coping and learning (Allen, 1981). One of the main functions of the faith community nurse is to foster dialogue between these two processes. The following discussion offers several examples of how this is done.

Shortly after her second miscarriage, Diane visited the faith community nurse, and asked to talk about mixed feelings that she was having toward both God and herself. Diane was 33 years old, and had a fulfilling and successful career. She desperately wanted to be a mother, and felt angry and hurt that her plans were not working out. She wondered if God was punishing her for waiting so long to have children.

In the same week, the faith community nurse was asked by the minister to visit a family who was struggling with issues related to end-of-life decisions. John's father was terminally ill with cancer, and could be moved into their home to live his last days. John and his wife, Marion, wondered about their ability to manage his care in addition to their careers and the needs of their three children. They had many questions about caring for a family member in the final phases of a terminal illness, and about what God wanted them to do in this situation. It was a time of much questioning and searching. The faith community nurse was asked to work with the family as they made this decision.

In times of loss and changes in health status, or during the normal transitions in life, people need introspection and reflection. Lane (1987) describes this activity of the human spirit as an attempt to make sense out of current life situations. People living in times of transition need to look back on the past in order to give meaning to the present and hope to the future. This reflective process helps people feel comfortable with who they are, and to accept and incorporate the changes life has imposed on them. It gives them the ability to go on. This is one example of how faith community nurses can assist people as they seek to connect their faith issues with the day-to-day situations of their lives.

To effectively function as an integrator of faith and health, the faith community nurse needs to be knowledgeable about what the human spirit is, what spirituality and the human spiritual dimension are, and how spirituality and religion both differ and overlap. Practice in this area also requires that the nurse has carefully reflected on her or his own spiritual journey, and continues to learn, grow, and develop spiritually. Nurses require skills in assessing the spiritual dimension of people, intervening appropriately, and, if necessary, referring people to additional spiritual resources. Faith community nurses work in an environment where such interventions can be developed in collaboration with other members of the ministry team. Spiritual resources might include prayer, music, spiritual writing, worship, sacrament, healing touch, healing services, or meditation.

Faith community nurses also serve as integrators of faith and health in the lives of people who are not currently experiencing life difficulties. The nurse, in various ways, reminds people that strengthening their spiritual life is one way to become and stay more whole and healthy. Consider the following situation as an example: A faith community nurse works in a highly professional congregation where there is a shortage of little but the time to enjoy all that life has to offer. The Christmas holiday season is coming up, and the nurse senses that people will be going through the motions of attending many holiday functions, buying expensive gifts, sending expensive greeting cards, and doing elaborate holiday entertaining while overeating, and getting inadequate rest and exercise. In preparation for this holiday season, the nurse plans a mid-October workshop, titled "Finding Simplicity and Beauty in the Christmas Season." Using guest speakers, discussion groups, and quiet time for reflection and meditation, those who attend are equipped with ideas about how to keep the holiness of the season without sacrificing their own health and well-being.

These are just a few of the many situations that faith community nurses deal with on a regular basis. Many faith community nurses have been drawn to this type of nursing practice because faith communities offer a unique context in which to speak with people about the deeper issues of life that have an impact on people's health. Although physical concerns may initially be the reason for visits to the nurse, there are often deeper psychological and spiritual issues at the root of the concerns presented. Faith community nurses spend much of their time working with people who have experienced loss of all types. Some have lost family members through death or divorce, and others have lost jobs, their health, or the familiarity of friends and community because of a move to a new location. In the faith community setting, people are free to discuss with the nurse all types of doubts and fears, even those related to changes in faith or lack of faith in these times of transition (Westberg, 1990b). Faith community nurses realize that questions and doubts regarding faith can prove to be the stimulus for further growth in faith, and thus greater overall health if the opportunity is used to its fullest.

∽ Health Educator

Health education is appropriate within a faith community setting, because there is often a close link between how people care for themselves as whole persons and how they view their health through the filter of their faith tradition. Many strive to be good stewards of what they have been given. People within faith communities often want to be healthier, and the faith community nurse can assist them in finding ways to achieve this goal. As a health educator, the faith community nurse increases awareness of how health issues and faith issues relate.

Faith Community Nurse as a Teacher

At times, the faith community nurse serves as a teacher when she or he functions as a health educator. Congregational members and their friends and neighbors are often responsive to workshops, seminars, and small group discussions on various topics related to health and health promotion. Frequently, it is the faith community nurse who, through ongoing community assessment, identifies the need for a particular class or seminar. Organizational skills are needed to plan the event and ensure attendance of people who could benefit. At times, members of a health and wellness committee may assist with identifying needs, advertising, and facilitating the session. The nurse may involve others expert in certain areas to actually conduct the sessions, leaving the nurse free to organize and conduct individual and family follow-up sessions as needed after interest has been expressed in the classes. Classes presented to congregational members and others are often only an entrance into the lives of the people (Boss & Corbett, 1990); many faith community nurses remain available after teaching sessions to meet individually with people who may want to talk privately about their particular concerns related to the topic presented. Follow-up sessions with individuals and families may take place during home or office visits.

Being aware of the principles of teaching and learning, and knowing what facilitates and blocks learning, will contribute to the success of any health education program. Furthermore, knowledge of the process of teaching and learning is basic to good faith community nursing. This includes knowing how to assess learners' needs, plan appropriate sessions, conduct sessions, and evaluate the effectiveness of the teaching. Faith community nurses need to be aware of differing styles of learning, as well as individual uniquenesses. Knowing the learning needs of various age groups and age-appropriate teaching strategies will also be essential to effective health education. For example, a presentation during a children's sermon would be quite different from a session with a group of teenagers or a meeting with a group of seniors.

The faith community nurse, as a health teacher, needs an understanding of how objectives are developed and used, so that sessions will be organized effectively. Objectives serve to guide content and process, and can be used as the basis for evaluating the effectiveness of the session. The nurse also needs to learn how to assess and use appropriate learning resources to aid learners. Although a variety of printed

material and videos are available to supplement health education sessions, nurses must assess the appropriateness of materials in terms of
the level of education needed to understand them, cost, and congruence with the intended objectives. Finally, the nurse must be attentive
to the physical and psychological environment that is optimal for
learning. For example, a group of teens might learn better sitting in a
circle on a carpeted floor with ample popcorn available than in a classroom setting with tables and chairs. Most learners will respond better
to a learning environment that encourages them to share their learning
needs early in the session, rather than one that imposes a totally pre-
planned session on them.

The activities of nurses serving as health teachers include conducting parenting classes for members in a congregation with many young
families, or inviting a local pharmacist to speak to a seniors group
about medication safety. In another congregation, senior members
may benefit from invited speakers addressing the topics of learning to
write journals or create scrapbooks as reflective strategies for increasing spiritual health.

Health Education in Faith Communities

We view the function of a health educator as being more than only
a teacher. Health education involves one-on-one work with people at
teachable moments, as well as the ongoing sharing of health promotion information with such groups as church committees. It also
includes making sure that current health-related information is available to congregational members, their friends, and their families
through the use of bulletin boards, pamphlet displays, articles in
newsletters, and inserts in bulletins. Sermons, children's stories, and
other opportunities to speak to groups are other ways to accomplish
health education. Health fairs conducted within faith communities
provide an opportunity for health resources in the larger community
to present their services through presentations, discussion groups, or
poster displays.

✑ Personal Health Counselor

Faith community nurses spend much of their time in activities that
could be considered personal health counseling. As a personal health

counselor, the faith community nurse assesses the health needs of individuals, families, and groups. Faith community nurses offer private sessions to assist people in modifying lifestyles, adjusting to short-term illness, coping with chronic illness, and dealing with other health concerns. Although some visits occur in the church, faith community nurses also visit congregational members in hospitals, homes, and nursing homes to provide a link with the faith community. The nurse assists people to express feelings, identify the health issues they are facing, identify possible solutions for dealing with their own health issues, and evaluate the effectiveness of newly learned coping strategies. The availability of the faith community nurse at informal settings makes access to her or his services easy. For example, during the coffee hour after the Sunday worship service, a parishioner might express a need, and the nurse respond with a suggestion that they meet sometime soon in the nurse's office. At other times, the nurse may follow up with health counseling on the telephone, during a home visit, or in a quiet and private corner of the church sanctuary. Availability and flexibility are most critical to carrying out this role effectively (Boss & Corbett, 1990).

Faith community nurses are sometimes involved in cocounseling with faith group leaders. The advantage to this is that the perspectives and expertise of two disciplines can be combined to give parishioners a richer counseling experience. Since most faith community nurses are female and many faith leaders are male, there is also the potential benefit of different gender perspectives. In particular, enriched marital and family counseling experiences have resulted in combining the expertise of a male clergyperson and a female nurse.

It is interesting to note that Westberg (1990b) found that health counseling was sought by three main groups within congregations: the elderly, parents of preadolescents and teenagers, and men over 40. The issues that the elderly brought to the parish nurse included medications, difficulties in communicating with their doctors, and the need for somebody to help them cope with the complicated healthcare system. Parents of preadolescents and teenagers needed assistance with issues related to drugs, alcohol, and sexuality. It seemed that in the case of men over forty, a physical complaint often served as a pretext for discussing deeper anxieties in their lives. Also, these men admitted that they were more open with the nurse than they were with their doctor. They were grateful for the opportunity to share their real issues.

✦ *Referral Agent and Liaison*
With Congregational and Community Resources

To become knowledgeable in the function of referral agent and liaison with congregational and community resources, one of the first tasks that a faith community nurse undertakes is a comprehensive community assessment. This involves looking at the resources and needs within the congregation, as well as becoming familiar with the resources that exist outside of the congregation. This assessment is ongoing, but once the work has begun, the nurse is in the position to fulfill the role of referral agent and liaison with the congregation and community.

As a health referral agent and liaison with the congregation and community, the nurse determines the health resources available within and beyond the congregation, refers people to appropriate community resources, and assists persons in understanding and using the healthcare system. For example, during the sharing of a meal following a Buddhist temple worship service, the faith community nurse might learn from the friends of a longtime senior member that she has stopped attending worship because her arthritis limits her ability to walk. The nurse telephones later in the week, makes a home visit, and prepares resources that the woman may consider in dealing with her decreased mobility.

In another faith community, at the coffee hour following a worship service, a middle-aged woman approaches the faith community nurse because she has read the bulletin insert about October being breast cancer month. In the insert, the nurse mentioned mammograms and breast self-examinations as ways to detect breast cancer. The woman says she has never learned to do breast self-exams, and, though she was 50 years old, had never had a mammogram. The nurse promised to call on Monday with some possible community resources to address the woman's interest in breast cancer screening programs.

In our current complex healthcare system, people are often in need of someone who can assist them to understand the system and access the appropriate services with minimal difficulties. The faith community nurse is in a perfect position to offer this service to people within the faith community and in the surrounding community.

In addition to knowing both what resources are available in the community and beyond and how to access them, the skilled faith community nurse will need to know when to refer people, and how to determine the appropriateness of various resources for specific situations. The nurse will also need the ability to recognize the factors that promote or hinder people's receptivity to referrals and to assist people to make their own decisions regarding the use of various community resources. Finally, the nurse needs to follow up with people regarding the effectiveness of the resources offered.

Conducting an ongoing community assessment keeps the faith community nurse aware of new resources in the surrounding community, and, through the exchange of information, makes the health ministries of the church known to those agencies. Wonderful partnerships in this two-way communication process have developed as a result. An organized, user-friendly filing system containing community resources is of great value, not only to the faith community nurse, but also to other ministry personnel. As part of the community assessment, the faith community nurse will determine the main age groups and special health needs present within the congregation. Since it would be impossible to gather information about all potential needs that might arise, this information will give the nurse a point from which to begin gathering information about community resources. It is far more practical to begin with resources that are most likely to be needed within the particular congregation. Grounded in the particular needs of the local faith community, the nurse then makes ongoing efforts to connect the local faith community with the larger community.

ᡒ *Trainer of Volunteers*

When we speak of the faith community nurse as a trainer or facilitator of volunteers, we are referring to her or his function in relationship with a congregation's health ministries. It is important to recognize from the beginning that a faith community nurse is not hired to carry out a health ministry in isolation. Facilitating volunteer activities is one way to ensure that the health ministry belongs to the broader congregation. The faith community nurse recruits, educates, coordinates, evaluates, and recognizes the activities of volunteers within faith community health ministries.

It has long been recognized that the church is not only a gathering place, but also a place of deployment; it is not an agency to be served, but a work force to be deployed. Although a ministry focuses partly on nurturing the lives of congregational members, the preparation of people for missions and ministries is equally important. Churches cannot exist without the contributions of volunteers. Indeed, faith communities operate largely on volunteer services. People want to be occupied with meaningful, challenging tasks, and want to be more than receivers in life. In most churches, however, the volunteer work force is small. This is largely because people have not been asked, motivated, and directed into useful volunteer congregational activities. Many members, therefore, have decided to channel their volunteer interests elsewhere (Feucht, 1974).

Carrying out a successful, intentional health ministry requires many caring and dedicated individuals who are committed to serving others. These volunteers often provide the only link between people in the faith community and those who are elderly, ill, and in other difficult life situations. Although some recipients of volunteer ministries are elated to experience this caring, others openly express anger and disappointment about their life circumstances to the volunteer. Serving in a health ministry in such situations is not easy. The faith community nurse brings to this type of situation the professional skills and leadership that can motivate, encourage, and give support to people as they go about these important activities with limited training (Boss & Corbett, 1990).

As the coordinator of volunteers in a faith community, the nurse will need to be aware of the health ministries and resources that already exist in a congregation and within the larger community. When the faith community nurse determines that needs exist and there are no resources, the church might have an opportunity to fill a need by developing a new health ministry or broadening an existing health ministry. A clear mission statement and position description are needed when a new volunteer health ministry is developed. People are more likely to volunteer when they have a title, know the purpose of the position, and the nature of the work to be done. They also like to know how much time will be required of them, and for how long they need to commit themselves to the task. Few people volunteer for something that has an indefinite term. Each volunteer has a right to know to whom they will be reporting in this volunteer position, as well as to whom they may go to seek guidance, direction, and support. They may also want to know if financial and other resources are available for doing the volunteer work.

The faith community nurse needs to be skilled in seeking out good volunteers. Personal invitations often produce the best results. Using talent forms and recommendations of others on the pastoral team may be ways to locate appropriate volunteers. In the area of health ministries, it is important that volunteers are easily able to meet, be open in conversations, and establish good rapport with people. Furthermore, they need to be people who can be trusted with confidential information. In searching for good volunteers, it is important to know what motivates people to volunteer. It has been shown that people volunteer because they have a desire to help and to feel needed, and because they want to learn new things. They also seek personal renewal and a sense of meaning, and often want to give back to an organization that has helped them. Some seek the sense of satisfaction that comes from being part of a community; these people respond best to a personal request from a staff person or another volunteer, and they like having clearly defined roles and responsibilities (Briggs, 1987; Gould, 1994; Murrant & Strathdee, 1995).

Once volunteers have been recruited for a health ministry, it is important to train and support the volunteers in their ongoing roles. Reasons that volunteers give for continuing in their positions include personal growth, self-actualization, support and satisfaction, and feeling a sense of purpose and accomplishment. It has been determined that the factors leading volunteers to terminate their positions include the requirement of too much time, feelings of inadequacy, a lack of clarity about the work, finding little sense of accomplishment, feeling taken for granted, feeling burned out, having health problems, and completing the project (Chevier, Steuer, & MacKenzie, 1994; Omoto, 1995). Examples of volunteer health ministries in a faith community might include outreach ministries, transportation services, youth peer-support groups, foster grandparent programs, friendly visitor programs, or conducting regular worship services in a long-term care facility. Knowing what motivates and keeps volunteers will help the faith community nurse to recruit capable individuals to these programs and to understand when volunteers feel the need to discontinue their services.

✍ *Developer of Support Groups*

Social support refers to interactions with family members, friends, peers, and health care providers for the purpose of communicating information, esteem, aid, and emotional help. It "occurs as a by-product of people's ongoing interactions" (Stewart, 1995b, p. 93). It is well known that people who experience social support in their lives are healthier, no matter how health is measured (Federal Provincial and Territorial Advisory Committee on Population Health, 1994). Faith communities have a long history of providing social support to people. By their very nature, they are communities of people who share in similar religious values and beliefs, and who come together to support one another in those beliefs. The role of the faith community nurse within a congregation will be to formalize some of the social support that already exists within the community.

Cutrona (1990) describes five types of social support: emotional, esteem (appraisal), tangible (instrumental), informational, and social integration. The sources of social support have been identified as lay sources (partners, spouses, family members, friends, neighbors, coworkers, and volunteers), self-help groups, and professionals (Stewart, 1995b). All types of social support can be made available to people within a faith community setting. The unique capabilities of the faith community nurse can provide not only the self-help group concept of social support, but also a broader view of social support within and beyond the faith community. As the examples to follow will demonstrate, the role of support group coordinator interfaces with many of the other functions of the faith community nurse.

At times, tangible or instrumental social support might be specifically set up through the faith community nurse when a person or family experiences a particular need. For example, a transportation system for getting a homebound person to chemotherapy appointments might be arranged through a faith community nurse; or, a family experiencing the crisis of a premature newborn might temporarily benefit from the instrumental support of a team of members taking turns to provide meals and child care for the family. Much of this type of social support comes forward voluntarily when needed. The nurse's role might be that of coordination, and of recognizing and thanking people who contribute their support.

At times, the request for social support comes from external sources. For example, a home care nurse may seek the assistance of a faith community when her patient, a member of that community, is in need of assistance that goes beyond what can be provided in the existing healthcare system. In the case of a congregational member choosing to die at home, for example, other church members may supplement home care services by taking turns relieving a caregiver, tired from ongoing care. A faith community nurse would work with nurses or other health professionals in the community to set up the additional services required to support the family in need.

Emotional and informational support might be supplied by the faith community nurse or other members of the ministry team, but the nurse may also furnish it by referring people to established self-help support groups in the broader community. These therapeutic groups provide assistance in dealing with various special situations, such as major illnesses, physical conditions, or a life crisis. The groups serve to prevent or reduce the effects of the stress that accompany the difficulties members share. Examples include alcohol addiction, obesity, divorce, and grief and loss (Newton, 1984). Faith community nurses are knowledgeable about the reputation of established community support groups. They also bring skills in facilitating support groups on an ongoing basis or initiating self-help groups that will carry on without the nurse. Such group facilitation is a skill that requires a great deal of knowledge and practice; if a faith community nurse feels limited in these skills, cofacilitation of a group with someone more skilled might initially be helpful. For example, a faith community nurse might cofacilitate a cancer support group with a faith community leader skilled in group leadership. Although this may appear to be a duplication of services provided in the broader community, the faith community setting is inviting to many people who seek to be informed and strengthened by their faith tradition in times of physical illness.

✑ Health Advocate

An important role of the faith community nurse is that of health advocate. As a health advocate, the faith community nurse works to provide resources that are in the best interest of people from a whole-person perspective. Sometimes the role of health advocate requires that the nurse listen and support clients in doing what they can do on their own, and sometimes it requires being the voice of a client who seems to have none (International Parish Nurse Resource Center, 1998). People often face healthcare situations and settings that are frightening, confusing, and unfamiliar. They might feel like ships needing guidance in unfamiliar waters, and will benefit from a professional working with them to navigate the unknowns of the system and to clear the path of obstacles (Kosik, 1972).

To be a successful health advocate, the nurse needs to understand the culture and uniqueness of the people being represented, so that she or he can communicate from their frame of reference. In addition to offering support, guidance, and intercession for others, the role of health advocate includes helping people learn to navigate the system better themselves. Finally, the nurse advocate works to make the system more responsive to client needs in the future (Kosik, 1972).

Although advocacy is identified as a faith community nursing function, making a system more responsive to the needs of individuals or groups can sometimes become the work of an entire faith community. Advocacy can mean that people within a faith community come together to bring about positive change in our social systems. This takes a major commitment on the part of the congregation, and requires leadership from someone like a faith community nurse or faith group leader as members work to promote social justice (Boss & Corbett, 1990). In the role of health advocate, the faith community nurse may also serve as a mediator, helping to interpret another's point of view in situations where an individual or family feels "up against" a system. In these times, there is usually not one side that is right or wrong; there are just miscommunications that require a neutral third party to act as a mediator (Boss & Corbett, 1990).

Examples of a faith community nurse serving as a health advocate include nurses assisting a parishioner evicted from an apartment to find appropriate and affordable housing, or organizing the faith community in political action to make known the needs of a disadvantaged group of people. Likewise, the nurse might attend a medical appointment with a parishioner who does not feel understood by her family physician.

∽ Summary

We have described the seven functions of a parish or faith community nurse. Just as the nurse strives to foster faith and health in the congregational context in her or his own unique way, this professional integrates the seven functions into the nurse's uniqueness. The description of functions draws attention to the fact that being a faith community nurse requires both broad-based and specialized education, ample nursing experience, and comfort in addressing the spiritual dimension of people. Furthermore, the ability to work independently and as a collaborative team member is essential to the work of the faith community nurse.

11

Components of Optimal Nursing Practice Within a Faith Community

Professionalism, Spiritual Maturity, and Self-Care

Joanne K. Olson

There are many factors that contribute to a successful faith community nursing program, including a congregation that truly sees its mission as that of health and healing; faith group leaders who understand, and are willing to work in partnership with, other professionals to promote the full potential of health ministries; and a nurse who is well prepared for faith community nursing. In other words, there must be a faith community ready to move in new directions, faith community leaders ready to offer leadership in the development of health ministries, and a faith community nurse ready to carry out the role effectively (Olson & Clark, 1999). The combination of these three components provides the potential for a flourishing new adventure in conponents provides the potential for a flourishing new adventure in congregational life. In this chapter, however, the focus will be on the factors that relate directly to the nurse.

A focus on wellness and personal growth has long been central to the essence of faith community nursing. It is no coincidence, then, that Westberg (1987) emphasized that the personal qualifications of a parish nurse were extremely important to the success of a parish nursing program. To be instruments of health and healing in others, nurses are required to demonstrate relational abilities, professionalism, spiritual maturity, and commitment to practicing self-care. Previous chapters have focused on the relational abilities needed for faith community nursing; this chapter will focus on professionalism, spiritual maturity, and self-care.

Often included in the requirements for being hired as a parish nurse are the following items:

- A knowledge of the healing/health ministry of a congregation
- Practice from a holistic health perspective
- Excellent communication skills
- Knowledge about principles of teaching and learning
- Knowledge about health promotion, health services, and community resources
- Participation in church and community activities
- Knowledge of and compliance with a code of ethics for nurses
- Active membership in a professional organization
- Continual growth and learning through formal and informal professional development (Westberg, 1987)

In this chapter, we will consider three components of optimal nursing practice in a faith community: (a) preparation for professional practice, (b) spiritual maturity, and (c) self-care for one's own well-being and as a model to others.

✒ *Professional Practitioners as Faith Community Nurses*

What does it mean to be a professional practitioner? How does being a professional practitioner contribute to optimal nursing practice within a faith community?

An occupation is usually considered a profession when it meets certain standards. These include (a) being relevant to social values (i.e., the knowledge of the professional practitioner is used for the benefit of society); (b) having the commitment to society demonstrated by a code of ethics; (c) possessing a theoretical framework on which professional practice is based; (d) possessing a formal base of knowledge that is complex, guides practice, and is continually expanded through research; (e) controlling, by members of their own profession, practice and education standards for the admission of new practitioners into the profession; (f) requiring a lengthy period of education and supervised practice before independent practice begins; (g) having a form of licensing or registration required prior to practicing in the profession; and (h) having a lifelong learning commitment by members working in the profession (Caplow, 1954; Flexner, 1910; Ross Kerr, 1996b). Professional organizations have developed for the improvement of standards of practice and education, and for the monitoring of professional conduct (Ross Kerr, 1996b).

Although nursing, as a whole, meets the requirements for a profession, it is up to each individual nurse to carry out her or his practice in a professional manner. To be truly effective in the role of faith community nurse, a nurse needs to be recognized as a professional, equal with and able to communicate with other professionals on the ministry team and in the community.

Educational Preparation

How, then, does the individual practitioner act or function to demonstrate that she or he is a member of a profession? First and foremost, the professional faith community nurse has undergone a long and rigorous preparation for the position. The basic nursing education is, preferably, a baccalaureate degree in nursing. In addition, several years of nursing experience in various health care settings is an important asset. Known for an emphasis on physical, emotional, mental, social, and spiritual health, baccalaureate education programs prepare practitioners to view people holistically. These programs develop the knowledge and skills needed by nurses working with individuals, families, groups, and entire communities. Compulsory and elective non-nursing courses offer students a general education, further assisting them in understanding people and the complexity of health and health promotion. Skills in leadership, critical reflective thinking, and the utilization of research findings, also highly emphasized in university nursing programs, are needed in the practice of faith community nursing. Finally, in these university nursing programs, students often have opportunities to work collaboratively with members of other health disciplines in their formative student years. This opportunity offers interdisciplinary team-building skills that will enhance faith community nursing practice.

Faith community nursing occurs in a unique setting, often without another nurse on the ministry team. These two factors—the unique setting and the independent nursing role—require additional educational preparation. Such courses can be obtained for credit at some universities, and other courses are offered on a continuing education basis. Of note in this regard are the curriculum development activities of the International Parish Nurse Resource Center (1997/1998). It is highly recommended that faculty-supervised nursing practice be a significant part of the courses that prepare nurses for the role and functions of faith community nursing. Additionally, courses in clinical pastoral education and theology will be valuable to the practice of faith community nursing.

Continuing Education

Knowledge in the nursing profession is continually updated through research and practice developments. It is critical, therefore, that an active professional nurse engage in lifelong learning; this is especially true for a nurse in the faith community setting. Because faith community nursing involves two professional bases of knowledge—nursing and theology—it entails keeping current with two professional groups. In some locations, nurses have developed faith community nursing interest groups in order to meet some of their continuing education needs; furthermore, parish nursing conferences are held at both national and international levels. For a nurse working in an independent nursing role, such as faith community nursing, it is of particular importance to interact regularly with other nurses for support and information sharing.

Professional Association Membership

For legal purposes and to maintain professional standards, faith community nurses must be currently licensed to practice as registered nurses in the state or province in which they are working. Some faith community nurses practice on an unpaid basis, through an arrangement agreed to by the individual and the faith community; the nurse must be licensed, nonetheless, and the congregation should go through the same hiring process and commissioning ritual that would be conducted for a nurse hired for a paid position. Retired nurses, health professionals not licensed as registered nurses, or nurses not currently holding active registration may not be considered parish nurses or faith community nurses. Their skills, however, are valuable, and they should be encouraged to contribute to the faith community's voluntary health ministry being coordinated by the faith community nurse. Although limiting use of the title *faith community nurse* or *parish nurse* to a registered professional nurse may seem restrictive, we believe that the complexity of this emerging nursing role requires the depth and quality that comes through broad-based, professional, academic education that is recognized through a professional registering process.

As a profession, nursing is autonomous in setting its own standards for practice. When working in collaboration with other professionals, nurses carry out their own nursing assessments, interventions, and evaluations based on the knowledge gained in years of formal and continuing education, as well as from work experiences. Membership in a professional nursing association links the faith community nurse to standards of nursing practice, a professional code of ethics, and, in some cases, professional liability coverage. It can also make available journals, continuing education, updates on current research, and networking opportunities. As an independent practitioner, each faith community nurse is responsible for following the standards of practice for the province or state in which practice occurs. These standards usually carry an obligation to document and keep confidential the assessments, interventions, and evaluations of the nursing care provided. Faith community nurses are guided by the nursing profession's code of ethics, as well as codes of ethics that might exist in the congregation or the sponsoring faith group body in which she or he is employed.

✍ The Faith Community Nurse as a Spiritually Maturing Professional

The successful faith community nurse feels a sense of calling to use her or his professional nursing knowledge and skills to serve others through a ministry. Spiritual maturation is a developmental process that runs parallel to physical, mental, emotional, and social development (Moffatt, 1996). As a process, maturing in all areas of human development needs to be ongoing. For the faith community nurse, spiritual maturation is especially central to holistic growth and development. The characteristics of a spiritually maturing person are, first and foremost, that this person understands the central role that the spiritual dimension plays in achieving wholeness for self and others. Second, the spiritually maturing person is aware of her or his relationships with self and others, including divine or transcendent others, and knows that fully experiencing, reflecting on, and learning from these relationships continues throughout life. Ongoing development means that at times, even cherished beliefs need to be released so that they can be transformed and changed. When assessing a potential faith community nurse candidate for involvement in the process of spiritual maturation, it is important to remember that personal piety is not the same as spiritual maturity. Personal piety, which stresses personal devotion at the expense of deeper theological and biblical principles (McBrien, 1981), may even serve as a barrier to the spiritual maturation process.

∽ The Faith Community Nurse as a Model of Self-Care

Caring for others in the congregation in health-promoting ways is important, but can only be done if the caregiver is also promoting her or his own health. Nurses have a reputation for giving endlessly, both at work and at home. In moving nursing practice into faith community settings, we have entered a culture that also has a long history of rewarding people for unlimited giving of themselves. The effectiveness of the faith community nurse will be significantly diminished if that nurse is tired, overcommitted, run-down, and stressed. Furthermore, the faith community nurse's skills in effective self-care can serve as a role model to clergy and others with whom she or he works on the ministry team. A successful faith community nurse is able to recognize the signs of physical, psychological, emotional, and spiritual distress in herself or himself, and knows when changes need to be made in the way life is being lived. The physical body tells us, through muscle tension, headaches, and illness, that we are living in stressful times. When we worry, feel depressed, or experience low self-esteem, our mind is telling us that something needs to be changed. Our spirits, too, cry out when the stress of life becomes too much. We feel like life has no meaning or purpose, and that there is an emptiness about what we do. We may feel hopeless and that God is far away.

At the 1998 Westberg Parish Nursing Symposium in Itasca, Illinois, Dr. Abigail Ryan Evans (1998) spoke about a prescription for health. She titled her presentation *Prescription for Health: Healthy Living, Holy Lives.* The main point of her presentation was that, in order to be effective health ministers, parish nurses need to practice what they preach and model healthy living. She defined healthy living as nourishing the inner spirit, acknowledging the transcendent in our lives and in the work, enriching our minds, and caring for our bodies as the temple of the divine. She talked of stress being caused by four things: (a) lack of self-understanding and low self-esteem, (b) workaholism (when we have low self-esteem we may justify our existence by overworking as a type of compensation), (c) the loss of a spiritual center or the following of false values, and (d) other people or life events over which we have no control.

Included in Evans's prescription for holy lives is becoming part of a faith community to provide the milieu for good health. In such a supportive community, health can be enhanced by love and support, rather than judgment or retaliation. Using Psalm 127 as a basis, Evans (1998) spoke of healthy living from the perspective that our physical health is affected by our spiritual well-being and our religious beliefs and practices. When she spoke of spiritual well-being, she argued that to achieve it one must affirm that one lives a life in relationship to God, self, community, and an environment that nurtures and celebrates wholeness.

Brian P. Hall (1982, 1991) identifies twelve resources for self-caring in ministry. They are as follows:

- Knowledge of God
- Knowledge of the self
- Contemplating others
- Time management
- The body
- Sacred texts and prayer
- Relaxation

- Nonattachment
- Meditation
- Work delegation and support
- An intimacy system
- A peer support system

Although these twelve ideas are to be credited to Hall, we wish to develop them in two ways. First, we will summarize Hall's descriptions of each type of self-care resource. Then, we will discuss selected self-care resources in more depth as they apply to the faith community nurse.

Knowledge of God refers to one's own experience of the divine or grace, as well as one's response to this experience. Knowledge of the self is one's basic self-understanding, informed through one's experience of woundedness and joy, in a lifelong process of learning and of serendipitous discovery. In going beyond the self and contemplating others, one recognizes and appreciates the innate goodness of others and the importance of integrity in human interactions, and one acquires the skills needed to foster meaningful relationships. Time management includes all that is involved in not only the strict management of time, but also the struggle to balance work and play in life. The body refers to the promotion of one's own physical well-being through rest, diet, and exercise. Reading sacred texts and developing an active prayer life are activities that nourish the soul and give us opportunity to spend time with the divine in whatever ways may be meaningful to us.

Relaxation is important, because when we relax we reduce the anxiety and tension in our body, mind, and spirit. As this happens, we become more present to the moment and to those around us. Nonattachment is a process of one-centered-ness and deep concentration that keeps us focused in the present. Meditation is the experience of waiting in silence for the divine to speak. Determining boundaries and limits, and recognizing the need for work delegation and support, are critical to people in care giving or ministry positions. One type of support is an intimacy system: a close and personal support relationship with a friend or family member. A peer support system is important as well; this is a system of persons at your professional level, possibly coworkers but not intimate friends, with whom one meets regularly to share ideas and receive feedback in a nonthreatening environment. Let us now look at some of these self-care strategies in greater detail.

Knowledge of God

Self-care involves reflecting both on the gifts of God in our lives and on how we respond in faith to these gifts (Hall, 1982, 1991). In the experience of clinical pastoral education, for example, there is opportunity to focus on activities that assist the faith community nurse in gaining these skills. Through ministry reflection, students learn about themselves in relationship with self and others, including divine or transcendent others. Peer and supervisory contacts support this intense self-growth process. Others learn more about their deity through reading, journaling, meditation, or prayer. At times, the assistance of a spiritual director or guide is helpful in tracking one's spiritual journey and getting to know the divine better.

Knowledge of Self

Telling stories about one's own life is one way to assist in getting to know oneself. It is important to ask, "Where is the divine or God in this story?" At the same time that one is learning about self, one is also learning about the divine. Being open to learning about all aspects of oneself and the divine allows one constantly to grow in greater depth. As a result, the skills of listening, communicating, and caring that one develops help not only oneself, but also others, to know who you really are. As others learn who you are, this is reflected back to you, and the ongoing cycle of self-knowledge and growth occurs.

Contemplating Others

Increasing one's ability to establish and maintain satisfying relationships is a powerful way of doing self-care. Seeing goodness and gifts in others, and contemplating God's love reflected in the love given by others, can be a self-care strategy. It is uplifting to take time away from working with others in human "doing" long enough to reflect on others as human "beings." This is especially true of those with whom faith community nurses share ministry work. Committing to team ministry means meeting regularly to share, plan, seek feedback, support, pray with, and encourage each other in the shared ministry.

Time Management

Countless books have been written on the topic of time management. Time is a commodity where no favors have been shown; we all receive the same 24 hours every day, and the same 168 hours every week. It is in choosing how we use the time that illuminates differences between people. We all struggle with questions of how to balance work with play, and time for others with time for ourselves. Stephen Covey (1994) indicates that being more efficient, as many time management strategies suggest, is not the answer; rather, the approach of deciding which things are important in life, and then going after them is the solution. He encourages us to remember that "the meaningful life is not a matter of speed and efficiency. It is much more a matter of what you do and why you do it, than how fast you get it done" (Covey, 1994, p. 12).

Effective time management also involves knowing our boundaries and limits. Likewise, knowing what we are capable of doing and what does not fall within our skill set may lead us to seeking assistance from others. Knowing how to balance work with relaxation is key to survival in faith community nursing. It is also critical to learn early that the role of the faith community nurse is to help others, not to rescue them; it is important to know where one's responsibility ends and another's takes over. Learning to say "No" assertively is not only self-preserving, but, in the long run, helps others also. By not taking on commitments one cannot keep, everyone will benefit. Remember that when people are asked to add a new obligation to their life, they have a right and a responsibility to themselves to think about it before responding. When thinking about a new commitment, one must consider that, to take on a new responsibility, something needs to be given up. What will be sacrificed for this new commitment?

The Body

Keeping oneself physically healthy is an important self-care strategy. Peak physical health contributes to mental, emotional, social, and spiritual health. Included in good physical health are good nutrition, being at an appropriate weight for height, getting adequate sleep, engaging in regular physical activity, avoiding tobacco and other harmful drugs, and limiting alcohol use. Our body lets us know when it is not being treated properly. Feeling easily fatigued and frequent illnesses are two examples of messages from our physical bodies that some changes in lifestyle need to be made.

Sacred Texts and Prayer

Many faith traditions have sacred texts. These are a focus of study, inspiration, and proclamation. The divine can communicate through these sacred texts and can nourish spiritual well-being. In addition, other spiritual readings can offer new perspectives and ideas for living deeper spiritual lives. Prayer, too, can be seen as time spent in relationship with the divine; this can sometimes mean talking and sometimes listening. In most faith traditions, prayers of thanksgiving, praise, confession, petition, and intercession can be found. In all of these types of prayer, there is active acknowledgement that the divine is present and powerful in our lives. Through prayer we create an openness in ourselves through which the divine can be known in nature around us, in people we encounter, in the situations we face, and as a divine other who transcends the here and now (Nouwen, 1995).

Meditation

A specific way of spending time with the divine is through meditation. Practices of meditation have been incorporated into many faith traditions. They emphasize a discipline of inner calm, unity, and receptivity that results in new ways of being in relationship with the divine, self, and others. "Meditation is communion. Meditation is accessing the Divine" (Moffatt, 1996, p. xv).

An Intimacy System

Human beings require intimacy for survival. Anyone wishing to grow spiritually must share intimately with at least one other person on a regular basis. This involves the open sharing of fears, hopes, joys, and possibilities. An intimate relationship needs to be reciprocal in nature, with both persons sharing equally. Self-care involves recognizing this need, feeling normal about having this need, and finding ways to meet one's intimacy needs.

A Peer Support System

Professional people are members of several peer support groups. First, they belong to a group of coworkers. To feel support within one's group of coworkers, one needs to be able at times to delegate work and obtain support when needed. For coworkers to be part of a network that contributes to self-care, they need to meet two criteria: First, anything that one person does can, if necessary, be delegated for a limited period of time to someone else; and, second, each member of the team has experiences of both giving and receiving support (Hall, 1982). A second source of peer support is from people who are at similar levels professionally, but with whom one does not work on a daily basis. As a self-care strategy, these people can supply us with feedback, encouragement, and new ideas for our work. Because they are not our coworkers, they can be helpful in a nonthreatening way. Formal professional organizations or informal groups can serve to meet these needs for professional contact.

✍ Summary

Although there are many factors that contribute to successful nursing practice within a faith community, the nurse herself or himself is one of the most important factors. In this chapter, we have considered how nurses prepare for professional practice within a faith community, and how they practice self-care physically, psychologically, emotionally, socially, and spiritually. Good self-care maintains health and models methods of health promotion for others in the faith community.

PART IV

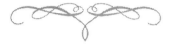

PROMOTING HEALTH IN TIMES OF TRANSITION

12 ✍

Living in a Time of Transition

Margaret B. Clark

When people experience change or transition, they respond first with *story*. Think of the times you have heard people tell over and over to stunned friends and relatives about their last memories of a loved one's life. In another vein, as nurses, consider how many times you have listened to new mothers giving precise and detailed descriptions of their birthing experience. These are stories of *transition*. What we find, in this regard, is that stories of change and transition are about one's relationships with the divine, other persons, or oneself.

Ministering within a faith community in times of transition will require of both nursing and pastoral professionals familiarity with *theology*. In this book we describe theology as an activity of *reflection and celebration around experiences of being in relationship with* the divine, others, and self. Being able to foster reflection and celebration in the lives of faith community members who are experiencing change can promote health and growth. Furthermore, it has been said that "theology proceeds by analogy" (Main, 1982). In analogy we seek likeness through comparison of things that are different; in a time of transition, we will spontaneously observe or study unfamiliar persons, places, and things to find out how they are like something with which we are more familiar. Indeed, the search for similarity in times of change is very basic to our nature. According to the Hebrew scriptures, our need for analogy commenced with the divine-human relationship. In Genesis, the creator declares, "Let us make humankind in our image, according to our likeness," and then goes on to create humankind "in the image of God" (Gen. 1:26-27 NRSV). Ever since that time, we humans have been reflecting on what it means to be "like God" (Gen. 3:5 NRSV). Across a multitude of cultures and faith traditions, we hear stories about the relationship between creator and creature. In studying these stories, various scholars have developed conceptual understandings about the world, heavens, gods and goddesses, heroic figures, and sacred places or objects. These are the disciplines of cosmology, theism, and heroism (Bowker, 1997; Campbell, 1968, 1988; Eliot, 1976; Hamilton, 1940; Leeming, 1990).

We suggest that a story is the first line of response to change, and the starting point of transition. *Webster's Ninth New Collegiate Dictionary* (1991) defines *change* as "becoming different," and *transition* as a "passage from one state, stage, subject, or place to another." Although more will be said about these concepts later, we all know what it is like to experience change. Perhaps it is a special family outing to the pet store where we pick out a new puppy. It may be the vacation trip when our car is hit by a drunk driver; our plans are radically changed, yet we marvel at the fact that no one was killed. Likewise, it may be the miraculous experience of becoming a parent or grandparent, where a new human life is held in our arms for the first time. Transitional events like these need to be talked about. In fact, it is in the telling and retelling of such stories that we begin to process and come to terms with their meaning for our lives.

This chapter will introduce the concepts of transition, worldview, paradigm, and filter. In light of our belief that story is the starting point of transition, it seems fitting that we begin this chapter with a fictional narrative, in which we see the anonymous narrator viewing the divine-human relationship in two ways: as a mechanistic and a relational approach. These differing points of view, alluded to in Chapter 6, are important inasmuch as they inform a person's perspective on not only the divine-human relationship, but also human-human interaction and human-object relationships. As such, they shape a person's ability to cope with change and make growthful transitions.

⌒ *A Story About Waiting in a Time of Transition*[1]

Arriving early for Matthew's birthday supper, I found a place to sit and wait. Nine-year-old Matthew appeared content to play with his toys in one part of the room, while his mother, Sarah, rehearsed for the evening performance of *Pilgrimage Theatre* in another part of the room. In her role as a faith community nurse, Sarah was working with a group of artists and musicians in the faith community who wanted to choreograph images of wellness through the media of ballet, ballroom, jazz, and rock dance motifs. Together they designed a theatrical collage of vignettes drawn from life experiences within the faith community that depicted a movement from illness to wellness. Tonight was the premiere performance.

From my place of waiting, I was able to observe both Matthew and Sarah in their different activities. My superficial observations grew into a more serious reflection as I began to see connections between what Matthew and Sarah were doing in their separate corners of the room and the idea of *worldview*, which had been introduced in a foundations of theology course I was taking. The instructor of that course had talked about the influence of philosophy on theology, and how the creator-creature relationship between God and humans has been described differently as a result of these philosophical influences. I began to ask myself, is it possible to see differing metaphors of the God-human relationship in the activities of Matthew playing with his toys and Sarah dancing her dance? And, if so, how might these metaphors be depictions of distinct worldviews that have been influenced by differing philosophical approaches? Suddenly my experience of waiting became a reflective event charged with curiosity and a search for meaning. I observed more keenly.

In Matthew's corner of the room, there seemed to exist a particular kind of relationship between the boy and his battery operated toy car.

As a metaphor of creator and creature, Matthew was creator and the toy car was his creature: Matthew put the car together and installed the batteries, and the final design was a reflection of his creativity and skill. The car was also something that could operate independently from him. Thus, when Matthew set the command button to "On," the car was able to function without him. It zoomed about on the floor at a distance from Matthew, who now became an observer of his creature. When he tired of playing with this toy, the car continued its movement even after Matthew shifted attention to other toys. Thus, in my observation, Matthew and his toy existed independently of one another; even though Matthew was "creator" and the car was "creature," once the car was set in motion it no longer needed to stay in relationship with its creator in order to operate.

I wondered, is it possible to see in the toymaker-toy relationship a metaphor of the relationship between God and humans? If God is the creator and human beings are God's creatures, is there a type of reasoning that parallels the "On" button and enables humans to function independently of God? Is this what René Descartes meant when he exclaimed, *cogito ergo sum* ("I think, therefore I am")? Is there some way that the exercise of human autonomy and free will can result in a human condition that no longer needs to stay in relationship with God? Is this the toy saying to the toymaker, "I no longer need you in order to remain in existence"? My mind was spinning and my heart raced as I let these thoughts take shape. I knew I needed to go back to my textbooks in order to explore this toymaker-toy metaphor in greater depth. I could see a connection with philosophies that grew out of the Renaissance and Enlightenment periods. For the time being, however, I had a sense of discovering something about a particular worldview in this metaphor. Now, how might this compare with what Sarah was doing?

In Sarah's corner of the room, a very different activity was taking place. I observed a woman using various ballet steps and movements to express herself through dancing. As a metaphor of creator and creature, Sarah was creator and the dance was her creature. It was Sarah who put the steps together and expressed them in continuous, graceful motion. The image of wellness portrayed through this dance was a reflection of Sarah's creativity and skill. Unlike Matthew's toy, however, Sarah's dance was not able to "run" on its own. Her dance depended on her, the dancer, for existence. Thus, in my observation, the relationship of dance to dancer was more organically connected than that of toy to toymaker. That is to say, even though Sarah as "creator" could exist apart from the dance as "creature," the dance could not exist apart from the dancer. Its existence was essentially dependent on Sarah to dance the dance. What a thought!

Again, I wondered to myself. How can the dancer-dance relationship be a metaphor of God-human relationship? If God, as creator, is the dancer and human beings, as creatures, are the dance, then the essential human condition is one of dependency on God. Just as the dance cannot exist apart from the dancer, human beings cannot exist apart from God; there is an essential and enduring connection between the two. This sounded both philosophical and theological in origin. I remembered hearing about the "principle of contingency" in metaphysics, and the "argument of cosmology" in my foundations of theology course. I also remembered stories from the Hebrew and Christian scriptures that spoke of the God-human relationship in terms of a dependency, such as sheep to shepherd, vine to vinedresser, infant child to parent, and so forth. In the dancer-dance metaphor, a very different worldview was in evidence than that found in the toymaker-toy relationship. I had a sense of being on the edge of important insights, and could see in Matthew's toy and Sarah's dance the possibility for further learning about worldviews. It was exciting even to think about!

Suddenly I was pulled out of my daydreams with a gentle touch on my cheek. I looked up and there was Matthew, a knowing twinkle in his eye and a mischievous smile on his lips. "We're ready now. I can't wait for you to see the place we're going for dinner! Mom says we can even have ice cream sundaes for dessert! And I get nine candles to blow out!" I got up from my chair, tucked my observations away for a time when I could reflect on them further, and joined the celebration.

∞ *From Story to Reflection*

The story of Matthew and Sarah invites reflection. Although it is tempting to go back into the story to identify the analogies and analyze their meaning, we have chosen a different approach. This story is used in teaching about nursing within faith communities; reading the story and discussing its meaning can yield significant insights. Our analysis, however, is not what matters; rather, it is the reader's response to this story that will awaken deeper levels of understanding. What if we allow the story to serve as a sort of "everyday life experience" that can change us? What if we choose to reflect on it as a type of "critical incident" from which to learn? What if it could become a container (Rutter, 1993) or holding environment (Maley, 1995) through which to better appreciate the network of relationships that arise in times of transition? What worldviews, paradigms, and filters can be found in the story? What methods of theological reflection or social analysis can be used to explore various aspects of the narrative better? And, what does the story say to us about ministering as a professional nurse within faith community settings in times of transition? It is important to point out that the experience of observing Matthew and Sarah changed the narrator of the story. Likewise, reading and reflecting on this story can change us. As we pay attention to how the storyteller processes the experience of observation, and to the ways we are processing our experience of reading and reflecting on the story, we will recognize that we are in the midst of the phenomenon of transition.

It all begins with relationship. Our narrator enters the scene, and this sets in motion a series of events that reveal different ways of being in relationship. There are the preexisting relationships between our narrator, Matthew, and Sarah. The story provides little information about the nature of these relationships, but there is a sense of comfort and warmth in their dealings with one another. Then, there are relationships connected to the day's events: Matthew's birthday party and the premier performance of *Pilgrimage Theatre*. Next, our narrator has a relationship with the room in which observations begin to occur, which leads the narrator to recognize the relationships between Matthew and his toy, and between Sarah and her dance. These two relationships point toward a theological reflection on the creator-creature relationship, and refer to some of the philosophical and theological principles influencing various perceptions. Finally, there is suggestion of a relationship between the narrator and various outside classes, books, concepts, and so forth.

As the reader reflects on this network of relationships within the story, questions may surface to guide his or her approach to the story. In time, it may be possible for the reader to entertain some tentative assumptions or insights about the narrative, and to point out different analogies and layers of meaning suggested through the images and actions portrayed. The phenomena of change and transition are evident at each stage of response to the story, as both narrator and reader employ processes of reasoning, feeling, curiosity, rumination, and tentative judgment in coming to terms with an event from everyday life that has caught their attention and imagination.

We are trying to show, through these reflections, that stories are containers for reflecting on the network of relationships that arise in times of change and transition. As we come to appreciate the containing or holding function of story, we increase our capacity for exploring the meaning of altered relationships brought about through developmental and situational change. Furthermore, since faith is understood as being in relationship with, as suggested in an earlier chapter of this book, and change is understood as something that affects *how* we are in relationship, we may want to consider a possible connection between faith and change. More will be said of this in later sections of the book.

∾ A Theory of Transition

We touched on the dictionary definition of *transition* earlier. We now wish to develop this further. According to *Webster's* (1991), a transition is a "passage from one state, stage, subject, or place to another," and also a "movement, development or evolution from one form, stage or style to another." In these definitions, we can recognize a distinction between *change* and *transition*. That is to say, if change is the experience of being in a motor vehicle accident in which there are injuries, then transition has to do with how this accident and these injuries are perceived within the context of one's overall life. William Bridges (1991) highlights this difference in his insightful text *Managing Transitions: Making the Most of Change.* He says that change is situational and external, whereas transition is internal, something he describes as a "process people go through to come to terms with the new situation" (p. 3). Thus, although changes happen and seem most often beyond our control, internal transitions in response to change are amenable to being shaped by the assistance of helping professionals, such as pastoral leaders and faith community nurses.

In the previous quotation, Bridges uses the word "psychological" to modify "process." We believe this modification limits the full scope of what is being described. That is to say, in order to appreciate transition as a passage, movement, development, or evolution, we must consider the *whole* person. Transition is as much a physical, intellectual, emotional, and spiritual process as it is a psychological process of coming to terms with change. Furthermore, transition goes beyond each new situation to a consideration of the *context* within which the situation occurs. Again, we look at the example of a motor vehicle accident. The accident and injuries may occur while on the way to work, during a summer holiday, or while running an errand on the weekend. No matter what the setting may be, a person will be affected by the sights, sounds, smells, emotions, ruminations, inspirations, and conversations that occur both internally and externally. Thus, transition enables movement from one's personal experience to the interpersonal and social realms of response to change.

In light of this broader perspective, we propose transitions to be both *processes* through which people come to terms with new situations in their lives, and *conduits* or *passageways* through which people move as these situations are viewed in relationship with all that has gone before and all that lies ahead in their life story. In the "big picture" of a person's life or a culture's existence, how, then, does one continue to become whole and healthy? How does one grow as well as learn from change?

Exploring different approaches to living in a time of transition is our theme in this section of the book. Building on earlier work, this chapter will revisit the terms *worldview, paradigm,* and *filter,* inasmuch as these concepts have an impact on times of transition. Subsequent chapters in this section of our book will discuss characteristics of transition and the types of transition that may occur within faith communities. Finally, we will reflect on the healing potential of transitional events, as well as on the nurse's role in promoting health during such times of transition.

⌐ Worldviews and Paradigms

The story of Matthew and Sarah, as seen through the eyes of the narrator, depicts two different approaches to the relationship between creator and creature. The metaphors of toymaker-toy and dancer-dance are introduced in relationship with the notion of worldviews. Building on references made to worldviews in previous chapters, we now want to approach the concept at three levels of experience. First, a worldview is one's total experience of creation as perceived through human consciousness and freedom (McBrien, 1981). Second, it is any theoretical framework used to speak about one's reality (Bosch, 1996; Rahner & Vorgrimler, 1965). Finally, it is a particular way of viewing the phenomenon of concern within one's professional discipline (Parse, 1987). What all three of these approaches have in common is their focus on *personal* experience. Although our lives are shaped by culture and tradition as well as circumstances and events, each person arrives at a particular worldview out of the uniqueness of their life story. Worldviews are held by individual persons. They flow out of the processes of perception, reasoning, understanding, and decision making, which constitute our ability to find meaning in our experience of created existence (Lonergan, 1972). People's worldviews give expression to their fundamental relationship with all that surrounds them.

By contrast, a paradigm is understood as a constellation of concepts, values, perceptions, and practices shared by a community, which forms a particular vision of reality that is the basis of the way the community organizes itself (Capra & Steindl-Rast, 1991). The important point of distinction here is that paradigms are *community* constructs. As soon as a person picks up a penny or a standard deck of cards, they are immersed in the domain of paradigms. Why is this so? Joel A. Barker (1992) tells us it is because both the penny and the deck of cards come with "a set of rules and regulations (written or unwritten) that establish or define boundaries and describe how to behave inside the boundaries in order to be successful" (p. 32).

Looking at the penny, for example, one sees on the front side a figurehead that indicates whether the coin belongs to Canada, the United States, or some other country. The Queen's image reminds Canadians that their roots return to a paradigm of monarchy. Abraham Lincoln's image reminds Americans that, in the United States, there is a paradigm of an executive office called the Presidency. In another vein, because of its assigned worth, a penny will not buy very much. One would not be successful if one tried to use a single penny as a down payment on one's dream home; the penny's assigned worth would limit such an attempt. Likewise, there are certain expectations associated with the standard deck of cards. One should be able to count out 52 cards, and to arrange them in four piles of 13 cards each, with two of the piles (hearts and diamonds) being red in color, and two (spades and clubs) being black. Certain values are assigned to each card, although in the context of a particular game, the values of the cards may change. All these structures help people to play with the cards and have fun.

So, what is a paradigm? When we look up the word in the dictionary, we discover it comes from the Greek *paradeigma*, meaning "model, pattern, example" (Barker, 1992, p. 31; see also *Webster's*, 1989). Paradigms come to us in all sorts of shapes and sizes. A classic example of a paradigm is the wheel. It is a model or pattern that emerged quite early in human history. When set within diverse contexts, the wheel has taken on a multitude of purposes and meanings. Thus, we speak of wagon, bicycle, and car wheels. At the same time, we can also speak of a potter's wheel, a roulette wheel, a wheel of cheese, a wheel of fortune, a wheeler-dealer, and so forth. In each expression, the basic paradigm is present, but the meanings change in connection to different aspects of social activity. Thus, paradigms become contextualized, assigned worth in relationship with other entities, and subject to the phenomenon of change.

༺ Paradigms and Filters

Paradigms flow out of everyday life experiences, and find expression in social mores, expectations, and interactions. In a manner of speaking, paradigms "filter" our life experiences, and help us to organize these experiences meaningfully. Furthermore, paradigms align with beliefs, values, and attitudes that derive from a variety of sociocultural sources. In Western Christianity, for example, feminine images of God are not common, but the image of Mary as Mother of God is familiar. In Hinduism, on the other hand, both masculine and feminine images of God are visible. Likewise, when speaking of relatives in Anglo-Saxon cultures, *grandfather* usually refers to the biological father of each parent, and one would expect to have only two grandfathers. In Aboriginal cultures, on the other hand, *grandfather* has both spiritual and familial significance; one may, for example, refer to the "grandfathers" when speaking of sacred rocks, spiritual mentors, or adopted providers. Thus, we see that a great deal of variation in paradigms derives from the filtering activity of social expectations and from cultural context.

Although we have referred to the term *filter* in several previous chapters, we now wish to look at this concept more closely. According to *Webster's* (1991), it is a word that came into English usage during the 1500s. Its primary application has been in the scientific design and operation of devices used to separate or purify liquids, gases, and other such elements. In the last hundred years, filtering has been used to describe the way a person perceives reality. In North America, for example, we sometimes hear it said that a person is "viewing the world through rose-colored glasses." This illustrates how a person can filter her or his perceptions of the world in a predominantly positive manner.

It is through the behavioral sciences of psychology and sociology that our understanding of the term has expanded more recently. Most personality theories include discussions of both human consciousness and the filtering activities of the unconscious (Goleman & Speeth, 1982; Herink, 1980). Likewise, social learning theorist Paulo Freire (1970/1993) addresses the relationship between filters and social awareness when he distinguishes between the "submerged consciousness," which actively assimilates knowledge without questioning; the "naively critical consciousness," which sees connections at first glance, but does not go so far as to see the big picture; and "critical consciousness," which has an ability to question and critically reflect on assumptions existing within a personal, institutional, or cultural way of life. Learning skills of questioning and critical reflection are important in the work of faith community nursing. That is to say, it is important to have some awareness of both the paradigms that are operative in a faith community setting and the filters that coexist with these paradigms, inasmuch as they influence what is seen, as well as what is not seen.

In this book, we define filters as learned attitudes, values, and beliefs formed in the context of everyday life that affect or color the way we approach new experiences. Relating this definition to the literature on paradigms, any data that exists in the real world but *does not fit* one's paradigm will tend to be filtered out. Likewise, data that *does fit* one's paradigm not only makes it through the filters, but is also concentrated by the filtering process and given greater weight or value. Thus, what may be perfectly visible and obvious to persons with one paradigm, will be invisible to persons with a different paradigm. This is referred to as "the paradigm effect" (Barker, 1992, p. 86).

Burley-Allen (1995) describes the influence of filtering on communication processes, stating that the "socialization process results in our listening through filters" (p. 39). She goes on to list assumptions, beliefs, values, attitudes, memories, expectations, interests, prejudices, strong feelings, past experiences, and the physical environment as some of the forms these filters take. Finally, she suggests that one way to gain greater consciousness of how our filters may be acting as blind spots in relating with others, is to question our beliefs.

An exercise offered to nurses studying about nursing within faith communities has been helpful in this area of questioning beliefs. The nurses are asked to complete the following sentence: "A belief I hold about the faith community as a context for my nursing practice is. . . ." Then, they are asked to consider the following questions in relationship with the belief statement they have formulated:[2]

How does this belief match what is actually happening in my faith community?

How does this belief limit me?

How does it feel to hold this belief?

How is this belief helpful to me, and what do I get out of holding this belief?

How would it feel to let go of this belief?

How would my life change if I were to let go of it?

How does this belief affect my practice of nursing?

Discussions based on this exercise have resulted in consciousness raising and energized communication, as filters are identified, and worldviews and paradigms revealed.

Successful faith community nursing rests on an ability to communicate effectively. Growth in communication among faith community nurses, pastoral leaders, and those who are the focus of their collaborative ministry endeavors calls for an exploration of filtering processes. Although the questioning of one's beliefs, values, and assumptions may involve a departure into uncertainty and doubt, it can also lead to deepened and broadened perspectives on healing and growth. In this regard it may be helpful to return to the notion of theological reflection as a way to self-knowledge, learning about others, discovering the collective story of a faith community, and doing social analysis when engaging in the work of questioning beliefs. Indeed, as the questioning of beliefs arises in self, others, the faith community, and society at large, those who are equipped with a variety of tools for theological reflection are in a position to do the work of journeying from doubt and confusion to renewed and intensified faith and clarity. In coming to terms with situations or circumstances that give rise to questions and doubts about personal and communal experiences of being in relationship, meaningful passageways to growth and health will be discovered. These passageways of transition are forged as the question-raising situations can be viewed in relationship with all that has gone before and all that lies ahead in a person's or community's life.

The challenge of living in a time of transition is that one must remain in relationship with the processes people go through to come to terms with new situations (Bridges, 1991). Staying in relationships that are conflicted, confusing, or severely stressed can be demanding. For example, the physical, emotional, and spiritual sufferings of war-traumatized children may endure in their bodies, minds, dreams, and memories for years. What beliefs about the faith community as context for ministry will need questioning when a faith community nurse joins a congregation's international relief mission and encounters real, live war-traumatized children? In another vein, a distraught mother who has lost an infant child may need to work her way through many layers of complicated grief before she feels that healing has occurred. How can the faith community nurse accompany this woman as she questions cherished beliefs and values that no longer fit? Likewise, the middle-aged man whose job is eliminated through organizational restructuring may need to struggle with a crisis of identity and purpose before he has energy to reenter the workforce. What forms of supportive presence on the part of a faith group leader or faith community nurse will enable him to enter his disillusionment and discover renewed meaning for his life? Finding answers for questions like these will involve an evaluation of one's worldview, paradigms, and filters.

ᘇ *Summary*

This chapter introduced the concept of *transition* and the important role faith communities can play when living in a time of transition such as our own. It also discussed the value of story and relationship in distinguishing between change and transition. Furthermore, our chapter proposes that transitions are, first, processes through which people come to terms with new situations in their lives, and, second, conduits or passageways through which people move as these situations are viewed in relationship with all that has gone before and all that lies ahead. The task of approaching situations both comprehensively and holistically is aided when individuals and groups become aware of the *worldviews, paradigms,* and *filters* that influence their perceptions of reality. Finally, if one is ministering within a faith community, it is important to be cognizant of how one's own worldview interfaces with the worldviews of others. Likewise, individuals, groups, and the faith tradition as a whole all need to be appreciated in the light of differing worldviews, paradigms, and filtering systems.

Coming to know the individual stories of congregational members, as well as the collective story of a faith community, can provide ministry professionals prepared in nursing and/or theology with an opportunity both to question beliefs about and to foster dialogue on topics of faith and health. Faith communities are locations where inter related conditions for faith and health coexist. Sojourning, through ambiguity and obscurity, in search of how these conditions give meaning to one's life requires endurance and perseverance. Remaining in transition requires that we bring a vision of faith and health to our worldviews, paradigms, and filters. Grounded in such a vision, we will participate in "weaving the web of life," and will contribute to an awareness that "all things are connected" (Chief Seattle, quoted in Gass, 1992).

Notes

1. The author wishes to recognize Ronald Rolheiser, O.M.I., for first introducing the images of toymaker and toy, as well as dancer and dance, to the author as metaphors of divine-human relationship during a class at Newman Theological College in Edmonton, Alberta.

2. The author wishes to recognize Frank Kimper, Presbyterian minister, for first sharing these questions with the author during a workshop at Angela Center in Santa Rosa, California.

13 ☙

Characteristics of Transitions

Margaret B. Clark

Nurses who minister within faith communities are in frequent contact with the characteristics of transitions. In this chapter, we discuss these characteristics in a variety of ways. First, we describe them; second, we break them down into components, and then develop them as both stages in an individual's sojourning and phases in a community's life cycle. Finally, the elements of space and time will be introduced in relationship with the characteristics of transitions; that is, space and time are important insofar as these two concepts create the primal boundary system within which human activities occur. For the faith community nurse, observing human movement within space and time is an aspect of whole-person assessment.

Nurses know that visible behaviors often point to invisible thoughts, feelings, longings, secrets, coping mechanisms, and hopes. It is within this invisible domain that transitions occur. Fostering life choices among members of a faith community will have implications for planning and decision making by spiritual leadership teams, including faith community nurses. Drawing out from persons and societies the deep resources that can inform their capacity to choose both quality of life and quality of death in times of transition is an activity of healing, health, and wholeness. The faith community nurse needs a breadth of both knowledge and skill to promote the capacity for health improvement and the inquiry necessary to mobilize potentials and strengths in service of healthy development. To assist pastoral leaders and nurses within faith communities in their tasks of both faith renewal and health promotion, the current chapter attempts to describe and reflect on some of the global and local characteristics of transitions faced by individuals and larger communities.

৩ Describing the Characteristics of Transitions

We said in the previous chapter that change is something that happens to us, whereas transitions are phenomena we participate in. Since transitions are often complex and multidimensional in nature, our participation in them will naturally be a combination of both conscious and unconscious involvement. We all know what it is like to hear shocking news or be affected by an unexpected catastrophe. Such events evoke many different forms of physical, emotional, mental, and spiritual adaptation. It takes time to adjust. Eventually, however, there is a process of coming to consciousness regarding the significance of the occurrence. This movement from adaptation to conscious participation in dealing with change is what we call *awareness*. Furthermore, we propose that transitions get underway with an awareness that some life-altering change has occurred. Participating in a transition proceeds with assessment of one's *ability to respond* to the change. It develops and expands through the *making of choices* as a result of the change. Finally, it takes on meaning through the *making of connections*, as the implications resulting from a change are woven together with all that has gone before, and all that is as yet unknown about one's life. What we arrive at are four elements of participation in the process of coming to terms with new situations. These four elements constitute what we are calling the characteristics of transition. In the present section of this chapter, we wish to summarize our own understanding of these characteristics, and indicate some ways in which they connect with the ministry of faith community nursing. In a subsequent section, we will introduce the writings of several transition theorists in order to expand on our perceptions through the language and insights of others.

Awareness, the first characteristic of transition, implies a shift in consciousness. John Newton's song "Amazing Grace" captures this shift poetically when he writes, "I once was lost, but now I'm found; was blind, but now I see" (North American Liturgy Resources, 1977). The shift being spoken of as *awareness* is something that activates both sequential consciousness and depth consciousness. In other words, Newton's experience of "amazing grace" first enabled him to move from not seeing to seeing. It then went on to help him differentiate the particular kind of not seeing he had been immersed in as a form of blindness. Awareness enables a person to break open the parts of an experience, and then reflect on both the whole and its parts.

Thus, a faith community nurse can observe congregational members talking about transitional phenomena in terms of (a) what existed previously, (b) the events that occurred to change a situation, and (c) the resulting conditions subsequent to that change. An example of this would be stories about the construction of a church building. It is not uncommon to hear someone say something like, "That brick section over there existed before the fire." The person might then go on to describe not only how the fire occurred, but also when new sections of the building were constructed after the fire. This is sequential consciousness. In addition, however, as the faith community nurse fosters a relational climate in which the promotion of inquiry is operative, she or he will also be able to observe the congregational member reflecting on nuances of meaning, as well as on significant details hidden within each phase of the sequence. For example, in the story of the church fire, the parishioner may go on to talk about how her younger brother died while fighting the flames. This, in turn, may lead to stories about the meaning of her family life with this brother prior to the fire or ways she has continued to remember him through a memorial stone built into one of the new sections of the church. This is depth consciousness. The characteristic of transition we call awareness calls forth both sequential and depth consciousness. It is therefore important for nurses working within faith community settings to be alert to communication emanating from both aspects of awareness.

In addition to awareness, transitions proceed with an *ability to respond* to changes that are perceived to be life altering. How many times have ministry professionals witnessed a sharp distinction in coping abilities among people who encounter similar traumas or tragedies? There are those who appear to respond with a bevy of abilities, and those whose aptitude for response is more limited. Having greater or less capability is not the issue; rather, the value lies in assessing and affirming people's existing resources in order to provide appropriate ministry support during times of transition. Nurses come to faith communities with skills in holistic assessment. In the face of life-altering change, it is important for faith community nurses to assess the strengths and potentials available to individuals, families, and groups. These are the resources for response that can guide faith community members in their life transitions.

A depressed teenager, for example, may ask to speak with the nurse about volunteering for a health ministry project. In the course of their conversation, the young man talks about his disabled sister, injured in a motor vehicle accident when they were both quite young. Ever since the accident, most of the family's attention has been directed toward this sister. What the conversation eventually leads to is the young man's anger toward his sister, parents, and himself for limiting their family activities so rigidly. As the teen becomes able to access his anger, he feels some of the locked-up energy of his depression release. Likewise, he gains a new ability to respond to the trauma of the motor vehicle accident. He sees how he and his whole family have been focusing on disablement. His sister has suffered physical disabilities, but he and his parents have also been disabled in emotional and spiritual ways. As he can break open these complexities, he becomes increasingly free to recognize additional options in his personal and family life. It is the nurse's attentiveness to the young man as a whole person, combined with skills of inquiry and accompaniment, that call forth from the teenager a previously untapped ability to respond to the life-altering accident that affected his family many years earlier.

This leads us to a consideration of how transitions develop and expand through the third transitional characteristic: *the making of choices*. When a person is traumatized, a first level of response springs from the need to survive. Choices at this point may be quite limited. For example, the middle-aged man who experiences a heart attack must seek immediate medical assistance to survive. After this first level of response, however, there will be a need for the making of choices by the man, his family, healthcare professionals, and the man's faith community as a part of his support network. Physical choices may include a need for bypass surgery, or the recommendation of a diet and exercise program that radically affects lifestyle. Emotional and intellectual choices may arise with regard to moderating hours of work, renegotiating the terms of financial obligations or debts, and learning how to share feelings more directly. Finally, spiritual choices may derive from unresolved guilt, disappointment, or disillusionment. Remaining in relationship with this man as he and his family discern their choices, and then act on these choices, can be a very important aspect of a faith community nurse's functioning. Knowing how to listen to the man's questions as they emerge, discussing alternatives through the provision of appropriate informational resources, and facilitating implementation processes are important nursing ministry skills; each skill will further the man's overall response as his transition develops and expands through the making of choices.

Finally, there is the characteristic of transition that we call *the making of connections*. This occurs as the transitional event takes on meaning in light of its relationship with all that has gone before and all that is as yet unknown about a person's life. For example, while listening to a woman speak about an experience of imprisonment and starvation, a faith community nurse might notice how the woman was involved in the making of connections. This congregational member nearly starved to death while she was doing missionary work a number of years earlier. After a period of reflection, the woman decided to focus attention on nutrition. She contrasted the starvation experience with basic healthy eating patterns developed from childhood. She then went on to university, and acquired a degree that prepared her to work as a nutrition expert in dietary planning and practices related with near starvation conditions. Eventually, she wrote a series of publications, rooted in both reflection on her own experience and the vast scientific knowledge she had acquired subsequent to that experience, on the topic of eating for survival when in wilderness or draught conditions. Because she was able to make connections between her trauma and her creativity, this woman's whole life changed in ways that were meaningful and of benefit to others.

These, then, are what we understand to be the characteristics of transitions. Although other authors will use different terminology to speak of these basic elements, we believe such differences contribute to an expanding base of knowledge. As faith group leaders and faith community nurses delve more deeply into this mix of language and meaning, it is hoped they will feel more equipped to minister in the face of transitional phenomena and events. Let us turn now to the writings of William Bridges (1980, 1991); Lawrence Cada, Raymond Fitz, Gertrude Foley, Thomas Giardino, and Carol Lichtenberg (1979); and Brian P. Hall (1986, 1991).

✍ Components, Stages, and Phases of Transitions

A number of writers have developed theories of transition. The insights of William Bridges (1980, 1991) stand out because of his emphasis on the personal and work-related changes that affect individual lives. In another vein, theories developed by Cada et al. (1979) and Hall (1986, 1991) draw attention to communal and organizational transitions. A brief summary of various authors' theories follows, and Figure 13.1 encapsulates these different theories, along with their core theoretical elements. As faith community nurses and faith group leaders read through these ideas they may wish to reflect on some of the ways faith and health activities are in evidence. Likewise, in the light of transitional theory, they may consider how health assessments, educational programs, community action groups, social structures, and the resources of our many faith traditions might be brought into relationship with people in ways that will accompany them through transitions. Are there contributions that faith communities need to make in expanding the body of knowledge that is being developed around the topic of transition? How might the collaborative efforts of faith community nurses and faith group leaders be reflected in these contributions?

Personal Transitions

William Bridges has written two books on transition theory that have gained popular attention and contribute a great deal to the topic of personal change: *Transitions* (1980) addresses ways that change affects a person's family and social realms, and *Managing Transitions* (1991) deals with a person's response to change in the work environment. Both texts discuss transition as a three-part psychological pro-

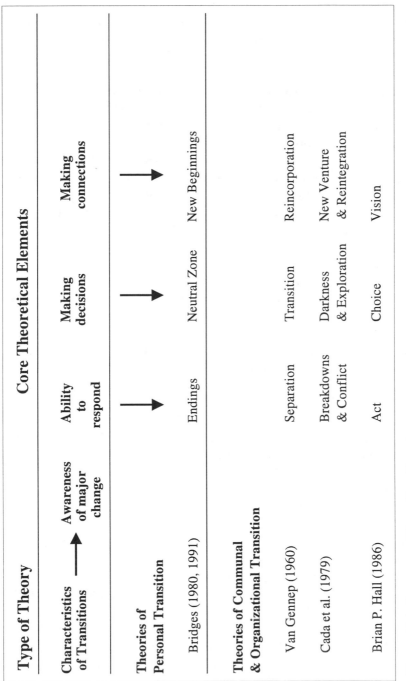

Type of Theory	Core Theoretical Elements			
Characteristics of Transitions →	Awareness of major change	Ability to respond	Making decisions	Making connections
Theories of Personal Transition				
Bridges (1980, 1991)		Endings →	Neutral Zone →	New Beginnings →
Theories of Communal & Organizational Transition				
Van Gennep (1960)		Separation	Transition	Reincorporation
Cada et al. (1979)		Breakdowns & Conflict	Darkness & Exploration	New Venture & Reintegration
Brian P. Hall (1986)		Act	Choice	Vision

Figure 13.1. Summary of Transition Theories

cess through which people come to terms with new situations brought about through change. The component parts of a transition, according to Bridges, are its *endings, neutral zone,* and *new beginnings.*

Endings. T. S. Eliot once wrote, "The end is where we start from" (Eliot, 1943/1971). This is because change imposes itself on a person's life in such a way as to create an ending, which differentiates a time *before* and a time *after* the change. Thus, people may speak of their life circumstances *before* the baby was born, *after* they were married, *before* the accident, or *after* winning a lottery. Each type of change precipitates not only the introduction of something new and unfamiliar, but also a number of losses related to what is known or familiar. Thus, there is an ending of that which existed before the change. At times, this ending may be subtle and barely noticed; at other times, the ending may be dramatic, and feel like a major upheaval in every aspect of a person's life.

Bridges (1980) distinguishes four aspects to the component of endings: *disengagement, disidentification, disenchantment,* and *disorientation.* With disengagement, a person experiences separation from the familiar world she or he has taken for granted. There is loss and mourning, a feeling of broken connections, and a sense of discontinuity. At such times, a faith community nurse may hear comments like, "My morning walks will never be the same since that was a special time I shared with her." By comparison, Bridges (1980) refers to disidentification as the inner side of the disengagement process. This is when a person experiences loss in the ways they refer to themselves. An example would be the young widower who looks around at his group of friends and is suddenly, painfully, aware that he is no longer part of a couple. Such shifts in identity can inaugurate disenchantment. For the young man newly widowed, identifying himself as a "widower" can seem unreal, with nothing making sense anymore. In tandem with disenchantment, disorientation comes as an experience of being adrift, without direction or purpose. Familiar locations seem disfigured by the glaring absence of a beloved other. In short, endings are a complex starting point.

The Neutral Zone. Bridges (1991) refers to the neutral zone as "a nowhere between two somewheres" (p. 35). For a couple who is trying to become pregnant, this may be the time between menstrual periods before taking a pregnancy test. In another vein, it may be the time of waiting after a medical investigation has occurred, but before the results are known. It may be the time between waving good-bye at the airport and receiving a telephone call letting you know your family has arrived safely at their destination. Likewise, it may be the period of time it takes following the death of a loved one before there is a desire to return to any form of festive social activity. Bridges (1991) identifies two important tasks for this period: "attentive inactivity" and "ritual-ized routine" (p. 114).

To begin with, the neutral zone plunges a person into emptiness. It is as if a vacuum has been created by the breakdown of old structures; one's reality no longer holds together, and there is chronic dread that everything is falling apart. An initial struggle in the neutral zone, therefore, is that of trying to escape emptiness and resist disintegra-tion. Attentive inactivity can enable a person to surrender gradually and gracefully to the process of inner transformation being crafted by the neutral zone. For example, a person can employ one or another of their five senses to be attentive: A person can feel grounded in the sound of a bird, the color of a passing car, or the smell of familiar foods cooking. Furthermore, attentive inactivity listens for paradox and cre-ates options. These will emerge as invitations and possibilities. Thus, loss can be a path to discovery, disintegration can lead to reintegration, and death can open into newness of life.

In support of attentive inactivity, Bridges (1980) describes ritual-ized routine as a way of "amplifying and making more real the essen-tial neutral zone experience" (p. 121). When people learn to surren-der to the emptiness, it is no longer terrifying. They then begin to catch their breath, and realize they can move around in the emptiness, since they are in a space and time that has been referred to as "in between." Ritualized routines can include spending time alone, jour-nal writing, or consulting with a spiritual adviser. These ritual rou-tines might also involve daily walks to a favorite coffee shop, placing telephone calls to people in one's support network, revisiting favorite home pages on the internet, reading passages from a sacred text, or similar activities that help to expand one's awareness. Things may continue to look different, but in the neutral zone they are no longer distorted or disfigured. This can be a time to take a long, loving look at one's total life span. What have been the roads taken and not taken? Where is there unfinished business? What desires of heart or spirit remain unexplored? Investing time in ritual-ized routine is an important part of journeying through the neutral zone. It allows for creative imagination, experimentation, and reorientation.

New Beginnings. The third component of transition identified by Bridges (1980) is that of new beginnings, which he describes as the inner realignment and renewal of energy that ripens gradually as a result of one's encounter with life-altering change. New beginnings cannot be forced; rather, they emerge with subtlety.

In new beginnings, one finds the stages of *reengagement, reorganiza-tion, reidentification,* and *enchantment* (Bridges, 1980, 1991). The initial ambivalence one feels at a time of new beginning requires reengagement. For example, starting a new job will involve getting through the first day. This can mean filling in forms, meeting new peo-ple, touring an unfamiliar setting, and being assigned a workspace. Once a start has been made, however, reorganization can occur, as the person settles in and learns how to function in the new work culture. Before long, there is a reidentification. Here, the person begins to see himself or herself as an employee of the new business; rather than speaking of "this firm" or "their hospital," a person speaks for the first time about "our company" or "our project." Finally, a person may experience the enchantment of discovery and cocreativity. There is a sense of reintegration and rebirth: A person comes home to herself or himself, and really likes the way this feels.

Although Bridges's theory focuses on personal transitions, his core theoretical components can be applied to individuals, groups or aggre-gates, and whole communities. Likewise, the identified elements of an ending, a neutral zone, and new beginnings do not necessarily proceed as linear stages. On the contrary, they tend to overlap and intertwine. In the face of these rhythms and variances, faith group leaders and faith community nurses are in an excellent position to foster both health and faith in times of transition. Listening, inquiring, accompa-nying, and supporting can take many forms. Thus, again, it is impor-tant for ministry professionals to draw on a variety of skills and theoretical frames of reference.

Communal and Organizational Transitions

A number of authors on transition theory make reference to the phrase "rite of passage." This term, coined by the Dutch anthropolo-gist Arnold van Gennep (1960), refers to the ways in which traditional societies structure major life transitions. According to van Gennep, rites of passage are made up of three phases: *separation, transition,* and *incorporation.* In separation, there is a symbolic death experience, which transports a person away from the old and familiar social context. Transition is a time of isolation and learning about additional types of support. Here the person must draw on both internal and external processes of coming to terms with their new situation or circumstance. Finally, with the ripening of inner/outer transformation, the person reenters his or her social order on a new basis. Although the language is different, one can see parallels with Bridges's endings, neutral zone, and new beginnings. What is different about rites of passage, however, is their source in the collective consciousness, rituals, and celebrations of a community. Originally, such rites were focused on the initiation and remembrance processes associated with birth, adolescence, betrothal, marriage, dying, and death (Van Biema, 1991).

In a different vein, Cada et al. (1979) address the topic of communal and institutional change. They speak of shaping the coming age of religious life through a threefold process of *disintegration, regrounding,* and *reintegration.* Although the focus of their work is the revitalization of religious communities within Christian churches, their theory offers a broad-based point of reference inasmuch as it proposes a communal or institutional parallel to van Gennep's rites of passage.

According to the sociological model offered by Cada et al. (1979), religious communities are organizations born out of a founding charism or vision that undergoes various phases of change. This is referred to as the organizational life cycle of a community. Parishes, congregations, and other types of faith communities can be studied using this model. It encompasses five stages: (a) the foundation period, (b) an expansion period, (c) a time of stabilization, followed by a time of transition that includes (d) a breakdown period, and (e) a critical period, during which time the community may move toward extinction, minimal survival, or revitalization. Building on this life cycle concept, Cada et al. go on to say that organizations and communities have vitality curves, which demonstrate their development and decline as social realities. Development occurs during the foundation, expansion, and stabilization periods; decline occurs within the breakdown and critical periods of the transition phase.

In this period of transition, we can recognize parallels to van Gennep's (1960) threefold model of separation, transition, and incorporation, and Bridges's (1980, 1991) vision of endings, a neutral zone, and new beginnings. Cada et al. (1979) situate the life cycle of a community as a "path of transformation" (p. 96). In tandem with van Gennep and Bridges, it includes three phases. First, the emergence of new questions among members of the community initiates a period of "breakdown and conflict" (Cada et al., 1979, p. 97).[1] This is described as a time of *disintegration*, in which there is identity diffusion, lack of grounding in relationships, and a feeling of powerlessness in the community's attempts to maintain direction and meaningful purpose. With the acceptance of contradictions, there is movement into a period of "darkness and exploration" (p. 101). Here, the task is that of *regrounding* the community within a new sense of identity, a new relatedness and commitment, and a new sense of purpose or meaning. This period is characterized by widespread experimentation and searching, which requires increased tolerance of diversity and pluralism within the group. As the period of regrounding gives rise to new insights and feelings of revitalization among a significant number of people in the community, there is movement into a period of "new venture and reintegration" (p. 104). This is where a critical mass of reenergized individuals converge to refashion a corporate or organizational identity, with shared relationships giving birth to new social structures and purposeful projects. In short, according to Cada et al. (1979), community transition runs parallel to personal transitions. Thus, what has been voiced by a number of theologians and social philosophers may also hold true with regard to theories of transition, in that the personal is also social, communal, political, and organizational (Graham, 1992; Russell, 1974; Thistlethwaite & Engel, 1990).

Interrelationships between personal and communal transitions, as developed in the theory of Cada et al. (1979), have contributed to the work of Brian P. Hall (1986, 1991) on personal and organizational transformation. Hall speaks of how individuals and organizations *act* out of an ability to connect internalized values and skills with language, consciousness, and image. He goes on to say that transitions invite *choice* by calling forth a number of mediating images that are intuited, but not yet visible. That is, a person may value health/healing/harmony (Hall, 1991), but lack the self-awareness and self-care needed to achieve this value set. With choice, the person imagines how a healthy life would look for them. These images of health form a *vision* toward which the person can aspire through the learning of concrete skills and capabilities. A task that exists for those who are living in times of transition, therefore, is to allow their mediating images to become visible in external and recognizable forms. Thus, as we contemplate the choice images that surface within our personal or collective consciousness, and discern the skills and technologies needed to mediate these images into life-promoting structures, we are participating in what Hall (1986) calls the *genesis effect.*

Again, personal transitions work in tandem with communal and organizational transitions. It is important, therefore, that faith community nurses and faith group leaders be attentive to the ways individuals and groups undergo change. It is likewise important that they be available to mark endings in a manner that "treats the past with respect and lets people take a piece of the old ways with them into their new beginnings" (Bridges, 1991, p. 31). In so doing, they will be helping faith community members to make the most of change.

↩ Contributions of Space and Time to the Characteristics of Transitions

In the previous pages, we have drawn from a number of authors to present theories of transition. We have also highlighted components of and stages within those theories. This approach seeks to provide the reader with an appreciation of the characteristics of transitions as these unfold in personal lives and social settings. Throughout our theoretical summaries, we have highlighted ways that personal and communal transitions parallel one another; this builds on our approach to the relational nature of transition. We now turn to a consideration of *space* and *time,* inasmuch as these are related with the characteristics of transitions.

Regarding space, we acquire, by virtue of our birth, specific physical, social, and cultural locations. Several contemporary theologians consider reflection on one's location, or context, to be "central to the theological task" (Thistlethwaite & Engel, 1990, p. 5), inasmuch as this type of reflection can link individuals and communities holistically. Physically, we inhabit distinct geographical regions, but we are also part of populating the entire planet. Socially and culturally, based on the conditions of our birth, we may be considered rich or poor as well as members of a particular majority or minority group. Regarding time, it has been said that we are born, we live, and then we die. This process is viewed by a number of faith traditions as the sum total of one's unique existence, and by other faith traditions as the manifestation only of a current incarnation. All of these elements associated with space and time have an impact on how people experience transitions.

In addition to their theological significance, nurses know that space and time are factors in nursing assessment. For example, in taking a health history, the nurse will ask about when a person first noticed changes in her or his health. The nurse may then go on to ask about what else was going on in the person's life at the time this change occurred. Such questions provide a basic frame of reference through which the nurse can better understand individuals or groups in a variety of contexts. Deepening one's appreciation of space and time as the primal boundary system within which human activities occur can assist nurses in observing human movement as an aspect of whole-person assessment. Likewise, nurses know that visible behaviors occurring in space and time point to invisible thoughts, feelings, longings, and hopes. As has already been said, it is within this invisible domain that transitions occur. Thus, we believe that a multidimensional assessment approach that is grounded in physical observations, but that also recognizes levels of invisible spiritual meaning, can aid faith community nurses in their ministry. Weaving together both visible and invisible aspects of the characteristics of transitions developed in earlier sections of this chapter can promote both faith and health in times of transition.

Space

Any one of us can describe ourselves by means of our location. In this regard, we often draw on physical, environmental, social, and geographical points of reference to indicate the space we are in. Thus, we may point to our heart when expressing certain feelings, or speak of our location in terms of family, neighborhood, sports team, political party, work environment, or faith community. On another level, we may situate ourselves by means of our citizenship, ethnicity, faith tradition, or global consciousness. Figure 13.2 depicts some of the contextual circles within which people are located. As part of their assessment process, faith community nurses may want to use this diagram with clients or families to start a discussion on the ways space may be affecting their experiences of transition.

It may also be of benefit for faith community nurses, building on information gained through observation and conversation, to explore

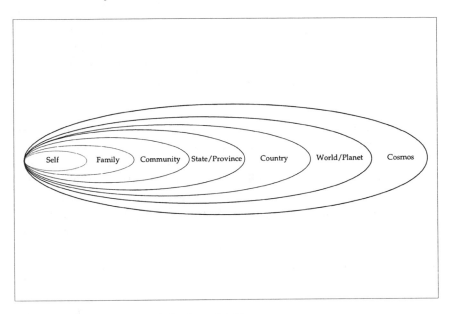

Figure 13.2. Contextual Circles of Self

how the dimension of space has been used in the symbols and icons of faith traditions. Most creation stories, for example, depict a particular type of space as the setting within which a shift from chaos to order or nonexistence to existence occurs. Thus, we hear about the heavens, waters of the deep, a cosmic egg, a formless void, an Above and a Below, and a garden in Eden. Likewise, there are geographic areas that serve as settings for purification or rest, such as the wilderness, the desert, gardens, and mountains. In a different vein, many faith groups speak of space in terms of directions, dimensions, orientations, levels, stories, and similar domains. Thus, Aboriginal peoples, for example, speak of the Four Directions on a medicine wheel, and Hindu believers refer to the levels of caste or *jati*. Another consideration, developed within Buddhist teachings, identifies space as a life element along with earth, water, fire, and air; it is part of both the outer and the inner processes that determine existence and function to form, sustain, or dissolve all manner of beings. Finally, space is a place where science and faith are in dialogue. The gravitational theory of Newton, the relativity theory of Einstein, or the more recently articulated chaos and quantum theories all deal with the intricacies of space as a primal boundary sys-

tem within which human activities occur. Space is something intimately linked with sequential and depth awareness, various responsive abilities, options for choice making, and a perspective on self as
well as others that allows for a making of connections.

Time

In addition to space, people are contextualized through time.
Although there are many ways to understand time, we would like to
distinguish two basic types of time that can be observed in faith community nursing assessment. These derive from two Greek words:
chronos, meaning incremental or linear time, and *kairos*, meaning seasonal or event time (Bowker, 1997; Vine, 1966). Thus, a person might
describe chronological experiences in terms of nanoseconds, minutes,
hours, dates, years, a particular century, or the millennium. On the
other hand, they may also speak about birthday celebrations, job pro-
motions, graduations, and bereavement experiences. These two kinds
of time exist in relationship with one another, and can provide information about time as a contextual element. Figure 13.3 depicts both
chronos and *kairos* time in relationship to a fictitious life story. Again,
this figure can serve as a tool to be used by faith community nurses in
developing parallel diagrams with clients and families.

As with space, faith community nurses may want to build on
information gained through observation and conversation in exploring the dimension of time as it relates with faith traditions. It is said
that religious understandings of time rest on the human awareness of
transitions in daily activities, the movement from birth to death, and
the unfailing rhythms of sun, moon, stars, and seasons (Bowker, 1997).
For example, although we in North America may be accustomed to
using the particular kind of calendar known as the Julian calendar, it is
important to be aware of the fact that at least six other types of calendars are in use around the globe. This is because systems of time were
at first derived from a faith group's cosmology. Thus, for example, we
have solar years and lunar years. There are also distinctions between
sacred time and profane time; thus we learn about religious festivals,
feasts, and fasts when being introduced to various types of calendar
years. Among Christian faith groups, for example, the central figure is
Jesus Christ, and there are seasons of Advent, Christmas, Epiphany,
Lent, Easter, and Pentecost. For Jews, whose calendar is fixed according
to the number of years since the creation of the world, festivals combine

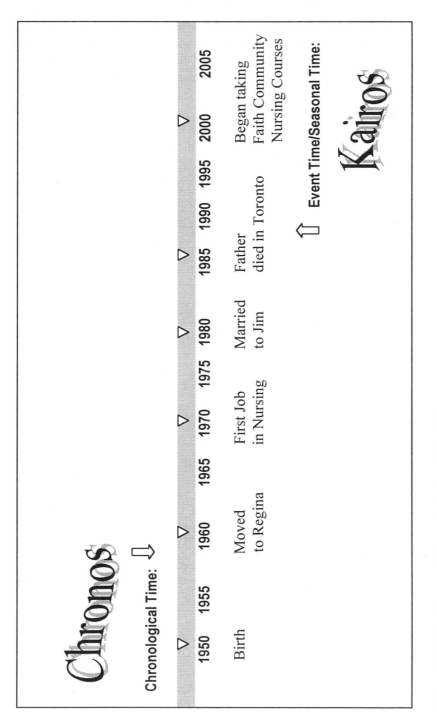

Figure 13.3. Continuum of Chronological and Event Time

agricultural cycles and commemorate events in their history of relationship with God. Among Muslims, who follow a lunar calendar,
major festivals and fasts are linked to the commands of the Qur'an or
to the life of Mohammed (Bowker, 1997). Finally, Wiccan believers
speak in terms of a Wheel of the Year and eight sabbat points, where
inner and outer turns of the wheel are said to meet (Starhawk, 1989).
Whatever the language or belief system, time is intimately linked with
both incremental and seasonal events in a person's or group's life. As
such, time is crucial to the transitional characteristics of awareness,
responsive abilities, choice making, and a capacity to make
connections.

ᴥ Summary

In this chapter, we have described the characteristics of transitions in a
variety of ways. Beginning with our own understandings, we then
went on to the writings of others. We introduced a number of theorists,
and talked about the components, stages, and phases of transitions. We
also looked at these elements in terms of personal, communal, and
organizational approaches to transition. Finally, we discussed contributions made by space and time in formulating various aspects of
assessment pertinent to the work of faith community nurses in relating
with groups and individuals during times of transition. Building on the
information developed thus far, we now turn to a theoretical consideration of transitions that may arise within faith communities.

Note

1. Cada et al. (1979) develop the idea of a "path of transformation" in
three sections: (a) a period of breakdown and conflict (see pp. 97-101), (b) a
period of darkness and exploration (see pp. 101-104), and (c) a period of new
venture and reintegration (see pp. 104-107).

14 ✑

Types of Transitions in the Lives of Faith Community Members

Margaret B. Clark

This chapter is about faith communities as places where transitional events occur. It is also about faith communities as settings in which people live out the struggles and joys of their developmental sojourns. In order to cultivate the renewal of faith and the promotion of health during times of transition, it is important for faith communities to recognize their unique contributions in support of transitional processes. Likewise, distinguishing between transitions that are developmental and those that are situational can enable both faith community nurses and faith group leaders to accompany congregational members with compassion and creativity. The pages of this chapter will address these topics. The introductory paragraphs draw attention to faith communities as places of enclosure and sanctuary; subsequent sections will describe differences between developmental and situational types of transition by means of both summary and in-depth reflection; and throughout we will present a number of theoretical and narrative resources.

We have said in an earlier chapter that the starting point of transition is story. We wish to add that event time, or *kairos* time, truly respects this important role of story in relationship with transition. As one author describes it, *kairos* time draws a person *inside* her or his story to a point of *awakening* (Neeld, 1990). It is as if the person connects with the story at a level of sacred awareness; that is to say, the person seems to see for the first time that the story is marked with certain features or qualities that do not need to "make sense," but that invite exploration and reveal meaning. We think, for example, of the story told by Viktor Frankl in his book *Man's Search for Meaning* (1959/1984). A young woman is dying in the concentration camp where Frankl was imprisoned during World War II. In talking with this woman, Frankl is struck by her optimism. He listens as the women tells him about the branch of a tree and its two blossoms, which are visible outside a window of the hut where she lies dying. The woman says that she talks with this tree, and refers to it as "the only friend I have in my loneliness." Struck by this unusual behavior, Frankl asks if the tree ever replies to her. The woman answers, "Yes." When Frankl inquires further about what it is the tree says to her, the woman replies, "It says to me, 'I am here—I am here—I am life, eternal life' "(Frankl, 1959/1984, p. 90). Stories like those of this woman touch deep spiritual chords. It is at such times of awakening that a faith community needs to be available to its members, just as Frankl was available to the woman.

A faith community can serve as a place where event time is honored alongside linear time. Indeed, faith communities need to reclaim their role as contexts within which to share reflection and celebration around experiences of being in relationship—our description of religion, provided in an earlier chapter. It situates religion as an outgrowth of faith, spirituality, and theology. Likewise, it suggests the role of faith communities as enclosures or containers around which both personal and communal transitional events can take place (Kidd, 1990; Rutter, 1993).

As an environment of enclosure and attentiveness, the faith community can do several things to support individual and group transitions. First, faith communities need to listen as stories emerge. Second, they need to respect the stories, and take them seriously as a starting point for transition. Finally, they need to dwell in faith—that is, stay in relationship—with the person or group who is entering the sacredness of event time with its seasons of discovery and possibility. On a material level, this may involve providing a quiet or festive sanctuary, a house of prayer, or a monastic center. On a relational level, it may be the availability of a listening ear and an ethic of confidentiality. On an intellectual level, it may mean engaging difficult questions arising from the person's or group's experience. And, on a spiritual level, it may involve the disciplines of empathic presence and respectful silence. In whatever ways possible, faith communities need to recognize and reclaim their role as contexts where significant experience is neither forgotten nor missed. This means giving serious attention to the transitional events that arise among individuals, families, groups, and communities. It all begins with relationship and experiences of being in relationship; as these experiences are shared, they will invite reflection and celebration.

ᥣᥩ *Developmental and Situational Transitions*

In this chapter, we will discuss transitional events as both *developmental* and *situational*. Developmental transitions grow out of the somewhat predictable experiences of change occurring throughout one's life span. This is what we mean when we speak of changes occurring during infancy, childhood, adolescence, adulthood, and old age. Situational transitions, on the other hand, grow out of our response to unexpected change. Here we may speak of how we come to terms with such things as getting lost, being in a motor vehicle accident, or winning the lottery. For the person who belongs to a faith community, each type of transitional event is experienced within that faith group context to a greater or lesser degree. Being attentive to this fact, one who is nursing within a faith community can serve as a liaison for the person, family, or group in connecting their experience with their stories, their stories with their transitions, and their transitions with the sacred domains of both faith and health.

We are aided in our understanding of developmental transitions by theorists within the behavioral sciences and theology who have approached these experiences of change from both chronological- and event-oriented perspectives. In this regard, we speak about theories of development. These theories imply that growth and maturity occur through both change and an ability to respond to change. They also highlight when an event or incident is age appropriate. Thus, Erikson (1963, 1968, 1980, 1982) writes about psychosocial crises, and Piaget (1952, 1954; see also Kegan, 1982) focuses on operations of logic. Freud (1953–1974) and Ferder and Heagle (1992) speak of stages in a person's psychosexual development, and Jung (1961) speaks about a process of individuation. Likewise, Kohlberg (1969, 1976) and Gilligan (1982) address the process of moral development, and Fowler (1981) and Ford (1988) concentrate on faith development issues. Familiarity with one or several of these theories can aid nursing professionals within faith communities as they seek to promote health development. Recognizing the transitional event underlying a particular chronological period will enable the nurse to invite inquiry as well as explore possible resources available to the person in coming to terms with each new phase of development.

Despite their helpfulness, however, a major limitation in developmental theories is that they are only mirrors of actual experience. They provide conceptual frameworks based on observation, clinical trials, and the condensation of many real-life experiences into abstract categories. Helpful though this may be to our knowledge base, developmental theories fail to capture the fact that not everyone's life proceeds in such a predictable manner. Thus, we need to reflect on events that are unexpected, unpredictable, and age *inappropriate.* What about the social experiences of intellectually gifted children who skip a grade or enter university early? What about the spiritual experiences of single parents? What about the emotional experiences of exhilaration and deflation resulting from the sudden gain or loss of wealth? What about the individual, family, or group transitions hidden within stories of domestic violence (battering, marital rape, incest, abandonment), as well as social and political terror (gang rape, bombings, hostage taking, captivity)? These are examples of what we call situational transitions.

Here, too, nursing professionals need to explore the literature, know their own levels of competence, and seek out resources that respond to these types of experiences. Individual and collective stories are an excellent point of entry in appreciating situational events. Examples of addressing situational transitions by means of narrative are provided by Lewis (1961), Meili (1991), Puleo (1994), and Vanauken (1977). A different approach is represented by the work of Joseph

Campbell. Campbell and others write about core concepts, such as the "hero's deed" (Campbell, 1968, 1988), and archetypes of the "hero" and "victim" (Wilkinson, 1996).[1] Learning about such concepts and developing a strong referral network will be important for the nurse in helping members of a faith community sort out some of the complexities emanating from experiences of trauma, unexpected violence, or disaster. On the topic of trauma and recovery, the work of Judith Herman (1992) is excellent for learning about the impact of traumatic stress, as well as about some important supportive skills needed by helping persons in order to foster recovery. Likewise, according to Kenneth Doka (1996), sudden losses brought about through heart attacks, stroke, suicide, homicide, motor vehicle accidents, and disaster events may complicate a person's ability to cope or grieve.

Situational transitions tend to breach the natural alignment between linear time (*chronos*) and event time (*kairos*). As a consequence of this rupture, a person may be overwhelmed by the experience. This can affect a person's or family's ability to come to terms with the new situation. Their natural coping mechanisms may split off from the rest of their lives. Without the support of health-promoting processes to help them come to terms with the traumatic or unexpected experience, these persons will face future developmental junctures with a tangle of unexamined beliefs, feelings, and reactions. In the science of psychology, words such as "complex," "delusion," "projection" and "introject" are used to describe some of the distorted filters or worldviews resulting from unexpected or age-inappropriate experiences that are still in need of transition.

Since nurses within faith communities do not work in isolation, it is important for there to be ongoing collaborative sharing among ministry professionals. With appreciation for their different types of skills and expertise, as well as referral resources that are external to the congregation, faith community nurses and faith group leaders can offer congregational members a quality of support that fosters the integration of faith and health in times of both developmental and situational transitions.

✿ Developmental Transitions in the Context of Faith Communities

There is a time-honored tradition within most faith communities that has served to connect developmental transitions with spiritual or religious meaning. The social expression most frequently used to describe this has been "religious ritual" (Bowker, 1997, p. 819). From the earliest of historical times up to the present, faith traditions all around the globe have played an important role in designing ceremonies related to birth and childhood, adolescence and initiation, betrothal and marriage, and death and remembrance (Cohen, 1991; Van Biema, 1991). Thus, when contemporary observers view the rituals of a particular faith tradition, they often recognize actions that are repeated in regular and predictable ways. Most of these actions are tied to beliefs, values, and attitudes reflected by the filters, worldviews, and paradigms operative within the religious culture. Often, the original meaning of an action has been lost or altered through historical overlays or additional levels of interpretation; what remains, however, is a sense of connection with the faith tradition's ancient roots. This connection enables a person today to experience affiliation or kinship with those who have gone before, as well as with those who are yet to come. Rituals bring *chronos* time and *kairos* time into relationship with one another. They create a context where experience, story, tradition, and ritual come together in offering support to the person whose life is in flux.

In considering a framework for discussing developmental transitions, we decided to draw on the work of Iris M. Ford (1988). Her approach highlights both spiritual and psychosocial development, which we believe complements the solid foundation nurses already have in the areas of physiological development and physical assessment.

Iris Ford's book, *Life Spirals* (1988), combines the faith development theory of James Fowler (1981) and the psychosocial theory of Erik Erikson (1963, 1968, 1980, 1982). Ford introduces the image of a spiral to describe developmental processes, inasmuch as the spiral is multidimensional.[2] For our purposes, the spiral communicates an approach to the whole person that involves making connections between both chronological- and event-oriented types of time. The spiral is also a concept used in theological reflection to portray both the possibility and complexity of divine-human relationship.

According to Iris Ford (1988), each spiral represents a certain "cluster of opportunities," and is fashioned by "maturation, experience, and previous opportunities" (p. 15). Spirals invite persons and groups to face what life offers, both the positive and negative, with an attitude of hope. Ford bases her approach to faith development on eight assumptions, two of which are especially significant in our study. The first highlights faith as something that leads a person "beyond self-actualization towards self-transcendency" (p. 18). This expands the notion of spirit as an exclusively human quality by viewing it as a dimension or capacity within our humanity that moves naturally beyond self to others (Goddard, 1995a). It is in light of such an understanding that Ford makes a second assumption significant to our study of transition: She says, "transitions are the times of greatest growth in faith, moving the person from within self to beyond self" (Ford, 1988, p. 18). In light of these assumptions, Ford introduces the idea of having a "faith gift" as part of each developmental phase. With this innovation, she contributes something unique to faith development theory.

Ford's model includes twelve stages. The first six have to do with self-actualization; the last six are oriented toward self-transcendence. Each stage is developed by means of four descriptive phrases, which give reference to each stage's (a) summary name, (b) chronological frame of reference, (c) psychosocial task, (d) form of enclosure or containment, and (e) faith gift. In the following paragraphs, we highlight each stage, together with examples of religious ritual from a variety of faith traditions.

Six Stages of Self-Actualization

In the beginning, between birth and about 6 months, there is *simple faith*. This emerges within one's family enclosure as an infant receives the faith gift of *trust*, and undergoes Erikson's (1963, 1980) psychosocial task of learning about trust and mistrust. Then, between the ages of about 6 months and 2 years, there is *initiative faith*, as the child struggles with the emergence of primitive feelings in light of Erikson's (1963, 1980) psychosocial task of distinguishing between autonomy and shame/doubt. Here, there is the faith gift of *joy* to aid the infant's exploration into his or her first great duality, that of "Yes! Yes!" and "No! No!" Third, between about 2 and 5 years of age, there is *literal faith*. Here, the child wrestles with limitations related to his or her needs. Erikson's (1963, 1980) psychosocial task at this point is that of making distinctions between initiative and guilt. The faith gift provided is *"okay-ness,"* and the child proceeds to develop a sense of what is "me" versus "not me," as well as what is "mine" and "not mine."

During these first three developmental periods of self-actualization, a faith community can provide support to both the infant and his or her family. According to Cohen (1991) and Van Biema (1991), soon after birth it is customary to name an infant. This is an act of inclusion, whereby the child becomes a member of the tribe, family, or community. Naming is often determined by familial custom, cultural heritage, or religious tradition. Sometimes rituals of naming and rites of spiritual initiation are combined. In Christian communities, there are christenings, blessings, dedications, and baptisms. In the Jewish faith, there are traditions of circumcision, naming, and *pidyon ha'ben*. Aboriginal parents often entrust the naming of their child to an elder, who may use sacred smudges and paints as a preparation before lifting the child high overhead and calling forth its name. Among Hindus, there is a ceremony of nomenclature. In Islam, there are special prayers into the right ear and the left ear of the child, as well as a ritual of circumcision for male infants. Other cultures have traditions of swaddling clothes, protective enclosure, and purification.

After a child has experienced the formative environment of family caregivers, and learned something about the language and symbols of that environment, he or she faces a second significant event of childhood, that of going outside the home to attend some form of school. According to Ford (1988), schooling initiates the stage of *learned faith*, at which time a child develops skills through which to encounter Erikson's (1963, 1980) psychosocial stage of differentiating between industry and inferiority. The faith gift at this point is *life stories*. The school-age child loves to listen to stories, and to picture these stories in his or her imagination. This is also a time when children learn to read and exercise computer skills, which can open additional paths for the child to learn through stories and images. Ford cautions, however, that although young children may be "taking in facts and situations, assimilating beliefs and values as seen through the lives of others" (p. 24), they do not as yet realize that what they read about may have implications for their lives. Children of this age are often unable to sort out "this belief" from "that belief," or "this value" from "that value." For the school-age child, thought processes are more mythic and literal than individual and reflective.

Here again, faith communities can serve to support the child's developmental transition by offering rituals of the loss of things associated with infancy. Within Hinduism, for example, there is the *mundan*, the first haircut. Likewise, according to Van Biema (1991), the American vestige of such a ritual may exist in the tooth fairy leaving money in exchange for a child's baby teeth. It is a time when children are eager to "show and tell." As members of faith communities listen to the stories of children during these years, they will be able to encourage the emergence of distinctive reasoning processes, beliefs, values, and early stages of moral development. Traditions of religious instruction, as well as reading and learning about passages from sacred texts, can aid children in this period of development.

The next major transition is referred to as a coming of age, or adolescence. It is a time of identity shift, when one moves from being a girl or boy to being a woman or man. In Ford's (1988) developmental scheme, this period includes two stages. First, between the ages of about 12 and 14, there is a period of *relational faith*. This is a time for initial departure from the family enclosure in order to become embedded in one's peer group and preoccupied with friendships. Peers and friends are needed for the sharing of mutual interests, as well as for talking about the deep and meaningful discoveries that are going on in relationship with self and others. The psychosocial challenge identified for this period is not one used by Erikson; rather, Ford draws on the work of Robert Kegan (1982) to describe it as a tension between affiliation versus abandonment. The faith gift for this stage is *forgiveness*. Friends can hurt each other, let each other down and not "be there" at crucial times. Forgiveness is an attitude of "give and take," which cultivates the value of self-acceptance and the acceptance of others.

Then, in conjunction with interpersonal growth and relational faith, Ford's second stage, occurring between the ages of about 15 and 21, is a time of *searching faith*. Here, the young person discovers that she or he is embedded in all sorts of cultural systems. There are such things as seamy and affluent sides of town, groups of socially or economically privileged and underprivileged people, and discriminations based on gender or racial differences. In the midst of all these contrasts and distinctions, the person encounters Erikson's (1963, 1980) psychosocial task of choosing identity versus identity confusion. The young person asks questions like, "*Who am I* as I meet others from different nationality backgrounds, sexual orientations, religious customs, cultural mannerisms, dietary practices, and dress?" "What if I try to be like you? What if you try to be like me?" "How do I know what is me and what is not me?" When these questions arise, they need to be taken seriously. This developmental transition will benefit from the *acceptance of difference,* this stage's faith gift. As one learns to accept one's identity, and to experience a degree of self-actualization, one has a base from which to reach out to others with confidence and care.

It is during the time of adolescence and young adulthood that societies have developed numerous rites of passage or rites of initiation. For girls, there is a physical signal of transition in the emergence of menstruation. Virginia Beane Rutter's book *Woman Changing Woman* (1993) includes a rich study of the Navaho puberty ritual referred to as the *kinaaldá.* It describes the processes of "containment," "transformation," and "emergence," through which a girl is ritually enclosed, adorned, and introduced to the mysterious powers of her womb as a container for life, creativity, and the cyclic rhythms of transformation between light and darkness, life and death. For boys, the ritual structure of passage into manhood tends to be more dramatic. According to van Gennep (1960), there are the phases of "separation," "transition," and "incorporation." In the description provided by Van Biema (1991), the process goes as follows. First, "isolate him from his normal society"; second, "disorient or confuse him with drugs or drums or lack of sleep or through some physical ordeal," and "subject him to indoctrination" about what it means to be an adult sexually, spiritually, and socially (p. 31). Finally, upon completion of such trials and tribulations, he emerges into manhood.

Whatever method a society or culture may choose, the developmental transition of adolescence and early adulthood is one also recognized by faith communities. For some Christians this, rather than infancy, is the proper time for baptism, insofar as the young person is now at an appropriate age to make his or her own faith commitment. Among other Christian groups, this is when a person receives first communion, celebrates confirmation, or makes an adult reaffirmation of baptism. For Aboriginal youth, adolescence can be an occasion for spiritual fasting and the sacred time apart from the rest of the community known as a vision quest. By contrast, within a number of Jewish communities, there is a time of celebration called *bar mitzvah* for boys and, more recently, the *bat mitzvah* for girls; at this time, the youth are surrounded by family and community in the accomplishment of religious responsibility. As faith communities are guided by youth leaders, they will be able to build on existing rituals and social activities in discovering new directions for the future.

Six Stages of Self-Transcendence

With growing security in one's adult identity, a person is now ready to explore the second half of Ford's developmental spiral through processes of self-transcendence. These highlight transitions related with commitment. The first, occurring between approximately the ages of 22 and 29, is a time of *reflective faith,* with its faith gift of *love.* This is when a person learns from mentors (Sellner, 1990; Whitehead & Whitehead, 1979/1982), and deals with Erikson's (1963, 1980) psychosocial tension between intimacy and isolation. Referred to as a time of discerning one's vocation, many young men and women experiment with roles and responsibilities that lead to dating, betrothal, and marriage. Others become disciples of a social or political ideal. Still others turn toward spiritual exercises and the interior landscape of soulmaking (Jones, 1985). In tandem with these aspects of commitment is the time of *serving faith,* with its gift of *caring.* This time period, around ages 30 to 39, is when Erikson's (1963, 1980) psychosocial stage of deciding between generativity and stagnation begins to flourish. It balances one's vocational commitments through development of occupational and professional accomplishments. In this spiral, a person is embedded in the stewardship of goods and resources. These may be material (e.g., money and belongings) or immaterial (e.g., time and skills). According to Ford (1988), generativity is "trying to make this world a better place for others," and conversely stagnating is doing nothing and "not caring" (p. 31). For many people, what makes the difference in the meaning of their life during this time of transition has more to do with inclusiveness, affirmation, and encouragement than riches or notoriety.

Faith communities have traditionally accompanied people in their early and middle adult years with the ritual of marriage and activities focused on family life. Many religious traditions have ceremonies for betrothal and marriage. This is seen as a time of movement within the community, and can involve a change of dwelling place, as well as of economic or social status. Thus, conventions such as the dowry or arranged marriages endure to this day in a number of societies. There is also emphasis given to marriage as an institution for procreation. Thus, rituals to encourage fertility and blessings for "many children" are included in wedding ceremonies. Finally, marriage is seen as a relationship within which two individuals can experience love and happiness as they join together their hopes and aspirations, and begin living together. Here, again, faith communities may sponsor social gatherings for newlyweds, young couples, new parents, and other such groups. They can also provide "schools" or classes for both adults and children to serve a mentoring role with regard to the various beliefs, values, and traditions of the group. Likewise, there are many outreach, administrative, and service options available through a congregation that can call forth the gifts and abilities of members in caring for the broader community. In short, there is no limit to the number of ways a faith community can accompany its members throughout these years when people reflect on and celebrate both success and disillusionment, companionship and loneliness, dedication and discouragement.

With increased years and accumulated life experience, a person becomes more aware of limitations and losses. In the language of Van Biema (1991), they are beginning to experience the developmental transition of remembrance. As life progresses, people begin to recognize that the spectrum of choices previously available to them is no longer there. For some, it is the time for "one more career move," testing out the pluses and minuses of an "empty nest," planning one's retirement years, or beginning to enjoy the grandchildren. For others, attention focuses more on how life has had (or not had) meaning and purpose. Adults in their middle years ask questions like the following: Who are the people that matter most? Are they close by or far away? What is my sense of accomplishment or failure? What have been the high points and low points along the journey? This series of questions is not to say that people begin to live in the past. Rather, they begin to remember, and remembrance is a sacred activity that calls the past into the future to be revisioned in the light of one's current reality.

In Ford's (1988) schema, there are three stages surrounding the events of remembrance. The first stage, which takes place between the ages of 40 and 55, involves *suffering faith,* with its gift of *accepting limits.* This stage parallels the eighth and last of Erikson's (1963, 1980) psychosocial tasks, that of pursuing integrity versus despair. Being able to look back at the vocational and occupational choices that have guided one's life with a sense of "I'm glad for the life I've lived" can involve a person in rich processes of thankfulness and recommitment. It can also precipitate a confusing form of restlessness and internal pain. Some people get stuck in the disillusionment and sadness of these feelings, deny their overall worth, and slip into a state of psychological despair. Others, however, allow the discomfort and restlessness to awaken them to new feelings and questions. This is the sort of experience described by Sue Monk Kidd in *When the Heart Waits* (1990), and what Ford refers to as the "other to within" transition (1988, p. 33); here, limitations are at first suffered, and then accepted.

With increased acceptance of one's limits, a person is more able to relax into what Ford (1988) calls a time of *liberating faith*, with its gift of *letting go*. Here, between the ages of 55 and 65, one can find the emergence of a balancing sort of wisdom—what Ford calls the psychosocial task of interiorizing versus separating. If one's self-worth is identified with one's job, physical abilities, accomplishments, or belongings, then one may feel devastated by some form of professional, family, or health setback. Discovering internal processes through which to make sense of change in one's older years can enable the letting go of cherished attachments while, at the same time, opening to their transcendent value.

This can lead to Ford's third stage in remembrance, occurring between ages 65 and 75, that of *renewing faith*, with its faith gift of *hope*. On the one hand, with a vision of hope, many people are able to expand their perceptions in later years; on the other hand, devoid of hope, some people narrow their horizons and withdraw. Ford refers to this as the psychosocial task of expanding versus constricting. It parallels the "universalizing faith" stage of James Fowler (1981), where a person identifies beyond the self with God (the divine) as a *felt reality*. Just as the first phase in this time of remembering involved movement from "other to within," this third phase involves a movement from "within to beyond" (Ford, 1988, p. 35). It prepares a person for life beyond the physical self or the limits of a particular life manifestation.

With growth in experiences of self-transcendence, a person moves into the final stage of development identified by Ford (1988). This is a time, from age 75 onward, of *resurrection faith*, with its gift of *peace*. In the context of our study, resurrection faith need not be limited to a Christian understanding of resurrection, important as this understanding is. Resurrection faith can also be seen as a faith that is restoring, reincarnating, and revivifying. Ford speaks of people in this stage coming to an experience of their life being "held together" by faith (p. 36). They enjoy things that others might discount or consider insignificant. Alternatively, they may also become preoccupied with fears. Questions arising at this time may sound like, "Who can I trust?"

and "Who do I fear?" Indeed, this tension of trust versus fear is the name Ford gives to the psychosocial task facing people in their final stage of self-transcendence. Physical vulnerability and even frailness can leave a person at the discretion or mercy of caregivers. It may or may not be a pleasant experience to live out the words of Christian scripture that says, "But when you grow old, you will stretch out your hands and someone else will fasten a belt around you and take you where you do not wish to go" (John 21:18 NRSV). As the faith gift of peace can be discovered deep within one's self, a person may find ways to receive the care of others. Eventually, all of life's faith gifts find their fullest expression in receiving as well as in giving. This, in turn, leads people to their final acts of self-transcendence: dying and death.

In the traditions of world religions, there are honors and rituals given to those who have reached their elder years. As we have suggested earlier in this section, the very term "elder" can have spiritual significance; indeed, in some traditions, to be an elder is to hold a religious office. In both ancient societies and contemporary cultures where honor is given to the extended family system, elders are looked to within the community for memories and wisdom. Elders are seen as sacred connectors binding one generation to another. In times past, one of the practical reasons for revering older people had to do with the fact that only a few reached old age. Today's society is different in this regard: With an increased life expectancy, together with growing numbers of men and women who qualify chronologically as elders, cultures around the globe are encountering a new spiritual reality. How will faith traditions draw on the mysteries within event time (*kairos*) to reflect on and celebrate the experiences of those who deal with not only the psychosocial but also faith development tasks of more advanced chronological ages? It is reasonable to believe that nurses within faith communities who appreciate the vital connection between faith and health will play a significant role in forging new religious rituals for tomorrow's seniors.

✑ Situational Transitions in the Context of Faith Communities

Throughout the writing of the previous section of this chapter, a niggling voice has repeatedly interrupted us with words like "but everyone knows life doesn't happen that way." For most of us, there are a number of unexpected events that significantly alter the kinds of predictable stages outlined by Ford, Fowler, Erikson, or any of the other developmental theorists. How often have we heard some variation of the expression "that person is seven going on seventy!" Such exclamations point to the rupture between event time and linear time in a person's experience. Furthermore, they underscore how some kinds of transitional events can "age" people far beyond their chronological years. This is the realm of situational transitions, which occur in the course of most of our lives. Some unexpected changes will be described as "delightful," others may be "disturbing," and still others will qualify as "traumatic." Healthy ways of coming to terms with unexpected change need to be encouraged by faith communities, who should be attentive not only to the change itself but also the process of transition precipitated by that change. Nurses who are able to bring their skills of health awareness to a ministry team will have much to offer in support of a faith community's response at times of situational transition.

At the core of unexpected change is an experience of loss. Someone's life is going along in a familiar way, and then, suddenly, everything is different. The change may be fortuitous or devastating. It may occur through chance, death, illness, violence, or a change in fortune. Whatever the circumstance, there is a sense that the person can "never go back to the way it was before." They are defenseless, vulnerable, caught off guard. All of their energies must shift abruptly to cope with the new reality. The circumstance of this new reality may be exhilarating, as in the case of people who have an experience of enlightenment or suddenly inherit money from a relative they did not know they had. On the other hand, the circumstance may be terrifying, as in the case of a person who is physically attacked or stalked. There is no way to explain reasonably *why* an event occurs; all a person can know is that something "happened," and now life is "different."

At the onset of most situational transitions, people cope. Approaches to coping may include a mix of physical, psychological, intellectual, and spiritual defense mechanisms. Such mechanisms are needed by the person in order to survive the initial phase of sudden change. Although some methods of coping may appear strange, they provide a signal to others that the person is experiencing significant stress. Listening to signals of survival within the context of a faith community can begin a process of being in relationship with the person who is commencing a situational transition. Indeed, before a person can hear the words, "How can I help you?" they need to hear words saying, "I am with you." Skilled, compassionate listening communicates *presence*. Knowing how to be truly present to another is an important intervention skill. It builds a foundation of trust; thus, it fosters survival as the first phase in a situational transition.

Of note, however, is that this notion of survival needs to be viewed holistically, including body, mind, and spirit. A helpful resource for nurses in faith communities as they begin to accompany people dealing with the onset of a situational transition is the book *How to Survive the Loss of a Love*, by Colgrove, Bloomfield, and McWilliams (1991). These authors write in a very readable manner, and speak about loss as a process of surviving, healing, and growing. Their practical approach is mixed with stories, poetry, and common sense. In addition, they view the concept of loss very broadly, including such things as success, which they see as a loss of striving, among their list of not-so-obvious losses.

As a person moves beyond initial coping and stays in relationship with the new situation, their level of response to the unexpected change will deepen. Now they are in a position to look back at the event and reflect on it. This is the time for nurses within faith communities to be available as receivers of story. Listening to stories is different from listening to signals of survival; it takes another set of skills. In addition to compassionate presence as a way of communicating "I am *with* you," the listener needs to engage with the person both verbally and nonverbally in a manner that says "I am *for* you."[3] In this regard, well honed interpersonal and systems awareness skills will support the faith community nurse in her or his empathic presence.

This is a time to "witness" (Herman, 1992, p. 180) the person as they "experience the experience" through remembrance. Stories serve as containers for viewing the event reflectively. Those who have written on the subjects of story theology (Crossan, 1975) and spiritual autobiography (Sullivan, 1991) know that there are "dark intervals" and "mysteries" to be found in the telling and retelling of stories. These dark mysteries can lead a person to deeply felt awakenings of rage, mourning, passion, enlightenment, meaning, and purpose. Of special note in this regard is the work of Jane Simington, who speaks of the searching power in story to take a person "down and under" to the dark core of truth in trauma. She then goes on to share the liberating power in story as the person moves back "up and out" into the light of that core truth's capacity to bring health and healing.[4]

In time, as the person is more able to integrate an unexpected change into his or her life, the nurse within a faith community can continue to accompany this person by means of commemoration. We often speak of an "anniversary of death." In addition to death, there are many transitional events that could benefit from rituals of remembrance. Among Aboriginal peoples, for example, the "give away" is a sacred sharing ceremony that honors both the dead and the living. By supporting people during and following their situational transitions, faith communities can serve as healing contexts within which to reflect and celebrate important life passages. Thus, unfinished business[5] can be revisited and worked through until, according to author Stephen Levine (1982), we can "just be with ourselves and others in soft openness" (p. 74).

ᴖ Summary

Nurses who minister within faith communities are continually encountering people whose lives are in transition. Listening to the stories of individuals and congregations, faith community nurses and faith group leaders need to exercise skills of inquiry in exploring possibilities and recognizing how worldviews, paradigms, and filters interact. Likewise, the nurse needs adequate familiarity with a faith community's context in order to know how best to draw on resources both within and outside this setting in responding to the transitional needs of individuals as well as groups. More will be said about this in the next chapter.

What has been attempted thus far in this section of our book is a presentation of various approaches to the topic of transition. We have emphasized that personal change affects social change, and, likewise, social change affects personal change. In addition, we have discussed how transitions occur within relationships. We all need to tell our stories, and to be seen at a level of what has value in our lives. This fact returns us to one of the original concepts discussed in this book, that of faith as being in relationship with. Faith is intimately connected with both the times of transition and characteristics of transition; indeed, faith is foundational in having the ability to engage processes for coming to terms with life changes. People of all faith backgrounds have a fundamental need to be in relationship with self, others, and the divine in order to mature individually and collectively. Likewise, a broad diversity of faith communities need to recognize and nurture the many resources available to their members through the stories, icons, sacred texts, and rituals of their faith traditions. Since faith communities are contexts within which to share reflection and celebration around experiences of being in relationship, they have much to offer in support of "choosing life" in times of transition.

Notes

1. Joseph Campbell (1988) speaks of the centrality of original experience to the hero's deed in the following quotation:

> Original experience has not been interpreted for you, and so you've got to work out your life for yourself. Either you can take it or you can't. You don't have to go far off the interpreted path to find yourself in very difficult situations. The courage to face the trials and to bring a whole new body of possibilities into the field of interpreted experience for other people to experience—that is the hero's deed. (p. 41)

Tanya Wilkinson, in her book *Persephone Returns* (1996), studies the complex relationship of "heroes" and "victims" through the theoretical framework of Carl Jung's psychology. In the following quotation, Wilkinson describes the emergence of both hero and victim archetypes in our culture. She believes that the one identified as hero (i.e., the one taking on a "hero persona") and the one identified as victim (i.e., the one taking on a "victim persona") share a common wound of unconsciousness. Both have become one-sided in their perception of a multifaceted issue related with human power, dominance, and vulnerability. Wilkinson writes,

> Adherents of the hero persona see themselves as heroic and see victims as morally deficient, but those adherents, in turn, are seen by victims as abusive. Adherents of the victim persona see themselves as outraged innocents but are perceived from the opposite side as, once again, abusive. Both sides maintain their identification with the chosen persona by projecting the shadow onto the opposing side. Interactions based on projection fail. Polarization is inevitable, and debate tends to degenerate into a competition for the moral high ground. . . . The constant use of quasi-moral and religious language, the processes of demonization and beatification, seem to indicate the presence of a spiritual issue, and one that carries a potent charge. The recurrent ideal images of pure victim and invulnerable hero hint at the activation of archetypal energies. (p. 12)

Wilkinson's book goes on to develop an approach to the hero/victim duality that seeks to integrate ego and archetype in a more whole and creative relationship.

2. The spiral is an ancient symbol (Walker, 1988) that, according to Schillebeeckx (1984), has received attention in recent decades from "Protestant philosophers such as Paul Ricoeur and Hans-Georg Gadamer and Protestant theologians such as Paul Tillich" (p. 103). One quotation worth reflecting on, in light of the nurse within a faith community as one who promotes inquiry, is the following reflection by Schillebeeckx (1984), in reference to what he calls the "hermeneutic circle," or circle of reflective interpretation. He writes,

> All understanding takes place in a circular movement—the answer is to some extent determined by the question, which is in turn confirmed, extended or corrected by the answer. A new question then grows out of this understanding, so that the hermeneutic circle continues to develop in a never ending spiral. . . . There is no definitive, timeless understanding which raises no more questions. (p. 104)

3. We express gratitude to Fr. Lawrence J. Murtagh, Margaret's first Clinical Pastoral Education (CPE) supervisor, for speaking about coming alongside others in pastoral relationships in such a way that we first let them know we are "with" them and "for" them before we try to "help" them.

4. We acknowledge the contributions of Jane Simington, R.N., Ph.D., who contributed these insights while teaching "Promoting Well-Being Within Faith Communities" at the University of Alberta, Edmonton, Alberta.

5. "Finishing business" is a chapter in Stephen Levine's first book, *Who Dies? An Investigation Into Conscious Living and Conscious Dying* (1982). In that chapter, he writes, "Finishing business means that I open my heart to you, that whatever blocks my heart with resentment or fear, that whatever I still want from you, is let go of and I just send love" (p. 73).

15 ✍

Health Promotion in Times of Transition

Joanne K. Olson

Faith community nurses promote the health of people whose lives are in transition. But, you might ask, isn't that the nature of nursing practice in all settings? Indeed, that is true. What then is unique about faith community nursing? We suggest that the word *broker* speaks to the uniqueness of faith community nursing. Usually associated with matters of finance, the term *broker* often means a "middle person" or "agent," a person who connects someone or something to someone else or something else. We introduce the idea that the faith community nurse is also a broker. The faith community nurse serves as an agent, connecting people in their times of transition with the rich healing resources available within the faith community. Simultaneously, the faith community nurse sees the needs of people whose lives are in transition, and the health-promoting potential of faith communities to which people are linked in varying degrees. While doing so, the faith community nurse also brings to light the needs of people living in times of transition, requesting and creating resources and approaches within faith communities that are health promoting in nature. One does not need to look far to discover people who have turned away from organized religious groups because they have not found these institutions to be health promoting. Sadly, some people even carry lifelong scars from hurts and pains that came about in the context of a faith community. The faith community nurse, together with other members of the ministry team, and indeed the whole faith community, can do much to both foster a healing reconciliation of past hurts and enhance the future health-promoting potential of faith communities.

In this chapter, we discuss health or wholeness as the goal toward which we strive during times of transition. We also look at health risks and health potentials as these exist in transitional times. Finally, we expand our previous exploration into the meaning of health promotion, and consider how faith community nurses promote the health of people whose lives are in transition. As a health-promoting agent of change, the faith community nurse will be discussed at both person-to-person and institutional levels of role functioning. Specifically, we highlight the value and healing power of presence and the importance of referral as strategies for being in relationship with people in times of transition.

ꙮ *Striving for Health and Wholeness in Times of Transition*

According to Reynolds and Lynn (1992), to be in an experience of transition is to encounter five health-related phenomena. First, there is a sense of being out of balance; second, transitions cannot be ignored; third, they impact our lives holistically; fourth, there are both health risks and potentials for health associated with transitions; and, fifth, there are relationship risks as well as potentials linked with transitional events.

Returning to our initial chapters, which focused on conceptual foundations of faith community nursing practice, we are reminded that it is toward health and wholeness that people try to move in times of transition. As professionals who accompany people during these times, we try to assist them as they move toward health and wholeness in their own ways and in their own time. Although health is a term used mainly in healthcare arenas, wholeness is a word familiar to faith communities. Health is viewed as a way of living, behaving, and developing. It is a social phenomenon learned in the context of relationships. Furthermore, it is a pattern of behaving, thinking, and acting that includes aspects of coping or managing a situation, as well as aspects of learning that are growth seeking in nature. The important element of this definition of health is that it is a social phenomenon that includes processes of learning in the context of relationships.

Like our definition of health, the experience of transition is also a social experience that includes elements of coping and learning. Looking back at the characteristics that define life in the midst of transition as a social phenomenon, we see a congruence between the experience of transition and health as defined in this text. First, we note that people do not enter periods of transition stripped of all previous coping abilities. We have mentioned people's natural attempts to deal with situations in ways to which they are accustomed. Second, we see that people in transition exist in relationship with others, and may at times put up barriers to experiencing the benefits of these relationships. In both the features of transition and the definition of health, emphasis is placed on people's uniqueness in responding to change. Finally, it is important to notice that people in the environments surrounding those in transition can have a profound effect on how people move through periods of transition. We reinforce this idea in our definition of health as a social phenomenon occurring in the context of an environment of other people. What, then, are the health risks and health potentials in times of transition?

✐ Health Risks in Times of Transition

In a book titled *Losses and changes: Finding Hope in Life's Difficult Times*, Randy Reynolds and David Lynn (1992) describe many of the health risks that exist in times of transition, including (a) isolating oneself, (b) suppressing expression of feelings, (c) moving too fast back into "real life," (d) making decisions too quickly, (e) neglecting physical care of oneself, such as rest, nutrition, and exercise, and (f) using coping mechanisms that give short-term relief. We will now briefly expand on each of these health risks.

All through life, we need other people. There is perhaps no time when this is more important than when someone has experienced a major change in life. Yet this often is a time when people run the risk of isolating themselves rather than truly being in relationship with others. Often, people isolate themselves for protection from more pain and disappointment. At times, people are embarrassed or ashamed of their reactions to change. Isolation, though, removes the potential of receiving support and affirmation, especially from others with whom the particular change is shared, and those who have had similar experiences.

Likewise, there is a second risk of suppressing the expression of feelings during times of transition. The main risk involved in the suppression of feelings is the building up of one change upon another. Unexpressed feelings, experienced during change and in the transition process, can follow us for years, like baggage weighing us down. When further changes come along, we accumulate new layers of pain and finally the unexpressed feelings overwhelm us, resulting in physical, emotional, or spiritual distress.

A third risk that people can succumb to during transition involves moving back into life too fast. In particular, people are at risk of this after significant losses, such as the death of a loved one or a broken relationship. Examples include parents who have experienced an infant death immediately becoming pregnant, or someone who has experienced a broken relationship immediately entering another relationship. The emphasis here is on allowing people to move through transition at their own speed, encouraging patience, and taking time to be cared for before taking on new commitments or responsibilities.

Closely related to moving back into life too fast is the risk of making decisions too quickly when experiencing change and beginning the transition process. Examples include those of a newly widowed person immediately selling a longtime family home or a newly divorced person moving to a new city. Although each person's needs and situations are unique and no outsider can determine the appropriateness of another's actions, it is worth wondering whether adequate time has been allowed for dealing with the recent change or loss when people are seen making sudden moves back into life or quick decisions that will impact the future.

People experiencing change and transition often neglect caring for themselves physically. Included in this self-neglect might be getting inadequate rest and sleep, neglecting nutritional needs, and neglecting exercise. It is believed that people who do attend to their basic physical needs will move through the transition process more effectively.

Finally, it is easy for people experiencing change and a process of transition to use coping mechanisms that give only short-term relief from the painful feelings. Some people overeat, use drugs or alcohol, blame others, and distance themselves from people by breaking societal rules (Reynolds & Lynn, 1992). The implication of seeking short-term relief through such coping mechanisms is that the real change is never dealt with, and, in addition, the side effects of one's short-term coping attempts generate new issues needing to be addressed.

There are, then, many possible health risks for people moving through a transition process and each has the potential to contribute to a person getting "stuck" during the process. This could involve dwelling on the change itself or holding on to painful feelings; both contribute to being unable to take steps toward the possibility of experiencing renewed life and feelings of joy. In the next section of this chapter, we examine the health potentials and possibilities that exist in times of transition.

ᴄ❧ Health Potentials in Times of Transition

In each of the theories of transition discussed in Chapter 13, there is a stage at the end that represents a new beginning, or a future filled with possibilities that can lead to reconnection and revitalization. Most transition theorists would agree that this time cannot be forced; it can emerge only when the work of earlier phases has progressed sufficiently, and there is readiness to say "Yes" to life again. This is when one opens to experiencing joy and new energy. It is not unlike the exaggerated feelings of wellness that one can experience after a sudden bout of flu or a cold. There is not only the physical sensation of feeling well again, but also a renewed appreciation for the state of well-being that may have gone unnoticed before the illness.

Many people express a heightened feeling of well-being even after coming through a very traumatic event. Likewise, they can easily identify the good that has grown out of the adverse conditions. It is these feelings of health, wholeness, and vitality that faith community nurses work toward uncovering when walking with people in times of transition. As Krauss and Goldfischer explain in their book *Why Me? Coping With Grief, Loss, and Change* (1990), it is at precisely these troubled times that people must grow inwardly. Like trees whose outward growth seems stunted in dry years, people's roots grow deeper in times of adversity. Said another way, people often find that a time of trouble is a time of growth (Krauss & Goldfischer, 1990).

Let us now revisit the concept of health promotion. If the faith community nurse is to promote health and wholeness during times of transition, we need to reconsider the meaning of the phrase *health promotion.*

ᴥ *The Nature of Health Promotion*

In an earlier chapter of this book, we discussed the concept health promotion. Although this phrase has changed and developed over time, as has the term *health,* we have chosen to use the definition of Labonte (1993), because it seemed to be most congruent with the purposes of this book. Labonte's definition includes activities or programs designed to improve social and environmental living conditions such that people's experiences of well-being are increased (Labonte, 1993). Labonte further developed his ideas about health promotion in a 1994 essay. He emphasized that health promotion is much more than simply planning programs. Rather, it should be viewed as a metaphor, a sort of lens through which professionals can reevaluate practices. His fascination with health promotion is for the way it acts as a lever for institutional or organizational transformation, which is not unlike our vision for faith communities as places of seeking both faith and health. Labonte (1994) suggests that institutions and organizations are not going to wither or be overthrown, but that they do need to be transformed. Health professionals, in his view, have a role to play in transforming all kinds of institutions into more health-promoting places.

Included in this view of health promotion is a plea to decrease our attempts at changing individuals, and to increase attempts at changing environmental conditions (Labonte, 1994). This means creating supportive environments that will remove the barriers that prevent people from making healthy choices. Labonte's (1994) view of health promotion also includes a focus not so much on developing people's personal skills as on listening to and hearing the experiences of people's lives. This parallels our earlier discussion about the importance of story as a container for transition and the place of therapeutic presence in the promotion of health in others. Labonte (1994) further encourages health promoters to work on understanding people's experiences in their own words, and then "negotiating mutual actions to improve those situations that people would like to alter" (p. 88). Labonte (1994) and Valvarde (1991) both use the words of Lily Walker, an Australian aboriginal woman, to describe the significance of mutual work in the process of health promotion. Lily Walker said, "If you are here to help me, then you are wasting your time. But if you have come because your liberation is bound up in mine, then let us begin " (quoted in Labonte, 1994, p. 88; see also Valvarde, 1991).

✑ Functions of a Faith Community Nurse in Transforming Faith Communities

In Chapter 10, we discussed the functions of a faith community nurse. We now revisit these functions in terms of how they can serve to facilitate the transformation of faith communities into health-promoting institutions. These functions, viewed in the light of health promotion in times of transition, take on new meanings. We recognize a two-pronged health promotion approach that is possible when faith community nurses serve as brokers between people in transition and faith communities. First, there are the efforts and functions that focus particularly on individuals and families. Second, there is the broad category of actions that serve to create a health-promoting environment within a faith community. We address both in this section of the chapter.

Being in Relationship With People in Transitions

Whether carrying out the faith community nurse's function of personal health counselor, health advocate, or integrator of faith and health, the primary feature of a helpful "being in relationship with" involves being a caring presence, as opposed to being one who focuses only on tasks needing to be done. The critical skills that constitute caring presence have already been addressed in Chapter 9. They are

worth revisiting, however, for it is these characteristics that contribute
to the nurse's presence with people and, as well, to the possibility of
promoting health when walking beside people in transition. As mentioned in Chapter 14, it is far more important to emphasize that "I am
with you" than "I can help you." This message is conveyed through
skilled, compassionate listening. This requires work at becoming
authentic and genuine, and work on dealing with one's own personal
issues concurrent with making efforts to focus on the issues of others.
It requires an approach of inquiry and questioning, more than of having answers. It involves an unhurried, patient approach. Furthermore,
it involves a nonjudgmental acceptance of whatever is being expressed
by the person experiencing change and transition.

Sometimes this "being in relationship with" occurs on a
one-to-one basis. At other times, support groups may be formed to
allow people in transition to be with others experiencing similar situations. At times, the faith community nurse may not be the person
directly in relationship with those experiencing transition; rather, by
facilitating volunteer work in the faith community, the nurse helps
others learn the skills needed to be truly present to those in transition.

Not to be overlooked is the responsibility of the faith community
nurse to serve as a referral agent for people and groups experiencing
transition. Although the faith community nurse may, at times, be a primary contact for individuals and families living in times of transition,
at other times, the nurse may be more involved in assessing who is the
most appropriate caregiver. Management of a strong referral system
that steers people to others who may be helpful is an important function of a faith community nurse. Included in such a referral system
could be faith group leaders and community professionals who spe-
cialize in working with people experiencing transition. It is most critical
that the faith community nurses view their skills and functions as part of
an array of all that is available within and beyond the faith community.

One final function of the faith community nurse that could promote health on a one-to-one or family basis is that of faith and health
integrator. Holstrom (1999) and Djupe et al. (1994) speak of this function as taking every opportunity to assist people in identifying more
deeply how their beliefs and values affect their health.

Working to Transform the Larger Faith Community

Let us now turn from working on an individual basis with people
in transition to viewing the faith community nurse's responsibility to

serve as an agent of institutional change. Considering health promotion as a lens through which faith community nurses and others reevaluate the practices of faith communities is in keeping with Labonte's (1994) full conception of health promotion. Looking at health promotion as an opportunity to facilitate a faith community's movement toward becoming more health promoting opens endless possibilities.

Such actions could take many forms within a faith community. First, the faith community nurse's very presence could serve to raise questions about whether certain faith community practices or messages are health promoting. For example, although most faith communities work to project an image of an unconditionally loving higher being—a health-promoting image—they sometimes have a reputation for promoting messages about sin and guilt; these latter messages may not be health promoting. At times, the message about sin and guilt is delivered in a less than health-promoting way; at other times, the feelings of sin and guilt result from the way people understand and interpret the messages being given. Let us consider, for example, a woman struggling to understand the message of her church, which says to her, "Forgiveness is required when you have been wronged by others." If the "wrong" experienced by the woman was physical abuse at the hands of a family member, she may confuse "forgiveness" with the idea of "condoning" what happened to her. In such a situation, the faith community nurse can serve as a broker, bringing the woman's misunderstanding to faith community leaders and helping the woman see that forgiveness does not mean condoning the abuse. Rather, forgiveness can entail letting go of "baggage" or "unfinished business," which prevents the woman from living life to its fullest. In a similar example, a church's message that marriage vows are for life may be taken to an extreme when a person remains in a marriage characterized by repeated incidents of abuse.

The very fact that nurses are not formally educated in theology may place them in a good position to raise questions about faith community doctrine. Is the doctrine health promoting? Are there ways of understanding the doctrine that could turn people away from, rather than toward, the faith community? Likewise, how can the doctrine be shared with people in their times of transition so that the health promotion potential within that doctrine can come through? In this way, a nurse can sometimes serve as an intermediary between people feeling distanced from the faith community in their times of transition and the faith community that wants desperately to offer its assistance and hope.

As members of a recognized health profession, faith community nurses bring important knowledge about the nature of professionalism to the faith community. Included here might be knowledge of the health-promoting benefits of establishing clear parameters for showing respect, observing confidentiality, and adhering to professional boundaries.

Finally, the presence of faith community nurses, by way of the services they offer, can do much to convert the faith community environment into an intentionally health-promoting setting. The development of health programs and support groups as a regular part of the faith community offerings would be examples of how this might be carried out. As well, there could be a more intentional linkage of the faith community to other health-promoting institutions in the community.

‿ॐ *Summary*

The basis of this chapter has been our belief that a faith community nurse has a vital role to play in the lives of people living in times of transition. We believe that the nurse can promote the health of people living in transition by serving as a *broker* who connects people in transition with the rich resources available within and beyond faith communities. We have developed our ideas by first reviewing the nature of health or wholeness as the goal toward which people strive during transition. Next, we considered the health risks and the health potentials that exist in times of transition. We revisited the concept of health promotion in light of what the concept means for faith community nursing. Finally, we reconsidered the functions of a faith community nurse in light of what it means to promote health both on an individual or family level and on a faith community level. In the next part of our book, we develop an in-depth example of one health situation arising within a faith community and a faith community nurse's health-promoting use of an inquiry process in her response. Although it is only one example, we hope it will serve to illustrate many of the ideas that we have put forth so far in this text.

PART V

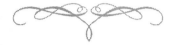

THE PROCESS OF NURSING CARE WITHIN A FAITH COMMUNITY

16 ✺

Promoting Inquiry

Assessment Processes

Joanne K. Olson
Margaret B. Clark

In the process of carrying out professional nursing practice, no matter what the setting, a complete and accurate nursing assessment is of prime importance. Good nursing assessment provides direction for planning, implementation, and evaluation, the next phases of nurse-client interaction. The main purpose of the assessment phase is to identify and obtain important information about the client and the client's concerns. Some definitions of nursing consider nursing to be the diagnosis and treatment of human responses to actual or potential health issues (Christensen, 1986a). It follows, then, that assessment focuses mainly on determining the client's response to health concerns or issues. Included could be biophysical, sociocultural, economic, psychological, or spiritual responses. Whether clients are individuals, families, or communities, assessment needs to occur in a multidimensional way, and be conducted by nurses who have a comprehensive knowledge base in assessing these various areas.

Data for nursing assessments are collected mainly in three ways: through (a) interaction, (b) observation, and (c) measurement. Interaction refers to verbal conversations with clients, other health professionals, or family members and significant others. During observation, the nurse gathers information by way of the senses (sight, touch, hearing, smell, and taste), and through written information. Measurement refers to the collection of information by way of instruments that give quantitative data. Examples of measurement information include blood pressure readings or height and weight measurements (Christensen, 1986a).

In this chapter, we address the assessment phase of the nursing process using the McGill nursing model as our guide. In particular, we apply this assessment approach to the faith community setting, considering the type of health issues that might be brought to the attention of a faith community nurse, how assessment is conducted using the McGill model, and what the goals of the assessment phase are. In addition, we sketch a summary of benefits of the assessment phase and highlight the essential features. Finally, we include an example of a nurse-client situation and the assessment related to that situation within a faith community.

✍ Assessment of Health Issues Within a Congregational Context

In the development of a professional nursing practice within a faith community setting, the unique functions of the nurse must be made obvious to people within the congregation (Holstrom, 1999). This is not an easy task for several reasons. First, it has not been common for nurses to hold staff positions within faith communities, and so people do not generally know about the type of health issues they could bring to the faith community nurse. Second, the stereotypical images of nurses and nursing, as described in Chapter 8, limit the range of issues that people initially bring to the attention of a faith community nurse.

A two-pronged approach to connecting with the needs of the congregation will likely be needed in the initial phase of establishing nursing practice in a faith community. As the nurse is conducting a complete assessment of congregational needs, she or he will also be finding ways to educate the congregation about the type of needs or issues that could be brought to the faith community nurse. It often takes up to two years from the time a nurse is hired by a faith community before most of the members of that community are aware of the services offered by this new staff member.

A congregational needs assessment may involve interviews with key congregational leaders, personal observation, and the use of both congregational data that is already available and survey information. The gathering of such data will assist the nurse in determining the health needs of a faith community, as well as the strengths and resources available within and beyond the congregation.

As part of the development of the McGill model of nursing, community health centers were established in Quebec, Canada, to provide a long-term family health service. This filled an identified gap that existed in the healthcare delivery system (Gottlieb & Ezer, 1997). It is worth noting that these centers were emerging at about the same time that Granger Westberg established "wholistic health centers" within U.S. faith communities (Westberg, 1990b). The Quebec demonstration sites aimed to engage clients and families in the pursuit of health behaviors and healthful living. Furthermore, they created a community environment in which health learning could take place using the resources available. This emphasis on learning was central to the development of the McGill model (Allen, 1982b). The project aimed to involve individuals, families, and groups in shaping the services that would fit a particular target group and the community at large. At the conclusion of the demonstration project, researchers reviewed the types of situations around which families sought nursing expertise. These situations emphasized the health promotion role of nurses, as well as the broad scope of situations with which nurses were prepared to intervene.

The research of Gottlieb and Allen (1997) can be helpful in assisting congregational members to learn about the types of issues that might be brought to a faith community nurse. Eight categories of health-related issues emerged in their research: First, people sought out nurses when their family was experiencing customary changes in family size, composition, roles, and relationships, including the introduction or loss of a member, or a transition to a new stage of growth. Second, families sought nursing expertise when learning to function in the social system; for example, assistance was requested when people were entering and utilizing the healthcare system, or planning for and adjusting to retirement. The third category of family situations involved interaction between environmental conditions and the development of healthful lifestyle practices; that is, people sought nurses when they wanted to alter their lifestyle to decrease destructive habits or incorporate new health behaviors, such as dietary changes for weight loss or when beginning an exercise program. Fourth, nurses were of assistance to people when they were experiencing biophysiological changes that accompany various stages of growth and development. Fifth, families sought the expertise of nurses to learn how to live with chronic illness or other long-term conditions in a healthful fashion. Sixth, nurses continued to be a trusted resource sought out for situations involving episodes of acute illness, injury, or uncertain health. Seventh, nurses were consulted when families were adapting to economic changes. Finally, nursing expertise was sought when families were trying to maintain interpersonal relations or resolve conflict (Allen, 1997b). Each of these categories can be explained in terms that would be easy for congregational members to understand. In the following paragraphs, we offer examples of situations that might occur within faith communities to warrant the assistance of a professional registered nurse.

Customary changes in family size, composition, roles, and relationships are times when individuals and families would benefit from the health-promoting interventions of a professional nurse. These situations could include the introduction or loss of a family member or the transition to a new stage of growth and development. These changes might arise because of marriage, divorce, the birth of a new baby, adoption, death of a family member, or when a family member moves away (Gottlieb & Allen, 1997).

It is important to note that faith communities are often the community institutions to which people and families turn when they are experiencing changes in family composition. Often these are not changes that require the services of another healthcare setting. Whether a family has regularly attended worship services within a faith group or not, they often turn to the local faith community when a marriage or birth is occurring, and many young adults find an increased interest in the support of a faith community as they begin to be parents themselves. I (Joanne) have often heard young parents comment that before the baby was born, their lives did not seem to have room for regular participation in faith community activities, but, now that they are parents, they have decided to return to a faith community, especially for the child's sake. Family deaths are also events in which the faith community is very involved. Again, even in families where there has not been regular participation in a faith community, the congregation with which they have had even a marginal affiliation might be sought for the purposes of funeral arrangements and grief assistance following the death. At times of change, people seek the stability of familiar spiritual roots and the support of others who can be found in a faith community.

In the second category of issues for which people seek the services of a professional nurse, it is easy to see that such needs readily surface within a faith community. Learning to function in a social system can include learning to access healthcare services for someone with a newly diagnosed chronic condition or adjusting to living in a new community. Faith community nurses have a wealth of information about healthcare resources within the community, and so might help a family new to the congregation locate a family physician, assist a new parent in connecting with the community immunization services, or work with a family seeking long-term care placement for a senior family member.

In terms of the interaction between environmental conditions and the development of healthful lifestyle practices, such health-related issues as attempting to alter eating or exercise habits or to make adjustments in lifestyle may arise. People might seek the services of a professional nurse for such things as weight management, nutritional counseling, the development of an exercise program, or for referral to programs to assist with cessation of smoking or dealing with addictions to drugs, alcohol, or gambling. Even after making a referral to appropriate programs for these lifestyle changes, the nurse can continue to work with the client and the family to support the progress that is being made. Likewise, the nurse can serve as the bridging link between the community-based lifestyle adjustment program and the faith community–based social support network.

Many health issues arise around the biophysiological changes that occur during normal growth and development. For example, sexual issues at all ages would be appropriate reasons to seek the services of a professional nurse within the faith community. The health-related issues that surround both men and women during the life stages of puberty, pregnancy, menopause, and aging may be particular causes for the faith community nurse to become involved with individuals, families, or groups. In a congregation with many middle-aged women, for example, the faith community nurse is in a position to design individual or small group interventions that focus not only on the physical but also on the psychosocial and spiritual changes of midlife women and their families.

Faith communities are filled with people and families learning to live with chronic illness and other long-term conditions in a healthful fashion. These chronic conditions might include such physical conditions as diabetes, arthritis, and cancer; there may also be chronic mental health conditions, such as recurring episodes of depression or schizophrenia. Nurses have expertise in helping family members learn to care for the ill or disabled family member, adjust to normal individual and family development when this is complicated by chronic conditions, and cope with children's reactions and family changes related to illness or disability. In terms of acute illness or injury, the nurse can be of assistance in referring families to appropriate medical care and in offering guidance and support in coping with medical interventions, such as diagnostic testing, treatments, and preparation for or follow-up after a surgical intervention.

Within faith communities, many families suffer silently through the adaptations that occur when a family experiences economic changes. Loss of work and other changes in employment status, by choice or through retirement, can be a difficult time that affects the health of an entire family. Nurses within faith communities can provide a safe place for people to receive individual or group support, as well as concrete assistance in terms of referrals.

Finally, nurses are often sought when people are dealing with interpersonal relationships, especially when trying to reach solution in times of conflict. These situations might include parent/child communication challenges, marital conflicts, or difficult relationships in the work situation. At times, the nurse would work alone with the individuals and families, and, at other times, the faith group leader would become involved in a cocounseling situation.

⌇ Assessment in the McGill Model

No matter what the reason for seeking the professional services of a faith community nurse, the assessment phase of the nursing process is where the relationship begins. Identifying the health issue *from the person's or family's perspective*, as well as the context in which that health issue arose, is the purpose of this phase of the nursing process. At this time, the nurse strives to place the health issue in the context of the person and the family as a whole, viewing the issue from physical, social, emotional, and spiritual dimensions. This requires skill in interviewing and observing for important data in all of these categories.

To obtain an overall profile of the health aspects of the situation, the nurse uses an exploratory approach to data collection, with observation and interviewing as the main sources of information. There is no predetermined assessment tool for the nurse to use when approaching a client or family in this situation-responsive type of nursing; rather, the nurse promotes inquiry, and seeks answers to the following questions:

- What is the client/family dealing with?
- What does the family want or what is it working toward?
- How are they going about it?
- What is their potential to develop and find healthier ways of living?
- What resources are they making use of and what others could be mobilized? What aspects of the broader context of family life might explain the family's present health behavior or situation? (Allen, 1997b, p. 169; Allen, 1986))

As the relationship progresses, and there is further promotion of inquiry, a variety of answers to these questions will emerge. The constancy of the questions, however, provides the continuity for the assessment as it continues throughout the nurse-client relationship.

↶ The Goals of the Nursing Assessment

First and foremost, the goal of the assessment phase of nursing is to establish a trusting relationship with the client and family (Grossman-Schulz & Feeley, 1997). The outcome of the assessment phase using the McGill model will be an understanding of what the family's health issue is, in the client or family's own words, and of the overall context in which the health issue has arisen. For us, an understanding of the overall context in which the person or family exists means seeing the health issue in light of the family, cultural, and faith filters through which the person or family views the world and, therefore, this particular issue. Furthermore, the nurse will assess the person's or family's health goals, as well as their readiness and motivation to invest time or effort in dealing with the health issue. Information will also have been gathered related to how this person or family learns best.

Involving the person or family in a learning process related to their health issues is central not only to assessment, but also to each subsequent phase of the nurse-client relationship (Allen, 1982a).

It is important to remember that the assessment process is ongoing; the information gathered about a person or a family evolves over time, and the process is never fully completed. Each time the nurse meets the person or the family, new information surfaces, and more clarity emerges around information previously gathered. Like working on a jigsaw puzzle, the pieces come together one by one, until finally a more complete picture begins to emerge. Also, like a puzzle that needs to be worked on over a period of many attempts, it would be almost impossible to learn all that is important about a person or a family in one sitting. In the process of leaving and coming back to the family over time, new data and patterns emerge that shed more light on the previous data and contribute to a holistic understanding.

The assessment phase is appropriately termed the exploratory phase (Warner, 1997), in that it is a time when the nurse guides the family into talking about how they have been dealing with the health situation at hand and whether their strategies are working. Sometimes the nurse asks a family to consider whether they have ever experienced a similar situation, and, if so, how they dealt with that situation. In this way, what persons and families have learned from their previous experiences comes into view. Throughout this phase, the nurse is looking for family and individual strengths that can be used as the collaborative work moves into the next stages. Part of the context information will also include determining how the family operates as a unit, who fills which roles in the family as a system, and how this family communicates, solves problems, and makes decisions (Warner, 1997). The assessment will provide the nurse with information about how to establish an environment that will stimulate, intrigue, and involve family members. As well, information about family priorities and how the nurse and family might work together to accomplish the family's health goals is gathered (Allen, 1997a).

✍ Benefits of the Assessment Process

Grossman-Schulz and Feeley (1997) studied supportive nursing actions, and determined that, in addition to establishing trust, the initial phase of the nursing process can be used to demonstrate many beneficial nursing behaviors. These include (a) encouraging the person to ventilate by exploring feelings so they become clearer, (b) helping the person to focus on the sources of the health issues or concerns, and (c) giving encouragement by instilling hope, putting the health issue in context, normalizing the health issue, and focusing on strengths and positive past behaviors. In all of these ways, the assessment phase can begin to be more than a time for the gathering of data. Already, therapeutic intervention is underway.

✑ Essentials of the McGill Model of Assessment

For many nurses entering faith community nursing practice, using the McGill model of nursing is a new experience. It is important, therefore, to highlight essential features in the assessment phase. The McGill model assumes that the nurse and client are collaborators in providing or seeking care, and this assumption of cooperation sets the stage for assessment. Such assessment takes time, and does not quickly move to planning and intervention. The exploratory approach serves not only to provide the nurse with information, but also acts as a means for clients and families to learn to reflect on themselves and their own behaviors. This, in the long run, helps individuals and families become stronger. It therefore empowers them to go through the same exploratory process when faced with new situations in the future.

✑ An Example of Assessment in a Faith Community: The Brown Family

Referral Information

The Brown family was referred to the faith community nurse by Rev. Jones, the head clergy of a suburban, mainline congregation in Edmonton, Alberta, Canada. When doing a routine pastoral visit to a family in the congregation, the minister learned that this family was dealing with the issue of caring for an aging family member, Mr. Brown's mother, who had recently come to live with the family from another city. The family had many concerns that they openly expressed to the minister. He explained the role of the faith community nurse, new to the congregation, and asked if the family would be open to a home or office visit with the nurse. The family was most appreciative and willing to meet with her, but had not thought about the nurse and the church as resources in dealing with this particular issue.

Several days later, Susan, the faith community nurse, arranged to make a home visit to the Brown family. During this initial visit, she began to get a picture of the issues facing this family. The nurse mainly used interaction and observation skills to gather important family health information. On this visit, Susan talked mostly with Mr. and Mrs. Brown; she also had a brief meeting with Mr. Brown's mother, Gladys. With the family's permission, she later interacted with the family physician and the intake nurse at the geriatric assessment facility where Gladys had been seen on one occasion. Observation skills were used to get a sense of the family environment and the quality of the family's interactions. No measurement information was collected during the initial visit. After establishing initial rapport with the family, Susan began the exploratory assessment phase of the nursing process by asking open-ended questions, listening carefully to responses, and observing nonverbal communication.

What Is the Client/Family Dealing With?

Nurse: The Reverend Jones told me that you were facing some major challenges around the care of your mother, Mr. Brown. Can you tell me more about that?

Mr. Brown: Well, she has lived in Toronto all her life, but recently we went there to bring her to live with us here in Edmonton. Neighbors in Toronto were constantly phoning us to say that she wasn't able to take care of herself. We knew her condition had deteriorated, but didn't know it was as bad as it was. Her apartment had a limited food supply, and she was becoming very confused. So, we brought her here several weeks ago and that decision has really changed everything for our family.

Nurse: In what ways has your family life changed?

Mr. Brown: Oh, we hardly leave the house in the evenings now, and even in the daytime my wife is restricted in where she can go and how long she is gone. We don't dare to leave mother alone at all. One day, for example, she filled a tea kettle to make a cup of tea, and then went to sleep. The teapot went dry, and the smoke alarm came on. We worry about her safety and the safety of the house.

| Nurse: | Yes, I'm sure the safety of both your mother and your home is quite a worry for you. [Pause] How has your life been affected, Mrs. Brown? |
| Mrs. Brown: | Except for phone calls, I really haven't been able to be in touch with any of my friends lately. Our kids are grown up, so Bob and I used to go out a lot. Now we don't even go to church together on Sundays. If we attend, he goes to the early service while I stay with Gladys, and I go to the late service. |

In just a short time, Susan has obtained a sketch of the family's primary health issue from the perspective of both Mr. and Mrs. Brown. She met Mr. Brown's mother briefly at the beginning of the visit. Gladys then went to bed for the night, so most of the visit proceeded with only Mr. and Mrs. Brown present. Without even asking specifically, the nurse is beginning to determine how the family is dealing with the situation at hand. The nurse then continues with her assessment.

What Is the Family Working Toward?

Nurse:	It sounds like you've made a lot of changes in your family life recently, and that you are both feeling quite frustrated about the restrictions that care of Bob's mother has placed on your lives.
Mrs. Brown:	You are quite right, but I don't want to sound selfish. We've had many good years together, and we owe our parents a lot, so we should do this adjusting when the time comes. After all, Bob's mother gave up a lot to care for her parents when they were in need. I know all of this in my head, but sometimes my heart feels differently.
Nurse:	How does your "heart" feel?
Mrs. Brown:	[Tears form in her eyes.] Oh, I feel angry and resentful sometimes. Sometimes I even cry quite a lot—my way of getting my feelings out I guess. I especially feel that way when Bob has to be away for days because of his job. Maybe if it was my own mother I would feel differently, but this is *his* mother.
Nurse:	So, you feel angry and resentful at times, and maybe somewhat discouraged. I also hear you saying that you feel guilty about feeling resentful. [Pause.] How are you feeling, Bob?

Mr. Brown:	Oh, I feel guilty because I see what this is doing to Sheila, and yet I can't be of much more help than I am because my work requires a lot of out-of-town travel.
Nurse:	So both of you are wanting some changes to occur. [Pause.] What is it that each of you want most for your family right now?
Mrs. Brown:	I guess I'd like for us to have his Mom placed somewhere where she could be happy and safe, and we could get back to our usual life.
Nurse:	What about you, Bob?
Mr. Brown:	I think I'd be happy if we could just figure out some reasonable ways to get some relief once in a while. Having mother in this condition is like having an infant in the house again.

Susan, the nurse, has now moved from identifying the issue to trying to determine what it is the family is working toward. She has asked about the health goals of the family, and noted that at this point Bob and Sheila have different perspectives on what they want for the family. She has also determined that the family is quite highly motivated to work toward some solutions to the health issue facing them. Next, Susan moves into trying to understand how the family is currently working on the health issue.

What Are the Family's Health Resources and Potentials?

Nurse:	Tell me about how you have tried to manage with the situation so far, and whether any of this has worked.
Mrs. Brown:	Well, as soon as we brought Bob's mother here, we made an appointment to see our family physician. She had a complete physical examination, and we shared with the physician the recent changes in Gladys's memory loss. It was Dr. Smith that put us in touch with the geriatric assessment clinic. Then, we took Bob's mother there, and they were helpful with doing a major workup on her. They say she has Alzheimer's disease, and that things will probably stay the same or get worse. They began to talk with us about placement, and we've gone to see some of the facilities they recommended. But at each place, she would be put on a waiting list, and it's the

	waiting that we find hard. How do we manage while we wait? We really don't know how to decide which place is best for Bob's mother.
Nurse:	So, you have used some community resources already, and, even though things are still uncertain regarding placement, you are coping the best you can. How have you been managing the home front while you wait?
Mrs. Brown:	Well, I have just changed my life all around, given up most of what I usually do. I don't know how long I can continue to do that though.
Nurse:	Have you as a couple ever had to deal with any situation like this before?
Mrs. Brown:	Yes, it feels just like when John was a newborn. He was quite fussy much of the time. I wasn't getting much rest. I couldn't get out of the house much, and it was pretty horrible. That was a long time ago, but I still remember how it felt.
Nurse:	How did you get through that difficult time?
Mr. Brown:	I remember that we decided that we would make time for us as a couple, no matter how hectic things were. Sometimes we had to get an adult friend in to take John for a few hours so we could get out, and sometimes we just stole a few minutes together over a cup of coffee in the living room. We sort of pretended we were "going out for coffee."
Mrs. Brown:	I forgot about those times, Bob. With the kids now grown up, we have been alone together a lot more, so I guess we haven't had to work at it. It helped me then to know that almost every day I would have a scheduled time when I could at least tell Bob what I was feeling, and he would listen even if he couldn't do anything else. I think another thing that I did was to focus on just taking one day at a time. And I did have some other friends who were going through similar situations at the same time, so we kept ourselves sane by talking to each other on the telephone.
Nurse:	Do you know of anyone else going through a similar situation with caring for an aging family member now?
Mr. Brown:	No, right now I can't really think of anyone. I haven't even said too much to my coworkers, because I felt it was kind of a private thing and that we should find ways to deal with it without telling everyone else about it.

This visit ended with the nurse summarizing what she had learned about the family, and with a joint decision that both the nurse and the family would gather more information. With permission already given by Bob and Sheila, Susan would talk to the family physician and the nurse at the geriatric assessment clinic. For their part, Bob and Sheila would make a list of the long-term care facilities that they had already visited, listing what they liked and did not like about each of them. The couple decided to try again setting aside daily special quiet time for each other, like they did when they went through the difficult time with John as an infant. Even when Bob is out of town, they decided that they could do this by phone. The nurse praised the family for their commitment to the care of Bob's mother, and also for their attempts to maintain their own individual health and their couple relationship through this difficult time. Before leaving, Susan asked if they would like to be remembered on the church's prayer chain. They did not feel comfortable with that, but said they would appreciate being remembered by the nurse in her prayers. She said she would pray for them, and asked for a specific focus for her prayers. They responded almost simultaneously, "That we somehow find the strength to get through this time of waiting." Plans were made to get together again in one week.

∽ An Overview of the Assessment

Let us look back now at the goals of a nursing assessment using the McGill model of nursing to determine if some of them were accomplished in this initial contact with the Brown family. The nurse's approach to the family was one of acceptance, empathy, and active interest in their issues. Grossman-Schulz and Feeley (1997) suggest that these three ways of demonstrating support are essential. Susan showed a nonjudgmental approach by allowing the family ample time to express who they were, what they were dealing with, and how they were feeling. At all times, she reserved her own personal opinions. She listened carefully to what they were saying, using well-developed empathy skills. She not only heard what they were saying, but listened to their feelings as well. Active interest and concern was expressed when the nurse set up a home visit with the family and made plans for a follow-up visit. Furthermore, she listened carefully to the family's explanation of how they were trying to deal with the situation, and agreed to carry out some further steps in the assessment process before their next meeting. Finally, concern, interest, and attention to spiritual needs were shown when she offered prayer in a nonintrusive and helpful way. Allowing the family to take the lead, Susan gave the family choices, yet let them know that her concern for them was not only as another individual, but also on behalf of an entire community of faith.

The nurse left this first encounter with a good understanding of the health issue with which this family was dealing. Furthermore, she was beginning to get a sense of the context in which this family's health issue had arisen. She had an understanding about how this family had dealt with similar situations in the past, what the family valued, the structure and roles of members within the family, and how Bob and Sheila communicated. There were many questions remaining, but she felt encouraged that they would be answered as time unfolded.

The family left this encounter feeling that the faith community to which they belonged genuinely cared about the real issues in their lives. Although the visit had not added any magical answers to their repertoire, they felt heard, and were stimulated by the questions the nurse asked.

The next day, at the church office, Susan shared with the minister that she had visited with the Browns, but reserved specific details of the visit for her nursing records. She also informed the minister that she would be working with the Browns in the future to try to find appropriate community resources and ways of dealing with the pressure they were feeling. She made a brief record of the information gathered on the first visit, and carefully placed it in a locked file in her office. Later that day, she telephoned both the family's physician and the nurse at the geriatric assessment clinic. Both telephone calls added to the assessment of the family. She discovered that Gladys Brown had been diagnosed with moderate Alzheimer's disease. From her nursing knowledge, Susan knew that this meant that Gladys Brown had obvious cognitive deficits, and would be disoriented to time and place. Gladys would require assistance in the complex activities of daily living, such as clothing selection, and would no longer be able to live independently or drive a car. Susan also learned that Gladys Brown was physically in good health, and that a nurse and a social worker from the geriatric assessment center were working on placement issues. Some of the main barriers to immediate placement included the fact that Bob's mother had recently moved from another province, and that many others with more severe Alzheimer's disease would need to be placed before her case could be considered. This additional assessment information was most helpful as the nurse made plans for the next steps in working with the Brown family.

In subsequent visits with Bob, Sheila, and Gladys Brown, the nurse learned more about their family. When helping the family complete a genogram (Friedman, 1986), Susan learned that Mr. Brown has one sibling. His sister, two years younger, is married, lives in Toronto, and has multiple sclerosis. She is therefore unable to participate in the physical care of her mother; she is, however, quite involved and connected by telephone. Susan also learned that Bob's mother has been a widow for 15 years. His father died suddenly of a heart attack. Regarding family roles, the nurse learned that the family has rather traditional male/female roles; Bob has always been the income earner, while Sheila has maintained the home and managed the care of their three children.

After becoming fairly comfortable with the family, Susan inquired about their faith and where it fits into the struggles of their life. She learned that both Bob and Sheila grew up believing that God expects children to respect, honor, and care for their parents even when that means sacrifice. They are not regular churchgoers, but continue to believe in a caring God. They used to attend church often when their children were teenagers and active in the youth group. They wanted their children to grow up with good values, but, now that their children are grown, the couple has been less regular in their attendance. They have a cottage on a lake two hours away, and find it is refreshing to go there on weekends. Lately, they have not been a part of any church committees or attended any of the church-sponsored activities. They had some difficulty answering questions about how they relate to God and how God relates to them on a daily basis. Mr. Brown said, "Well, we believe and everything, but we don't talk about our faith much if that's what you mean."

During the assessment phase with the Brown family, the faith community nurse learned about (a) the health-related issue that the family was dealing with, (b) what the family was working toward (i.e., family goals), (c) how the family was going about dealing with the issue, and (d) what resources were being used. In the area of resources, the nurse learned that in approaching spiritual resources and potentials, a strong belief in God is present but that the family is not comfortable speaking about their beliefs in religious language.

∽ *Summary*

In this chapter, we have introduced the idea of assessment as the first step of the nursing process. We situated our assessment in a faith community context, and discussed the goals of nursing assessment using the McGill model of nursing. We demonstrated, by means of a concrete example, the Brown family, how a nursing assessment could be carried out within a faith community setting. In subsequent chapters, we will address the additional phases of the nursing process using the McGill nursing model.

17 ᘓ

Promoting Potentials and Strengths

Planning Processes

Joanne K. Olson
Margaret B. Clark

I n the previous chapter, we introduced the ongoing process of assessment using the McGill nursing model. Following the assessment phase, which includes a determination of the health-related issues facing an individual, family, group, or community, the faith community nurse, in collaboration with the client, moves into the planning or working phase of the nursing process. In this chapter, we discuss the essential components of this portion of the nursing process when using the McGill model of nursing within a faith community. Included is an overview of the planning phase of the nursing process, documentation of the planning process, and an example of planning with a family within a faith community context.

✎ Planning Phase Overview

In this section, we review the purpose of the planning phase of the nursing process with a particular focus on how planning is carried out in the learning-oriented McGill model of nursing. As in all nursing processes, it is important to remember that the planning phase begins even as the assessment phase of the nurse-family relationship continues. In this regard, the phases of the nursing process in the McGill model can be compared to the overlapping components of William Bridges's (1991) theory of transition, as described in Chapter 13.

In a diagram used by Bridges, we see that even as the ending phase of transition is occurring, the person has already entered the neutral zone, and has begun to proceed into the phase of new beginnings. While living in the phase of new beginnings, the person continues to carry the elements of the ending phase. Similarly, the phases of the nursing process also overlap, with the next phase beginning even as the previous phase continues (see Figure 17.1). Assessment, for example, continues throughout the entire helping relationship, even though most of the assessment process takes place early in the nurse-client relationship. Likewise, most of the evaluation phase of the nursing process takes place near the end of the nurse-client relationship, but it begins on a limited basis early in the relationship. The terms more commonly used for the phases of the nursing process in the McGill model include the exploratory phase, which parallels assessment, the working phase, which overlaps with planning and intervention, and the discovery phase, which corresponds to intervention and evaluation. None of these phases is a discrete category; rather, they all occur simultaneously, with greater emphasis being on one or the other of the phases, depending on where the nurse and family are in their collaborative working relationship.

The goal of the planning phase of the nursing process is for the nurse and family to work together to begin testing out a plan that moves the client or family toward the stated health goals. Negotiation, flexibility, and collaboration are key concepts during the planning phase. Gottleib (1997) reminds us that the essential feature of this phase is the collaboration of the nurse and the client or family. Both partners are active and involved: The nurse functions as a facilitator, and structures the learning experiences, and the client or family functions as the participant and provider of direction during the process.

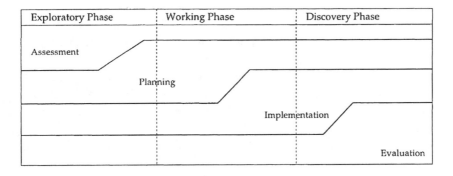

Figure 17.1. The Components of the McGill Model Nursing Process.

Source: This figure is based on a figure that orginially appeared in *Managing Transitions: Making the Most of Change,* by W. Bridges, 1991, p. 70. Copyright 1991 by William Bridges Associates. Reprinted with permission.

Together, the nurse and client discuss client and family goals for the future, and the ways by which the goals might be achieved. The clients know themselves best, so it is appropriate that they take the lead in identifying the manner in which goals can be realized. As a facilitator, the nurse must be sensitive to cues from the clients, and able to assist clients as they articulate their ideas. Plans can then be devised that will include relevant learning experiences for the client and family. At times, the nurse devises "homework" for families to carry out to gather more accurate information about the goals toward which the family is working. The outcome will be a plan tailored to meet the client's unique needs and learning styles (Gottlieb, 1997).

The planning phase of the McGill model nursing process is based on the assessment data that has previously been gathered regarding a client's health status, health-related issues or concerns, individual and family strengths, and available health resources. Although many nursing models use the term *nursing diagnosis* to identify the key client health concerns that result from the assessment process and that can be affected by nursing intervention, the McGill model does not. Rather, at the conclusion of the initial assessment phase in the McGill model, the nurse has determined the main health-related issues that face the person or family as they move toward health. Because nursing diagnosis terms have been developed *a priori*, and because they largely focus on client and family deficits rather than strengths, their use is not consistent with the assumptions on which the McGill model of nursing is based.

As in other models of nursing, collaboration with others is of key importance in the planning phase of the nursing process (Christensen, 1986b). In the McGill model, collaboration with the client or family is assumed because the model is based on this important principle of nurse-client interaction. Collaboration with others in a multidisciplinary team is also critical to effective planning. In the case of faith community nursing, it is especially important to include other members of the ministry team in appropriate parts of the planning. The nurse will need, as well, to seek out collaboration with health care professionals and agencies within the community.

The roles that the nurse plays in the McGill model reflect a learning approach. In the planning phase, the nursing roles of *coordinator/liaison, expert, focuser, integrator, negotiator, role model,* and *stimulator* are especially important (Gottlieb, 1997). Using the McGill model approach, nurses serve as a *coordinator* or *liaison* when they arrange appointments and set up opportunities for the families to explore resources both within the family and within the community. The focus here is always on assisting the family to learn to use the available resources. In the role of *expert*, information may be given to clients and families based on nursing and healthcare knowledge, but the manner in which the information is shared is collaborative. This means that there is an information exchange and a mutual exploration of the issues at hand. A nurse serves as a *focuser* when she or he sets up projects that will assist families to see their own patterns of behavior or their unique ways of dealing with situations. When serving as an *integrator*, a nurse highlights relationships between events and patterns of behavior within the family. The purpose is to help families transfer knowledge and skills from one situation to another. As a *negotiator*, the nurse becomes a partner in the planning process; both nurse and family discuss goals and devise plans specific to the family and to their style of learning. The nurse uses *role modeling* as a way of demonstrating a problem-solving approach. Finally, as a *stimulator*, the nurse asks provocative and rhetorical questions to invite the family to consider other points of view (Gottlieb, 1997).

In any planning process, it is important that the planners determine priorities, establish goals, and develop objectives that are the steps to achieving the larger goals (Christensen, 1986b). Likewise, in the McGill model, the planning phase is a time of strategic planning with the family to determine what the family's priorities, goals, and objectives are as they learn to deal with the health situation facing them. Working from a model of empowerment, the nurse plans care with the client and family, focusing on their strengths as a basis for action rather than highlighting the deficits that may exist. Documentation during this planning phase is key to successful collaboration with the family. We now describe the documentation process as it might occur in a faith community setting.

✍ Documenting the Health Work Plan

In addition to keeping records of what has been learned during the assessment process, the nurse needs to document the health work plan developed in collaboration with the family. It is important that this plan be developed collaboratively, and that the family verifies its accuracy. The plan can then serve as the family's road map in the process of working on health goals. Usually, such a health work plan is made up of four parts: (a) events in process, (b) goals, (c) tasks and activities, and (d) outcomes and responses. It is created to allow the nurse and family to track the health work process visually as they move toward their health goals (Laforêt-Fliesser & Ford-Gilboe, 1997). In the case of faith community nursing, this plan is developed and revised with the family during meetings in their home or in the nurse's office in the faith community.

The *events in process* are the health-related issues that the family is working on at the time. In the case of the Brown family, introduced in the previous chapter, learning to live with a dependent, senior family member was the event in process. Other examples of events in process that might be brought to a faith community nurse include learning to live life after the death of a spouse, learning to live in a new community, anxiety about upcoming surgery, depression following surgery for breast cancer, learning to live following loss of a job, learning to adjust to the needs of a family member with a chronic health condition, learning to live as a single parent following divorce, working toward a healthier lifestyle, or learning to live in a new culture.

Family or individual *health goals* are what the client wants life to be like in the future. Examples include such things as being able to resume some of the outside activities given up to care for a dependent mother-in-law, involving all family members in one family activity each week, learning how to pray, exercising four days each week, stopping smoking, or losing 30 pounds by Christmas. The experience of involving the client or family in the concrete action of writing the goals, rather than merely verbalizing them to themselves or to the nurse, is affirming, and serves to suggest commitment and motivation on the part of the client or family.

Once the health-related issues or events in process have been determined, and the family has identified the health goals toward which they are working, it is very tempting for a nurse to advise or suggest, rather than to structure activities that help individuals and families observe and think about their own situation. Various strategies can be incorporated to interest the family in health and to motivate them to search for their own solutions. Homework in the form of family activities, exercises, or the keeping of a journal are examples of such strategies (Laforêt-Fliesser & Ford-Gilboe, 1997).

In the previous chapter, the nurse left the Brown family with homework after her first visit. They agreed to make a list of all long-term care facilities that they had visited, and to identify what they liked and did not like about each of them. In addition, at some point during the assessment phase, the family completed a genogram (McGoldrick & Gerson, 1985) with the nurse's guidance (see Figure 17.2). This activity was helpful in showing the nurse who was a part of the Brown family. But even more important, the activity helped the Brown family consider the health status of each family member, review the recent and past life events that had occurred for other family members, and think about the relationships that existed between various family members. The activity provided information that would later be useful in brainstorming about possible ways to deal

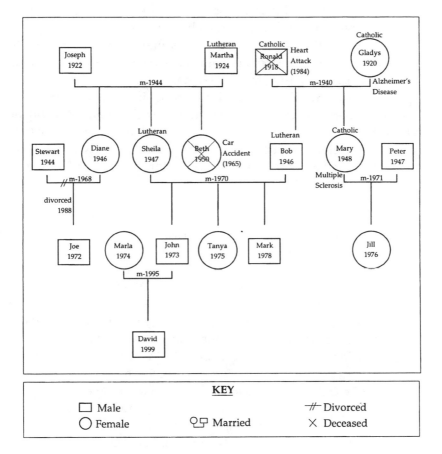

Figure 17.2. The Brown Family Genogram

with the health issue facing the family. The family had never before been involved in creating such a "picture" of their family, and decided to include it as a page in one of their family photo albums.

When the nurse moved into the topic of spiritual resources within the family, it was their decision to pull out the family genogram again. Using the drawing, they talked openly about which family members had been most influential to each of them as they developed their ideas of spirituality, faith, and religion. Bob Brown shared his experience of drifting away from his Catholic roots but finding renewed religious affiliations in Lutheranism following his marriage to Sheila. As a result, some ongoing tension has existed between him and his mother around faith issues. In turn, they talked about the values that they had hoped to pass on to their own children, and their joys and disappointments in that area of family life. By introducing the family to a way of collecting their own data rather than the nurse doing so with only limited family involvement, the data became family property, and served to stimulate the family to create new uses for this way of looking at their own family.

⌐ Continuing Assessment and Documenting the Brown Family Health Work Plan

As the faith community nurse continued to visit the Brown family over the course of several weeks, the planning phase of this collaborative relationship began to unfold. While continuing to gather data about the family and the health issues facing this family, Susan began to move the family into developing a health work plan. As the planning process unfolded, both the nurse and the family members had tasks and activities to complete; family members worked on becoming active participants in learning to live with Mr. Brown's aging mother, and the nurse took responsibility for structuring experiences that would help them learn more about their needs, goals, and problem-solving styles. At all times, Susan considered family and individual strengths, potentials, and resources.

The developed health work plan was used to track the Brown family's progress as they moved toward their own health-related goals. While working with the family on developing the health work plan, Susan was able to observe individuals and their interactions with other family members. This allowed her to see individual strengths and potentials, as well as giving her insight into how the family members related to each other and made decisions.

During several visits, the faith community nurse included Gladys Brown in the family-nurse interactions, and on several occasions she met individually with Bob's mother. During these interactions, Susan was able to gather further information about Mrs. Brown's functional abilities, and was able to assess her general health status. Knowing that cognitive impairments are often made worse by very treatable situations, such as dehydration and certain medication interactions, the nurse assessed these areas, and was reassured that Mrs. Brown was adequately hydrated and on few medications, which Sheila Brown carefully administered appropriately. Another part of Susan's assessment of Gladys Brown was a determination of her awareness of and feelings about her changing cognitive condition. Mrs. Brown at times was quite aware that she was forgetful, and realized that this was why she was living with her son and his family. At other times, she seemed totally unaware of where she was. The faith community nurse learned from Gladys that she felt some depression at times; she missed her Toronto neighbors and the many plants she had in her Toronto apartment. She told Susan that she is Catholic, and misses listening to Mass on the radio on Sunday mornings. In assessing Mrs. Brown, the nurse aimed to determine Mrs. Brown's level of functioning, identify factors that affect her level of functioning, and identify her response to her chronic condition (Miller, 1995). While the family works toward its goals, the nurse will serve as an advocate for Mrs. Brown, so that she can be assisted to function at her highest level of independence and have the highest possible quality of life.

Though this chapter focuses mainly on planning, the assessment information on Gladys Brown as an individual has been included here for several reasons. First, its inclusion here demonstrates that the planning phase can begin with the family even before all assessment data is collected; and even as planning begins to occur, new information is continually being gathered. Second, it is important to emphasize that, although the McGill model focuses mainly on family as client, the individual is not overlooked. Rather, the individual is assessed in light of the family, which serves as a background and context for a more complete understanding of the individual's present health situation. Finally, the focus on the individual was purposely left until later in order to emphasize the importance of first exploring issues from the family's perspective, rather than focusing on preidentified issues, diagnoses, or health-related concerns. Unless there are urgent individual needs to be dealt with, this assessment can occur as the nurse-family relationship progresses.

On her fourth visit to the Brown family, the faith community nurse shared a rough draft of what she perceived the family to be working on. After discussion, clarification, and further refinement, the Brown Family Health Work Plan emerged (see Figure 17.3), with the outcome/response portion left to be completed later in the discovery/evaluation phase of their relationship. It was designed to be a flexible working plan, one that would evolve and change as family needs changed and as new information developed. The main *event in process* was learning to live with a dependent senior family member who needs supervision and assistance with activities of daily living. Family *health goals* included (a) placement, (b) periodic relief and support, (c) learning to be patient while waiting for placement, and (d) learning more about how to effectively care for Mrs. Brown. The *tasks and activities* that emerged were shared between Bob, Sheila, and the nurse. Although placement of Gladys Brown at first seemed the highest priority, it was soon determined that little could be done to further the process along. Bob and Sheila felt they could participate in the process by continuing to visit suggested facilities, and then keep track of what they liked and did not like about each facility. The nurse agreed, with the family's permission, to contact the family physician and the geriatric assessment team. As well, she was in touch with professional members of the community who were working on Gladys's future placement.

At the same time that placement was being worked on, Bob and Sheila identified that there were other issues they could pursue. They desired periodic relief from their ongoing caregiving responsibilities, and were open to support from others who might be going through similar situations. They offered to continue finding ways to have quiet "couple time" each day, even if that meant only phone conversations when Bob was out of town. Bob was interested in learning more about the Alzheimer's Association that the faith community nurse had mentioned as a resource. Susan suggested that resources right within the faith community might be accessed, and agreed to talk with the congregational minister and the chair of the pastoral care committee about this. The nurse also offered to seek out several other couples she knew in the congregation who were dealing with a similar caregiving situation. Furthermore, Susan offered to contact several volunteers in the

Events in Process	Goals	Tasks/ Activites	Outcome/ Responses
Learning to live with a dependent senior family member	Placement of G. Brown in institution that meets her needs and those of the family	Bob and Sheila will list long-term facilities visited, noting likes and dislikes about each of them.	
		Nurse will contact family physician, and geriatric assessment team.	
	Family receives periodic relief from ongoing care-giving responsibilities and support from from others as needed.	Bob and Sheila will set aside quiet "couple time" each day, and by phone if Bob is out of town.	
		Bob will obtain information about the Alzheimer's Association's services.	
		Nurse will consult with congregational minister and chair of the pastoral care committee.	
	Be patient while waiting for placement and find some positive aspects to having Mrs. Brown in the home temporarily.	Bob and Sheila will identify ways to use this family "waiting time."	
	Learn more about how to care for a person living with a cognitive impairment.	Nurse will bring suggestions. Bob will contact Alzheimer's Assoc.	

Figure 17.3. The Brown Family Health Work Plan.

Source: This figure was developed from a figure in J. Laforêt-Fliesser and M. Ford-Gilboe (1997), p. 395.

church who might be able and willing to relieve Sheila of her caregiving responsibilities on a periodic basis.

From an understanding of transition theory and her inquiry into the family's health issues, the faith community nurse knew that "waiting" was difficult for this family, as it is for many others. She knew also that a time of waiting could serve as a "holding environment" or developmental "container" for positive psychological and spiritual growth. When this subject was brought up with the family, they were challenged by this opportunity saying, "We hadn't thought of it quite that way." They decided to spend some time addressing the positive aspects of having Mrs. Brown with them in a way that they never had before. Finally, the couple requested from Susan some practical help in living with Mrs. Brown: "There must be things that we can do to make our life and hers more pleasant while we wait for placement." Susan agreed to return with practical information about caring for someone with cognitive impairment. In addition, Bob suggested that when he contacted the Alzheimer's Association, he would also ask for such information.

After the initial planning was done, it was with some excitement that Bob, Sheila, and the nurse went about their agreed upon tasks. At each of the next visits, they discussed with each other what they had learned. The faith community nurse watched a family, at first overcome with the frustrations of what they had lost, now focusing on what they could learn from a difficult situation. She saw a family looking at what they could control about a situation that at first seemed to be controlling them. The planning process was truly collaborative, while being empowering for the family and rewarding for the nurse.

✍ Summary

This chapter has focused on the phase of planning as the second step of the nursing process. We have discussed the fact that the various phases of nursing process overlap, such that no one phase occurs as a separate event, and the goals of this planning phase were considered in terms of the McGill model. We highlighted the roles that a nurse would play within the planning, emphasizing the importance of documenting the plan of work with the family, and offering an example of a health work plan for the Brown family. The next two chapters will focus on the implementation and evaluation phases of the nursing process using the McGill model in a faith community setting.

18

Promoting Health Development

Implementation Processes

Joanne K. Olson

The implementation phase of the nursing process involves carrying out the plan as created by the nurse together with the client and family. Throughout this phase, the nurse continues to assess, modifying plans as new information is gathered or as the client and family situation changes. In this chapter, we consider the knowledge and skills required for a successful implementation phase, both in general nursing terms and specifically as implementation relates to the McGill model of nursing. We then follow the Brown family through the implementation phase of the nurse-family relationship using the McGill model as a guide.

◌ Nursing Knowledge and Skills Needed
for the Implementation Phase

Several authors have identified the skills needed to implement a nursing plan as *intellectual, interpersonal,* and *technical* (Fayram, 1986; Yura & Walsh, 1983). *Intellectual* skills are the ability to reason and understand. Also included are decision-making skills, particularly decisions about prioritizing actions and determining the timing of nursing actions. Finally, intellectual skills in observation are required as the nurse continues to gather data, and notes the client and family's reaction to the implementation of the developed plan (Fayram, 1986).

Interpersonal skills are required throughout the entire nursing process. Specifically, in the implementation phase, they are needed when communicating with clients and with other health care professionals and agencies. When making referrals, for example, the nurse must provide clear explanations and accurate information both in verbal and written form (Fayram, 1986). Excellent interpersonal skills throughout the implementation phase communicate to the client and family that they are genuinely cared for. In the case of a faith community nurse, the client and family need to feel they are cared for not only by the nurse, but also by the faith community that she or he represents.

In the faith community setting, there is limited need for nurses to practice specific *technical* skills, which involve the competent and safe performance of procedures. An example of technical intervention would be the administration of cardiopulmonary resuscitation in an emergency situation, or the taking of a blood pressure reading. Studies have shown, however, that it is difficult to separate the nurse's intellectual and interpersonal skills from technical skills. To carry out technical skills, the nurse needs knowledge about the following: (a) the principles and steps of the procedure, (b) the expected outcomes and possible complications, and (c) the legal and ethical aspects of the procedure. Because faith community nurses practice in an independent fashion, it is crucial that they take seriously the professional responsibility of being current and skillful in any technical procedures carried out.

During intervention, there is overlap of the nurse's intellectual, interpersonal, and technical skills. Intellectual decision-making skills, for example, are required when the nurse determines the appropriateness of making modifications to technical procedures. When performing technical skills, interpersonal skills are also important; they are used to support and give instructions to clients, and to obtain data about the client's reactions to the intervention (Fayram, 1986).

✍ Implementation in the McGill Nursing Model

When offering nursing care from a McGill model perspective, implementation is not a rushed step in the overall process. It is important that, rather than "zooming in" with concrete aspects of a plan, the nurse takes adequate time to allow the family to have a waiting period, which directs them toward achieving the best fit between the actions to be taken and the individual's or family's situation (Allen, 1997a). This phase is often termed the *working phase*. During this time, the client and family become occupied with learning about how to deal with health-related issues facing them, while the nurse works to structure relevant learning experiences for the family. Mainly, the nurse is working to create a learning environment that strengthens the problem-solving and coping skills of the client or family (Gottlieb, 1997).

Gottlieb (1997) describes a number of nursing roles that might be used in structuring learning experiences for clients and families. She has entitled these roles *focuser, stimulator, integrator,* and *awareness raiser.* Both the *focuser* and the *stimulator* roles involve helping the client and family to enlarge or clarify their health concerns, and to view their concerns within a larger context. The focuser role involves devising projects that help a client or family discover patterns of behavior and obtain an objective method of determining how they usually deal with situations. It involves assisting family members to carry out information-gathering assignments to improve the family's ability to gather their own information. As a stimulator, the nurse "asks provocative or rhetorical questions for the purpose of having the client consider a situation from another point of view" (Gottlieb, 1997, p. 112).

As an *integrator,* the nurse points out relationships between events and patterns of behavior, so that clients and families can move knowledge and skills from one situation to another. Specific strategies that assist clients or families to generalize their learning include relating and linking factors, pointing out similarities and differences between situations, and drawing parallels. In all of these ways, it is important that the client or family learn new skills in problem solving so that they arrive at a solution. Even though a nurse may possess "expert" knowledge about certain health-related issues that face a client or family, the manner in which this information is shared is always consistent with the collaborative nature of the nurse-client relationship in this nursing model. The nurse encourages clients to participate actively in discussions, seeking information for themselves, and applying the new information in ways that are uniquely relevant for that family. If the implementation phase has proceeded successfully, the nurse has structured learning experiences that have added to the client's and family's ability to solve problems. In addition to reaching some acceptable solutions to their health-related issues, the client and family have learned new ways of approaching future issues.

As an *awareness raiser*, the nurse assists individuals and families in bringing to consciousness the things that have been learned at an intuitive level. Within this overall strategy are included more specific tactics, such as summarizing lessons learned, identifying indicators of client and family progress toward health goals, and asking the client or family to review what they have learned. All of these strategies serve to increase clients' analytical skills, which are essential to effective problem solving (Gottlieb, 1997).

In short, the implementation phase of the McGill model is the time during which the nurse "steps back"and allows the family to begin working on the plan they have developed. They begin to test out, and work through, how the plan will actually work for them. The nurse's contacts with the family may be brief and less frequent during the implementation phase than they have been in the assessment and planning phases. The nurse takes on the role of "coach" in the family's health work, purposefully leaving the family on their own for a period of time in order that they might have the opportunity to test out new behaviors. The nurse makes it known that she or he is available, but also conveys to the family a belief that the family has the ability to carry out its plans. When they meet again, the purpose is to identify small achievements or outcomes, or to help the family change their plans if the situation changes or their original plans are not working. The nurse notes whether the family is able to incorporate the health work plan easily into their normal, day-to-day life. In addition, the nurse determines if the family is using resources available to them, discussing plans among themselves, remaining interested and challenged yet not overwhelmed, and is venturing out to try new approaches (Warner, 1997).

∽ Implementing the Plan: The Brown Family

Susan, the faith community nurse, visited the Brown family weekly for four weeks as the assessment and planning phases of the health work process were carried out. Once the Brown family health work plan was established, the nurse visited the family every two weeks to allow the family time to test out the tasks and activities to which they had agreed. Meanwhile, the nurse carried out her own tasks, and gave the family information as she uncovered it. She could be easily reached by telephone at the church office when the family needed to connect with her. When Susan did visit the family, she asked questions and made observations about the ease with which the family was incorporating health work into their lives, and whether any changes in the family situation necessitated a revision of the health work plan. She also looked for indications of how challenged, motivated, and satisfied the family was with the health work. Let us now look at each of the health goals determined by the family, and track the progress of that goal through the implementation phase of the health work process. Throughout, we will comment on how the nurse collaborates with the family on each health goal.

Placement of Gladys Brown

Initially, the family expressed a feeling of motivation regarding work on this health goal. Whenever Gladys Brown's name rose to the top three people on the waiting list of a particular institution, the family asked to be notified. Even before the nurse's first visit to the family, they had been contacted by several institutions. They had visited the institutions, and were beginning to identify what they liked and did not like about particular facilities. It was only after the faith community nurse asked, "What are you looking for in a long-term care institution?" that Bob and Sheila began to think further about the specific criteria they were using to place an institution on the "We like it" or the "We don't like it" list. The nurse's question had challenged them to develop a strategy of rating facilities in a systematic way. Other questions that had stimulated the family's thinking included, "I wonder what you would consider to be important if your children were selecting a facility for you to live in?"

Bob and Sheila proceeded to develop criteria for how they would evaluate the institutions. In doing so, they considered what they already valued in a long-term care facility. They wanted a facility that was relatively close to their home and had special programs for people with Alzheimer's disease, and they wanted to find a placement within the financial means of the family. With no previous experience in placing a senior family member, Bob and Sheila asked the nurse what else they should consider. Susan responded, suggesting one or two ideas that had been important to other families with whom she had worked, and then asked the family to think about where else they might get this kind of information. They remembered a woman with whom they had worked years ago through the local community league who recently had placed her mother in a nearby nursing home. They wondered if she might have some helpful information for them. They also knew that one of the ministers at the church was known to make visits to members in long-term care facilities. They wondered if Rev. Blake would have some ideas. They also decided that they would call Bob's sister and ask for her input. A search of the local library resources also resulted in one good book about placement issues.

Within less than a week, the couple had devised a list of criteria that would make the process of reviewing placement options much easier. In addition to what they had originally considered, they added the following questions to the list of things to be considered in their choices: Does the facility provide for spiritual care consistent with Mrs. Brown's valued Catholic traditions? How are the staff educated and oriented? What is the nursing staff to patient ratio on various shifts? What is the level of preparation of the staff? Is there ample opportunity for the family to participate in care? Does the facility have a multidisciplinary staff and approach to the care of residents? Does the resident have opportunity to bring in personal belongings, plants, and so forth? Are the accommodations private, semi-private, or wards? Are pets encouraged within the facility?

While the family worked on the placement issue on a day-to-day basis, the nurse remained in contact with the family physician and the geriatric assessment team to keep them apprised of any changes that she noted in Gladys or the family. In relating with the family, Susan was especially observant of whether the activities regarding placement were challenging the family, and whether at any time the family seemed overwhelmed by the tasks.

Getting Periodic Relief From Caregiving

Bob and Sheila made an agreement to set aside daily quiet "couple time," after remembering that this had been a good coping strategy when they dealt with a demanding newborn years ago. They decided to take turns planning the way in which they would spend their time together; some evenings they played cards or watched the news together. By asking a neighbor to come into the house after Gladys Brown had gone to bed for the evening, the couple was sometimes able to go for an hour-long walk. Sheila prided herself on being able to come up with interesting new varieties of coffee that the couple could share in their cozy family room; Bob was proud of his innovation when he arranged for a catered candlelight dinner for two on Valentine's Day night.

Bob took seriously his promise to obtain information about the local chapter of the Alzheimer's Association. Though there is no direct caregiver relief available through the organization, he learned that the chapter sponsors family support groups, which are established to provide families with information, emotional release, and encouragement to cope with the daily burdens of caring for a loved one with dementia.

The nurse discussed the need for temporary caregiver relief with the minister and the chair of the pastoral care committee. She learned that Janet, a church member with a long-term mental health condition that prevented her from working, was willing to be hired to stay with Gladys Brown. She was willing either to come to the family home or to have Mrs. Brown brought to her apartment several mornings or afternoons each week. The extra income would be a welcome supplement to Janet's limited social assistance. The faith community nurse also learned about a quilting group that had been operating at the church for a number of years. The woman who manages the group was willing to take Gladys Brown into the group to see if Gladys would be interested in quilting activities. At the same time, the group leader would assess Gladys's reaction to the group and her ability to remain focused on a project.

Bob and Sheila decided to investigate the resources that might exist right within their own family. The Browns' son and daughter-in-law live three hours away, but offered to come for a weekend if they were ever needed. They indicated that with their newborn, they were unable to get out much socially, and would by happy to care for both the baby and Gladys Brown on a weekend. John mentioned that he might actually enjoy spending some time with his grandmother; it had been years since the two of them spent time together. He recognized that caring for her in her current state would be a change from his last memories of his grandmother, but he was willing to give it a try.

Finding Support From Others in Similar Situations

In his research on the Alzheimer's Association, Bob learned about several support groups in various parts of the city. He located the one nearest to their home, and talked to the leader. The faith community nurse located two couples in the congregation who had recently been through a similar situation of arranging for placement of a senior family member; both couples were willing to meet with Bob and Sheila if that would be helpful. Susan also discovered that another church in the area was sponsoring a weekend workshop on caregiving. One of the guest speakers had just written a book about the spirituality of people living with Alzheimer's disease (Everett, 1996); another speaker was presenting information on community resources for people living with cognitive impairments. This information was shared with the family.

After the family health work plan had been drawn up, Bob decided to investigate Internet resources. He discovered a chat line for caregivers of loved ones with a cognitive impairment. He decided to try this resource as an option to small group support, because it fit more with his sporadic work schedule of being at home some weeks and out of town other weeks.

During Susan's first visit with the family, she had asked if Bob or Sheila knew any other people going through a similar situation with caring for an aging family member. Thinking that this situation was a private matter, Bob did not talk much to his coworkers about what he was going through at home. The nurse's question remained with him long after that first visit; later, Bob thought, "I wonder if I should be more open about what I am dealing with at home?" Several weeks went by, and then he decided to venture out and share. Over lunch one day, he discovered that several other employees in his company were dealing with similar situations. Even his immediate supervisor was quite familiar with the extra strains of such a temporary living situation. He offered to lessen Bob's out of town commitments for a time, if that would be helpful. Bob was amazed at the way in which his sharing was received.

One day, Sheila phoned the minister to thank him for his earlier visit and for his referral of the family to the faith community nurse. Following a lengthy discussion, Sheila suggested that she would now like to have their situation included on the prayer chain at the church. She commented, "At first, we were kind of embarrassed that we weren't easily able to deal with this on our own. We're beginning to see that this is a major change for our family, and that we may need all the help we can get. We also know that others might be suffering through similar situations, and as we share our experience and ask for God's help, others may also feel free to do the same. We're also beginning to see that God isn't at a distance with some magical answers but that God is here in every person that comes our way. Maybe God is using my mother-in-law to teach me something. This whole situation has made me think more deeply about who God is, how God works in us and through us, and how we are sometimes called to care for others even though we don't think we have the ability."

Finding Positive Aspects in a Temporary Situation

At first, this health goal was a challenging one to work on. It was easy to focus on all of the negative aspects of this temporary living arrangement. Bob and Sheila noted that when their son and daughter-in-law visited from a city three hours away, their newborn baby seemed to have quite a positive affect on Gladys Brown. On a recent visit, they had discovered that Gladys loved having the baby around, and seemed to be quite clear in her thinking while interacting with the baby. She enjoyed holding him and rocking him. While the baby was present, Mrs. Brown tended to reminisce more about when she was a young mother; stories were being told that no one in the family had ever heard. On one occasion, Sheila asked Gladys if she could tape-record her stories of when Bob and Mary were children. Gladys agreed, and family history was captured. The family also used the opportunity for a four-generation family photo. On another occasion, Sheila located old family photo albums, and discovered that this moved Gladys into sharing more stories about her life. Again, with her permission, a tape recorder was used to capture pieces of her life story.

There was initial difficulty in getting Gladys interested in the quilt-ing activities at the church. She seemed fearful of being left with women whom she did not know. Sheila stayed with her the first time, and it was during that session that the group leader discovered Gladys's attachment to and fondness for her great-grandson. A baby quilt project was thus initiated, and from that day forward Gladys was motivated to attend the quilting sessions when reminded that she was working on a quilt for her great-grandson, David.

Knowing that Mrs. Brown had left many of her own house plants in the care of neighbors and friends in Toronto, Sheila decided to use the waiting time effectively by inviting Mrs. Brown to be the caretaker of the household plants. The activities of watering, pruning, and fertil-izing the plants were organized so that Gladys could keep track of when each task needed to be done, which also served to keep Gladys more oriented to the days of the week. Finally, Sheila discovered that, on occasion, Gladys was able to assist with supervised meal prepara-tion, folding of laundry, table setting, and other such household activities.

Learning More About Caring for Persons With Cognitive Impairments

Bob discovered that the Alzheimer's Association was a good source of specific information about the care of a loved one with a cog-nitive impairment. He was sent a large package of information, from which he learned that the Association had a library. Bob and Sheila were able to use the library to check out helpful books and informative videos about this condition. Susan brought Bob and Sheila additional suggestions for living with someone who has a cognitive impairment. Many of the suggestions resulted from the nurse's research into the topic. Various nursing research articles and current textbooks con-tained up-to-date information.

Together, the nurse and the Browns discussed what they had learned from various resources. Earlier, Susan determined that Mrs. Brown was aware she was living with her son because of memory defi-cits. At times of cognitive lucidity, she was included in determining which activities of daily living would benefit from assistance and how this assistance could be implemented. The nurse stressed the impor-tance of trying only some of the things she was suggesting. She men-tioned to the family that each person is unique; what works for one person may not work for another, and what is effective one day is not necessarily effective the next day (Burgener, Shimer, & Murrel, 1993). Some of the suggestions made by the nurse were based on nursing research findings that indicate a decrease in environmental stimuli can lead to improved cognitive functioning, whereas an increase in environmental stimuli can lead to decreased functioning (Hall & Buckwalter, 1987). Environmental modifications that may be of help to people living with cognitive impairment, as well as to their caregivers, include using clocks, calendars, daily newspapers, and simple written cues for orientation to day, date, place, and events. Simple pictures or written cues may help with identifying items and places, such as the toilet, bedroom, and so forth (Miller, 1995).

The nurse took the opportunity to discuss ways in which to communicate with people with dementia. One study found that when the caregivers used relaxed and smiling behaviors, there was a positive, calming effect on cognitively impaired elders (Burgener, Jirovec, Murrel, & Barton, 1992). Bob and Sheila had read about the importance of not using demeaning or condescending tones of voice. Using simple sentences and presenting only one idea at a time was recommended. When a person does not understand a statement, the statement should be repeated using the same words. The use of positive statements, rather than statements that contain the word *Don't*, was suggested. When the person is able to make some decisions, she should be offered simple and concrete choices. An example would be asking, "Do you want the green dress or the red dress?" rather than saying, "What do you want to wear today?" It was also suggested that caregivers listen carefully for feelings the person is trying to express, and let the person know that you hear what they are feeling. It is important to ask only questions that you know the person can answer correctly. To avoid confusing the person, it is also important that nonverbal communication is consistent with verbal communication. Touch can be used to gain the person's attention and to reinforce feelings of concern. Good eye contact, pleasant facial expressions, and a relaxed and smiling face are encouraged when approaching the person with cognitive impairment (Miller, 1995).

Regarding safety issues, the family learned that it is suggested the person carry identification, as well as a telephone number of someone to call, if wandering is a problem. The family inquired about ways to secure doors if needed. Susan suggested that sometimes alarm devices can be used on doors to prevent wandering. She further recommended that the environment should be kept uncluttered; medications, cleaning solutions, and poisonous chemicals should be kept in inaccessible places (Miller, 1995).

One of the pamphlets received from the Alzheimer's Association emphasized the importance of keeping stress to a limited level for the person by reducing (a) fatigue, (b) physical stressors, (c) competing or overwhelming stimuli, (d) change of routine, (e) change of caregivers, (f) change in environment, and (g) demands to function beyond the person's ability. The pamphlet further encouraged planning and maintaining a consistent routine. Regular rest periods were recommended to compensate for fatigue and loss of reserved energy. The importance of providing unconditional positive regard was stressed, as well as the suggestion that caregivers remain nonjudgmental about the appropriateness of all behaviors except those that pose a threat to safety. The use of reassuring forms of therapy, such as music and reminiscence, were also encouraged (Miller, 1995).

The family decided, after hearing about some of these interventions, that they would incorporate more soothing music into their home environment. Sheila had recently purchased a set of classical tapes with relaxing nature sounds in the background. In addition, they would try to be more intentional about the ways in which they were communicating with Gladys Brown.

Putting Theory Into Practice

In relating to the family around their own identified health goals, the nurse served as a *stimulator, awareness raiser,* and *integrator.* As a *stimulator,* the faith community nurse asked provocative and rhetorical questions for the purpose of having the family consider the situation from another point of view. She asked them to consider themselves being placed in a long-term care facility, and then to think about what they would want their children to look for when they made decisions. Susan also asked the family to think about other people who were currently dealing with similar situations of family caregiving. In so doing, she stimulated Bob to venture out and share with coworkers in a way he had not previously done. In the role of *awareness raiser,* the nurse helped the family to bring to consciousness the things that they had known at an intuitive level, but had not previously stated in specific terms. The result was a detailed list of criteria for evaluating long-term care facilities. The beauty of the list was that the family developed it themselves; it was based on their needs and requirements, and on input received from outside sources. In the role of *integrator*, Susan pointed out relationships between events and patterns of behavior, so that the family could move knowledge and skills from one situation to another. For example, her questioning about how the family had dealt with previous difficult caregiving situations stimulated discussion about what it was like when John was an infant and how the couple had dealt with that situation.

✎ Summary

Throughout the implementation phase, the nurse structured learning experiences that enhanced the family's problem-solving skills. Focusing on the problem-solving process, rather than on solutions, empowered the family, as they realized that the solutions to their issues were right at their fingertips all along. They felt further empowered knowing that what they had learned in this situation could be transferred to new situations in the future (Gottlieb, 1997). In the next chapter, we will move into evaluation, the final phase of the nursing process.

19 ↶

Promoting Improved Health

Evaluation Processes

Joanne K. Olson

The final phase of the nursing process is evaluation. In this chapter, we discuss the purpose of this phase, as well as the roles of the nurse during evaluation. We then observe the faith community nurse walk through the evaluation phase with the Brown family.

↶ Overview of the Evaluation Phase

The evaluation phase of the nursing process is a planned and systematic comparison of the client or family's health status and the health goals they had hoped to achieve. It is ongoing and deliberative in nature, and its purpose is to evaluate the client or family's progress (Griffith-Kenney, 1986). Using the McGill model of nursing, the nurse and client or family reflect on their working together toward the family's health goals. This final phase of the nursing process is sometimes termed the *discovery phase*, in that the nurse and the family look back over their time together and link actions with consequences, thereby discovering what has been learned in the process (Warner, 1997). If progress is not being made as hoped, the partners discuss whether the goals themselves need to be modified, or if the methods selected to achieve the goals need to be changed (Allen, 1997a). The client or family, together with the nurse, may determine that there are a number of reasons that explain why the health goals are not being achieved. Likewise, there may be many reasons for altering the original plan: (a) a change may have occurred in the client or family situation, (b) plans may have been unrealistic for the time and resources available, (c) the client or family may not have had the ability to carry out agreed-to tasks, (d) the health issue itself may have changed, or (e) new resources may have become available.

It is in this phase of the nursing process that the *outcomes and responses* category of the health work plan, described in an earlier chapter, is completed. This is a reflective step, designed so that ongoing learning can occur as the client or family moves toward higher levels of health. It is the family that indicates when it is time to move to the final phase of the nursing process; they will either indicate that their health goals have been reached, or that they are satisfied for now with the existing situation (Warner, 1997). Since the whole nurse-family relationship has focused on a learning process, rather than on searching for solutions to specific problems, the outcomes of the nurse-family interaction will be process-type indicators. Included will be such indicators as the family's ability to develop new insights, find new approaches to gathering information, discover untapped personal or family strengths and resources, and improve on analytical skills (Gottlieb, 1997).

The main roles of the nurse in the evaluation phase of the nursing process are those of *reinforcer* and *pacer*. As a *reinforcer*, the nurse evaluates the effect of her or his presence on the family, and on their responses to the health issues. When the nurse notices changes in the family, she or he reinforces these by pointing them out to the family. This reinforcement supports the family's ongoing learning efforts. As a *pacer*, the nurse is sensitive to cues from the family that they are in need of a different learning approach. The nurse may sense boredom, frustration, or exhaustion, which are cues to the nurse that new experiences are needed to promote continued learning (Gottlieb, 1997).

✍ The Brown Family Reflects

As the Brown family continued to implement the plan they had developed for themselves, the faith community nurse visited the family every two weeks. One day, about two months after Susan's initial visit to the family, they indicated some changes in their home situation that signaled to the nurse that it was time to begin the evaluation phase, and to move toward termination. It was on a day in late March that Sheila said to the nurse, "I don't know if it is the longer days or the warmer temperatures, but I feel things have changed for us. Gladys's condition is much the same as it was, and we aren't much closer to placement, but somehow I don't let the situation get me down as much as it did before." The nurse then asked Bob how he felt, and he replied, "Yes, it seems we've made some changes or just gotten used to having mother here. Somehow it's not so bad." Comments such as these often tell the nurse that the family is ready for a different type of relationship, and that it is time to stop and reflect on what has been learned with the goal of terminating with the family in the very near future. It is reassuring for both the nurse and the family to know that termination, in the faith community setting, is not as final as it sometimes is in other healthcare situations. The nurse will continue to be available, and she and the family will see each other on occasion within the faith community context. The nature of the relationship, however, will not be as structured as it has been for the time that they were working together on specific health issues.

At this point, it is helpful for the nurse and family to return to the family health work plan to discuss the outcomes and responses that have already been noted regarding each of the family health goals (see Figure 19.1). The nurse encourages the family to focus on the process-type indicators, again by using a mode of inquiry and asking such questions as, What new insights have been developed? What have you learned about yourself or your family? What have you learned about finding information and resources that you needed?

Events in Process	Goals	Tasks/Activities	Outcomes/Responses
Learning to live with a dependent senior family member	Placement of G. Brown in an institution that meets her needs and those of the family.	See Figure 17.3	(1) Bob and Sheila developed criteria, based on what they thought was important, to use in assessing the suitability of placement sites. (2) Bob and Sheila learned much about what they want in a placement site. (3) Gladys Brown was not yet placed, but the family was less stressed. (4) Bob offered to be a resource to others in the congregation.

Receiving periodic relief from ongoing caregiving responsibilities and support from others as needed.

(1) Couple time worked well. Bob and Sheila were proud of ways they devised for being together.

(2) A woman from church to care for Gladys. It worked best for Janet to come to the family.

(3) Bob discovered an Internet support group.

Being patient while waiting for placement, and find some positive aspects to having Mrs. Brown in the family home temporarily.

(1) Sheila became close to her mother-in-law.

(2) Bob was satisfied with his mother's time with her new grandson.

(Continued)

Figure 19.1. Outcomes/Responses of the Brown Family Health Work Plan

Figure 19.1 *continued*

Events in Process	Goals	Tasks/ Activities	Outcomes/ Responses
			(3) Sheila learned to ask for help.
			(4) Bob and Sheila met new people in church.
			(5) They found the quilting group too difficult.
			(6) They discovered an opportunity to record family history.
	Learning more about how to care for a person living with a cognitive impairment.		(1) They learned how to communicate with Gladys.
			(2) They learned how to create a soothing environment

Let us now revisit each of the family goals, and listen to some of the conversation that took place as Bob, Sheila, and the nurse evaluated the nurse-family interactions over the past two months.

Placement of Gladys Brown

Although this health issue seemed to be the highest priority two months ago, it is not the main focus of the family now. Sheila summed this up by saying, "When Gladys first came to live with us, I was very anxious to have her placed. All I could see was how much her presence was changing our lives. I actually think I was afraid of caring for her. I didn't think that I would be able to take good care of someone who had Alzheimer's disease. I mean, she wasn't just my mother-in-law anymore. Now she had some kind of a condition that I thought I couldn't manage, because I didn't really understand what it was or how people acted. I was afraid of it."

Nurse: How do you feel about her placement now?

Sheila: Oh, I still want placement to occur, but I've learned that it isn't the most important thing.

Nurse: What is the most important thing now?

Sheila: I think it is more important that I get over feeling so incapable of dealing with this temporary situation. I'm working on that. [Pause.] I even think that Gladys's behavior has changed a lot since she first arrived here. At first, she was very confused. I suppose a move would do that to someone in her condition. Now, she seems more adjusted to our home and our routine, and not so confused. [Pause.] I wonder, too, if maybe my feeling more capable and relaxed has contributed to Gladys's settling down more.

Nurse: Bob, what do you see as you look at some of the changes that have occurred?

Bob: I think Sheila is much more calm and not so desperate as she was two months ago.

Nurse: What do you think has contributed to that?

Bob: I think we've made a real attempt to keep talking on a regular basis. When we are alone, I allow or even encourage Sheila to tell me exactly how she is feeling, even if I sometimes wished I didn't have to hear about it. I learned that I don't always have to *do* something to change her feelings. I tried to just listen and be there for her. I wasn't always the perfect husband, but I tried.

Nurse: How did you learn about the importance of being a good lis-
          tener?

Bob: Oh, I think I've always known that listening, rather than only
          doing, was important. Maybe your presence helped me feel
          the benefit of that personally. I came to value your visits not
          so much because you changed things for us, but because you
          listened carefully to what we were experiencing, and didn't
          try to fix what only we could fix.

Nurse: I believe in you and Sheila. I knew that you had what it takes
          to get through this time. [Pause.] Getting back to the place-
          ment issue, what did you learn about searching for place-
          ment sites for your mother?

Bob: Well, initially we would drop everything, and run out to see
          the next place that phoned to say mother's name was close to
          the top of the list. Taking some time to look at what we
          wanted in terms of distance, cost, and so forth, saved us from
          even having to visit some facilities. We could almost elimi-
          nate them from our list without a visit, based on distance or
          cost factors. It was interesting to think about what we
          wanted in a placement facility. Our family had never really
          talked about that before. Often, we would joke, saying,
          "Don't ever put me in a nursing home," or "When we're both
          in the 'old folks home' . . ." Now, we were really faced with
          some decisions around what is available and what we want
          for mother, and even for ourselves. It was a whole new world
          for us. I think we've learned a lot, and if ever you come
          across any other couples who are dealing with this issue, I'd
          be happy to tell them what we have learned.

Nurse: Sounds like you learned a lot about yourselves and about the
          process of placing a family member in a long-term care insti-
          tution. I remember the day when I sensed that you were both
          getting tired of running off to every possible facility. I'm glad
          that it helped to have you become more specific and focused
          in your search. And, actually, I had been considering some
          group sessions at the church that might focus on senior
          caregiving or placement issues. I'll keep your offer in mind,
          Bob. [Pause.] Sheila, would you like to add anything about
          what you've learned about placement?

Sheila: I think I shared with you my talk with the minister on the
          phone one day. I think that this whole placement issue has
          caused me to dig deeper, and try to think about why this was
          all happening to me. I believe everything happens for a rea-
          son. For some reason, Gladys wasn't supposed to be placed

immediately. God must have intended me to learn something from all of this waiting. So, in answer to your question, I haven't learned as much about placement as I have about myself. I think God was trying to strengthen me, make me work at something that initially I didn't think I could do. That made me find something in me that I didn't even know was there.

Finding Positive Aspects in the Temporary Situation

Nurse: You seem to be referring to the idea of working on finding positive aspects in this temporary situation, which was one of the goals that you set up for yourselves when we drew up this work plan. Maybe it's a good time to move down to that goal to see how you've progressed. In addition to some deep thinking about the "Why" questions, what other positive aspects of this waiting time have emerged?

Sheila: I think I've become closer to my mother-in-law. Or maybe we just have a better understanding of each other. Not that we haven't had our difficult times. I still find conflict occurring at times between me and my mother-in-law. Some of that, you know, goes way back to when Bob left the Catholic faith to marry me. I loved him very much, but couldn't see having our children raised Catholic, so I felt we could only get married if he would become Lutheran. She's always disliked that I encouraged him to make that change. He's been quite satisfied, but she's never forgotten that.

Nurse: In what way have these last weeks helped to bring the two of you closer?

Sheila: I think we've become closer because I took the opportunity of her living here to ask for her forgiveness for having hurt her all those years ago. It was a hard thing to do, but talking to you about how I might do that helped. I remember you suggesting that we all have the spiritual need to forgive and be forgiven. You talked about this need being almost as basic as air, water, and food. I hadn't thought about that before. I'm not sure that Gladys understood what I was trying to say, but I felt better after I told her what I felt I needed to say. I've always felt some guilt over the whole matter, and now I feel relieved.

Nurse: What about this living situation helped you initiate a discussion now?

Sheila: Oh, I guess we've never had so much time alone together before. I decided that if we couldn't be totally open and honest with each other, it would be quite a long and difficult time together. Also, I think I realized that she's getting older and more confused, and that maybe someday soon it would be too late to talk. I'd always regret that.

Bob: One of the unexpected benefits of having mother here, for me, was watching the bond that developed between my mother and my only grandson. It was an experience that moved me at a level deeper than I had expected.

Nurse: Can you tell me more about that?

Bob: Well, it was like my past and my present and my future all came together at once. That perhaps sounds strange.

Nurse: No, it doesn't sound strange. We all have another important spiritual need: the need to feel connected, especially with our past. You've expressed it beautifully.

Sheila: Another thing that I learned was how to ask for help. I had always thought I should do this kind of thing all on my own. I actually asked my son in Calgary if he could help out, and surprisingly he was willing. I also met several new people in our church that I had only known enough to greet before. For example, the woman who runs the quilting group is very nice. The quilting project was a bit too complex for Gladys's limited attention span, so it didn't really work out. She also didn't like being at the church without me, and would try to leave, so that became too difficult for the other women. But, I met some nice women there, and may actually take up some quilting with them once everything settles down.

Relief From Caregiving and Support From Others

Nurse: Another goal that you wanted to work on was that of getting some relief from caregiving, and finding some support from other people in a similar situation. What did you learn along the way as you worked on this health goal?

Bob: I found a support group on the Internet!

Nurse: I know, you mentioned that to me one evening when I was visiting. Tell me more about that.

Bob: Well, a nurse in Pennsylvania has a big research grant to place computers in the homes of people caring for family members with Alzheimer's disease. Her goal was to demonstrate that a virtual support group could be just as effective as a face-to-face support group. I decided to join the study. It was great! We would get online to chat about all kinds of things, like our frustrations, suggestions for dealing with the situation, and even addresses of agencies and associations that might be helpful.

Sheila: What I really liked about it was that you could chat with people at any time of the day or night, because you weren't ringing them up on the phone and waking them. I remember one night, I got up because I heard Gladys wandering. I got her settled, and then I couldn't get back to sleep. So, just to be funny (heaven knows you need a sense of humor about all of this sometimes), I got on the computer and typed in "HELP!—Is anyone else out there awake?" To my surprise, I got several replies in the middle of the night. I didn't feel so all alone.

Nurse: So you found that this type of electronic support was actually more useful to you than attending a local support group?

Bob: Well, we didn't even try a local support group, because I am out of town so much, and it isn't something that Sheila wants to go to alone. Nor is she able to get away on the evenings when it is held.

Nurse: Your "couple time" has worked as you wanted it to?

Sheila: Oh, pretty well. I found, as time went on, that we didn't need to connect every day in that way. We were a bit unrealistic in trying to set aside time for just the two of us every day. We are able to spend some quiet time together about three times a week. The best surprise was the catered Valentine's Day dinner that Bob arranged for us.

Nurse: That was quite creative, Bob. You should put that suggestion on the Internet chat box!
[Laughter.]

Nurse: How has the arrangement with Janet worked out?

Bob: Oh, she's a lovely person, and I'm glad that we can help her out with some income at the same time that she can help us out. We tried having mother go to Janet's apartment, and that just didn't work. Mother tried to leave. I guess the change in environment was too much for her. But, on several occasions, we've had Janet come here. That works much better. We'll probably continue to use her services as long as mother is with us. Somehow, I don't feel bad having Janet here, because there is mutual benefit.

Nurse: I can understand how you want to be benefiting someone else at the same time you are receiving a benefit.

Learning How to Care for a Person With a Cognitive Impairment

Nurse: The last item on the original list of goals you were going to
            work on, included learning how to care for a person with a
            cognitive impairment. How is that going?

Bob: Oh, we've learned a lot. I never realized how important fa-
            miliar surroundings were to a person in this condition. Once
            mother got used to our home, she seemed to settle down,
            and now our challenge is trying to take her places where she
            isn't familiar. Going to places like the grocery store is almost
            too much for her and us.

Nurse: What have you learned, Sheila?

Sheila: I discovered that there is a wealth of information out there, if
            you want to go looking for it. I almost found myself getting
            overwhelmed with it. I found it better for me to only learn
            what I needed to know for a particular day. I liked the work-
            shop that was conducted at the neighboring church. The
            woman who had written a book about the spirituality of peo-
            ple with Alzheimer's disease was most interesting. I also en-
            joyed hearing from the woman who shared various commu-
            nity resources and how to access them. We know now that
            we have a lot of control over how agitated and confused
            Gladys gets. We have learned how to communicate with her,
            as well as how to make our home a quiet, relaxing place by
            using soft music and pleasant fragrances. Each night, when I
            put her to bed, I play a tape of very relaxing classical music
            until she falls asleep. Then, I later use the same method to
            settle myself down enough to fall asleep. The tape automati-
            cally turns off! It's been quite a learning experience.

✍ Terminating the Nurse-Family Relationship

Nurse: It seems time that our relationship change. You've made a
            great deal of progress in terms of working on the health goals
            that you set for yourselves. You are always welcome to con-
            tact me again at the church office should your family situa-
            tion change. If it's OK with you, I will now meet with Rev.
            Jones, who initially put me in touch with you. I would
            like to generally update him regarding the situation, and let
            him know that, for now, we won't be meeting on a regular
            basis.

Bob: Sure, we don't mind you talking with the minister. He actu-
            ally has been in touch with us several times by phone, so he
            is probably up-to-date with what is going on here.

Nurse: Before I leave, I just want to take this opportunity to thank both of you for teaching me so much about how families work together to get through difficult times. It has been a pleasure coming to your home. Also, before I leave, I would like an opportunity to spend some time with Gladys. I brought the tape-recorded Mass from the neighborhood Catholic church, as I had promised. I would like to leave that with her. She can use my tape recorder for a while and can listen to the Mass whenever she wants.

Sheila: I'm sure she'd love to see you too. She has learned your name, and has become quite fond of you.

✑ Summary

For now, the relationship between the faith community nurse and the Brown family has ended. Perhaps the most important observation on the final visit came from the rich dialogue offered by Bob and Sheila. Their descriptions of outcomes and responses showed that the nurse's interventions were important to the family. This was not because Susan solved problems or presented answers to their questions, but because she guided their learning regarding how to live with a health issue affecting their family life. The *relationship* was health promoting in and of itself; within that relationship, the faith community nurse sometimes supplied information and promoted problem solving, but she did so in ways that fit uniquely with this family's needs, learning styles, and health issues (Ezer, Bray, & Gros, 1997). This approach served to strengthen the family by allowing them to find their own ways of dealing with situations. Some approaches they drew from their past experiences (e.g., the "couple time" idea), whereas others were recent discoveries (e.g., the Internet support group).

Throughout the evaluation phase, the nurse directed the evaluation to focus on a health and learning perspective, rather than allowing it to focus on illness. Furthermore, she continually highlighted learning rather than solutions. The nurse created a situation where the family has become self-reliant such that the termination phase was not difficult to implement. Bob, Sheila, and the faith community nurse have all learned and gained something valuable from this two-month relationship. The couple felt cared for by their church, and the church demonstrated, in a concrete way, that a faith community can be a health-promoting institution.

PART VI

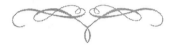

FAITH COMMUNITIES PROMOTING IMAGES OF HEALTH

20 ∽

Nurses and Faith Community Leaders Growing in Partnership

Margaret B. Clark

Throughout the various chapters of this book, we have made a number of references to the *relationship* that exists between faith community nurses and faith group leaders. In our current chapter, we reflect on the concept of *ministry partnerships*. We believe that ministry partnerships need to be both inwardly developed and outwardly expressed. That is, the inward-looking elements of a ministry partnership constitute its depth of *colleagueship*. These inward elements include a growing understanding of ministry as both a profession and vocation, of power as both caring and forceful, and of power differences as factors that invite ever deepening levels of communication. Outward aspects of a ministry partnership constitute its breadth of *collaboration*. These outward aspects include learning as a creative interchange between ministry professionals and those who are the focus of their ministry, establishing boundaries as places where care and influence encounter respect and limitations, and engaging in dialogue as a nuanced and creative integration of insights, words, and ministry actions. Various sections of this chapter address each of these approaches to ministry partnerships. Underpinning the ways we speak about their growth in partnership is our belief that faith community nurses and faith group leaders are companion pilgrims on a path of inquiry that seeks to foster health as integral to faith, and faith as integral to health.

There is a long history of relationship between faith communities and role-related healing activities. One author speaks of the *shaman* as the "world's oldest professional, and the personage from whom both the modern doctor and priest descend" (Achterberg, 1985, p. 12). In ancient China, there is the story of Miao, who disguised herself as a priest in order to administer healing wisdom to the king, who was also her father (see Eliot, 1976, pp. 193-197). The god Apollo, the myth of Asclepius, and the description of Hippocrates as "father of medicine" speak to shifts within Greek culture, which first saw healing as a divine activity, and only gradually included it as a mortal ability (Gordon, 1993, p. 311). In another vein, the role of women as healers has been studied more recently in order to recover ancient healing wisdom lost through an emphasis on the male-centered, Greek-instituted medical model (Achterberg, 1990; Sjöö & Mor, 1991). Indeed, countless men and women across various cultures and faith groups have borne witness for centuries to a mixture of tension and mystery in the linkages between faith and health (Achterberg, 1985; Bowker, 1997; Sanford, 1977).

Although the previous references serve merely as an introduction, they point to a field of inquiry where much has been written and a great depth of knowledge is available. With the recognition by faith community leaders that registered nurse professionals are *partners* in furthering the spiritual and religious purposes of their faith groups, deeper levels of colleagueship and collaboration in ministry can occur. This, in turn, will lead to an enriched and more effective dialogue on matters of faith and health.

✑ Ministry Partnerships

As we prepare to develop the concept of ministry partnerships, we believe it is important to ask a preliminary question: What have we said thus far on this topic? We believe that ministry partnerships are a particular type of relationship. Throughout this text we have spoken about relationships as outgrowths of an association, involvement, or connection that we become aware of, experience, reflect on, and celebrate. It is important, therefore, to inquire about ministry partnerships along similar lines. What kind of relationship is it? When and how is the relationship experienced? When and how is the experience of relationship reflected on? And, finally, how, where, and when are these relationships celebrated?

We propose that ministry partnerships between nurses and faith community leaders are a type of relationship that is both collegial and collaborative. That is, the faith group leader and faith community nurse partnership is composed of both (a) respect for and a willingness to learn across vocational and professional differences in background and language, and (b) the carrying forward of a shared ministry to others through holistic planning and practices that foster dialogue on matters of faith and health. Future sections of this chapter will address the topics of colleagueship and collaboration, but we turn now to the concept of *partnership*.

Discussions on partnership have surfaced in literature from the fields of history (Eisler, 1987; Eisler & Loye, 1990), sociology (Edelman & Crain, 1993; Montuori & Conti, 1993), theology (Ferder & Heagle, 1989; Russell, 1981; Whitehead & Whitehead, 1991), and psychology (Sanford, 1980). Eisler (1987) introduces a broad-based approach to partnership when she suggests that "underlying the great surface diversity of human culture are two basic models of society" (p. xvii). She goes on to describe a *dominator model* and a *partnership model.* The dominator model uses rank as the basis for distinction and differentiation. By contrast, the partnership model uses a principle of linkage to address differences. In partnership, diversity is not equated with superiority or inferiority; rather, diversity is valued as a cocreative and mutually empowering dynamic. Indeed, according to Eisler and Loye (1990), all interactions have the possibility of partnership, because interactions based on the mutual respect and empowerment essential for partnership can happen "with all kinds of people, in all kinds of different settings" (p. 10). We suggest that included among these kinds of people are faith community nurses and faith group leaders, and that the different settings include a multitude of faith community contexts. As the concept of partnership is better understood in professional ministry relationships, we believe a partnership model of relating can then extend from the ministry partners to congregational members, families, and groups.

Since partnership is a process rather than an outcome, it will continue to evolve as long as participants are committed to the work of constructing relationships in a partnership way (Eisler & Loye, 1990). This means that people learn how to do the following: (a) become *aware* of alternatives to dominance and subordination, (b) believe in the *value* of these alternatives, and (c) work within *concrete settings* to achieve greater mutuality and cocreativity. In this regard, ministry partnerships will be forged as nurses and faith group leaders stay in relationship with one another, even at times of conflict, confusion, and distress. In fact, it is to be expected that conflict and confusion will arise in these relationships, inasmuch as awareness, valuation, and practical achievements tend to occur when there is a healthy balance of both creative tension and comfortable respect.

In appreciating the notion of a healthy balance between what we call creative tension and comfortable respect, the following tool may be helpful. It was developed by Carol Pierce, Bill Page, and David Wagner (Pierce & Page, 1986; Pierce, Page, & Wagner, 1998) as a product of their many years of consultative work on valuing diversity and understanding power equity. These authors observed that in situations of value diversity, it was quite common for differently valued persons to be organized in relationships of *dominance* and *subordinance*. We see examples of this type of relating in such areas as role, race, gender, age, sexual orientation, ethnicity, religion, and life circumstances. Thus, depending on the social or cultural context, relationships of dominance and subordinance develop between young and old, men and women, in-groups and out-groups, and so forth. The question arises, however: What needs to be done in order to move beyond dominant/subordinate ways of relating, toward relationships characterized by an equal valuing of differences?

In this regard, Pierce, Page, and Wagner suggest (Pierce & Page, 1986; Pierce et al., 1998) that a *decision to learn* needs to be made. Both the identified *dominant* person or group and the identified *subordinate* person or group need to enter a transition of consciousness, which opens them to the possibility of valuing the self and the other *equally* across their existing differences. Thus, in the examples referred to earlier, both young and old need to be willing to learn from one another across their age differences, and men and women need to be willing to learn from one another across their gender differences. This transitional work can lead to experiences of what Pierce, Page, and Wagner (Pierce & Page, 1986; Pierce et al., 1998) call *equity*, which is a new type of relationship in which shared learning grows into colleagueship and collaboration, bearing fruits that are mutually empowering and supportive.

The tool Pierce et al. (1998) offer is a continuum of change that occurs in three phases. First, there is a phase of *role stereotyping*, then a period of *transition*, and finally the development of *power equity*. In role stereotyping, a great deal of unproductive conflict emanates from a need to control. Discordance and impasse are seen as a collusion of dominant/subordinate ways of relating. Pierce, et al. (1998) suggest that people in differing paradigms or in power-imbalanced relationships can move away from unproductive conflict by deciding to learn from one another across their differences. Communication at this level may be confusing, but it is far less conflicted than in situations of dominance/subordinance. In time, with continued commitment to processes of dialogue across various differences, there can be additional movement toward the quality of relationship that Pierce et al. (1998) identify as *colleagueship.*

Thus far, three applications of the continuum tool have been developed. These are the male/female continuum (Pierce et al., 1998), a sexual orientation and identity continuum (Wishik & Pierce, 1994), and a racial/cultural difference continuum (Thomas & Pierce, 1999). Additional applications are encouraged by Carol Pierce, who urges readers to add their own "perceptions and insights for other combinations" (Pierce & Page, 1986, p. 10). We believe one such combination could be that of faith group leaders and faith community nurses. We envision theirs to be a *ministry partnership continuum.* Although this continuum will need to be developed further over time and with the input of others in order to parallel the kind of detail provided in the three earlier applications, we suggest using the following diagram (Figure 20.1), which includes a depiction of relational elements within the McGill nursing model (Gottlieb & Ezer, 1997), insofar as these might serve to aid collaborative reflection.

Although we are tempted to avoid identifying categories of dominance and subordinance between nurses and religious leaders in the use of our ministry partnership continuum, we are aware that such an identification is needed for the continuum to achieve shared learning

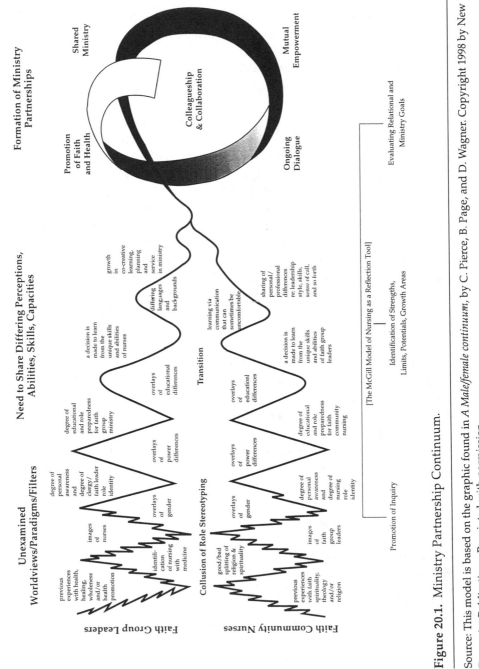

Figure 20.1. Ministry Partnership Continuum.

Source: This model is based on the graphic found in *A Male/female continuum*, by C. Pierce, B. Page, and D. Wagner. Copyright 1998 by New Dynamics Publications. Reprinted with permission.

and growth in power equity. That is, if we do not identify the areas of creative tension existing between nurses and religious leaders, we run the risk of not recognizing what needs to be learned by each profession in order for their differences to be seen as complementary in the service of others. Likewise, if this learning does not occur, there is risk of never arriving at experiences of comfortable respect and mutual empowerment in ministry provision. With this being said, therefore, we choose to identify faith group leaders in the dominant category and faith community nurses in the subordinate category. We make this choice based on the fact that, when carrying forward an intentional health-promoting ministry within faith community contexts, nurses are usually identified as "employees" or "staff members" in their role relationships with religious leaders or faith communities. Faith group leaders, on the other hand, are often identified as having the power to hire, fire, evaluate, promote, and so forth. Furthermore, nurses enter faith communities as newcomers to a setting where the main focus is faith renewal, rather than health promotion.

Looking at our continuum, then, we envision the *role stereotyping* phase, where conflicts are most likely to exist, as a place for the promotion of inquiry across differences in vocation, profession, background, and language. Here, it is important for faith group leaders and faith community nurses to examine their worldviews, paradigms, and filters. With movement toward the phase of *transition*, where a decision has been made to learn across differences even though a degree of conflict and confusion may still exist, there is a need for the identification of strengths, limits, potentials, and areas of growth. Here, it is important for faith community nurses and faith group leaders to articulate and reflect on their differing perceptions, abilities, skills, and capacities for working together in the making of choices relevant to a health-promoting and faith-renewing shared ministry. Finally, in the *power equity* phase, mutual empowerment and cocreativity begin to replace conflict and confusion. This is a place where nurses and faith community leaders can evaluate how well colleagueship and collaboration are working for them as they continue to develop their ministry partnership.

If this diagram is used by faith community leaders and nurses as a reflection tool, we believe it will support efforts being made to respect and learn from one another across vocational and professional differences in background and language. In particular, the continuum tool can help nurses and ministry leaders to (a) gain *awareness* of alternatives to dominance and subordinance, (b) explore how these alternatives are believed in and *valued*, and (c) develop *concrete actions* through which to ensure that their work together remains oriented toward mutuality and cocreativity. In another vein, use of this tool can provide a frame of reference for responding to the four questions raised at the beginning of this section on ministry partnerships. That is, faith group leaders and faith community nurses who spend time alone and together with this tool will be able to describe the kind of relationship they are in. They will also be able to speak about the ways in which they experience their relationship. Furthermore, use of the tool as a means of reflection on the relationship may prove especially helpful when conflicts or confusions arise. Is there a collusion of dominance and subordinance? Does a decision to learn need to be made? As various forms of impasse are worked through, it will be natural to celebrate growth in colleagueship through rituals and feasts. In these ways, professional ministry partnerships between nurses and faith group leaders will model the mutual respect, support, and empowerment of a partnership way of relating that can extend in widening circles of inclusiveness to faith community members, families, and groups.

ᴕ Elements of Colleagueship in Ministry Partnerships

In order for ministry partnerships to evolve, they need to be both inwardly developed and outwardly expressed. The inward-looking elements of a ministry partnership constitute its depth of *colleagueship*. We consider the following three elements to be directly related with the notion of colleagueship. First, there is *ministry*, as both a profession and vocation. Second, there is *power*, as both caring and forceful. Finally, there is the factor of *power difference*, which needs to be considered in order to deepen communication and explore mutuality.

Ministry
In our book, we define *ministry* as an orientation to serve others that is both representative of and carried out in relationship with a faith community's reason for being. It is endowed with and accountable to a public trust. In Chapter 1, we highlighted the professional nature of ministry relationships. As a profession, ministry is both

informed by a unique body of knowledge and governed by self-regulating norms. Thus, both theological and nursing knowledge are needed to inform a faith community nurse ministry. Likewise, standards of practice and codes of professional conduct drawn from both nursing and faith group sources are needed to support appropriate and beneficial faith community nursing interventions.

In another vein, Chapter 9 introduced the notion of ministry as a vocation. In addition to being duty bound and work related, ministry is also a gift; that is, it includes a dimension of spiritual or heartfelt inspiration. How many times have we heard about a person's restlessness and longing as they were being impelled by a sense of summons to serve others? We believe it is significant that both nursing and religious ministries are frequently spoken about in terms of response to a "call" (Fowler, 1991; Hall, 1991; Lane, 1987; Striepe et al., 1993; Whitehead & Whitehead, 1979/1982). Hall (1991) identifies "service/vocation" as a goal value. In other words, it emerges and thrives in those phases of personal or organizational development where the use of authority fosters both choice and union. According to Hall (1991), to operate out of the value of service/vocation means that one is motivated to use one's unique gifts and skills "to contribute to society through one's occupation, business, profession or calling" (p. 165). For faith community nurses and religious leaders, a vocation to ministry includes not only knowledge and skill, but also gift and grace. In this context, grace acknowledges the existence of a divine other who freely endows a person with abilities or gifts through which to perceive and foster unity and wholeness (Bowker, 1997). Grace given to nurses will advance their whole-person, health-promoting gifts. Grace given to religious leaders will support their whole-person, faith-renewing gifts. Grace given to ministry partnerships between faith community nurses and faith group leaders will empower them in their collegial and collaborative efforts to further an integration of faith and health in the lives of individuals, families, groups, and social structures. An ongoing exploration of how ministry is understood, in both its professional and vocational dimensions, will foster growth in ministry partnerships.

Power

The way power is used in the face of differences or diversity will affect whether or not equity and colleagueship can be achieved.

Although power has been the focus of massive investigation, as well as significant insight (Toffler, 1990; Whitehead & Whitehead, 1986; Wink, 1984), we use the term *power* here to mean that one has as an ability to influence others. In this regard, power occurs in relationships. Each difference observed in a relationship can provide a point of reference for measuring both power and vulnerability. In her workshop manual on ethical conduct in ministerial relationships, Marie Fortune (1992) supplies an excellent list of *sources of power* and *sources of vulnerability* based on the categories of role, age, gender, sexual orientation, race, ethnicity, life circumstances, and the like. Each category describes a difference that is also a resource through which to relate with others. Faith community nurses and faith group leaders, for example, provide ministry interventions out of differing abilities; thus, each type of ministry has unique resources related to its role, through which it exerts influence or power.

Fortune (1992) also says that power and vulnerability are relative and contextual; that is, "to speak of a person 'having power' or 'being vulnerable' is a misconception; a person has power in relation to another person in a given context, and is vulnerable in relation to another person in a given context" (p. 38). It is the affinity between resources and power that is crucial here: "Those who command greater resources than others have power relative to them; those who command fewer resources are vulnerable relative to them" (Fortune, 1992, p. 38). The resources nurses have available to them with regard to whole-person, social, and community assessment skills, for example, give them a certain type of "skills power" in relation to faith group leaders and faith community members. At the same time, a spiritual leader's ability to draw on resources within his or her faith tradition to encourage reflection and celebration around experiences of relationship with the divine, self, and others gives that leader "religious power" in relation to the faith community nurse and faith community members. There are also vulnerabilities in power that can parallel these strengths. For example, since clergy are often male and nurses are often female, there can be a power imbalance between them in relation to gender. On the other hand, if a rabbi, imam, priest, or minister working in North America has come here from another country or culture, this religious leader may be at a power disadvantage in relationship to the nurse who is familiar with the language, customs, and culture of the local faith community. Many variables need to be taken into consideration when assessing sources of power and vulnerability.

A final point we would like to make in this section is that power resources can be influential in ways that are both caring and coercive. In the language of Mayeroff (1971), caring is intended to be a *selfless* kind of influence. Furthermore, Hall (1991) writes about care as a type of physical and emotional support that is both given and received. In another vein, however, the Christian scriptures draw attention to a close affinity between care and anxiety. As it says in 1 Peter, "Cast all your anxiety on him, because he cares for you" (1 Pet. 5:7 NRSV). This is born out by formal definitions, which indicate that care can mean a "troubled or burdened state of mind" (*Webster's*, 1989; see also Vine, 1966). Anxiety has a way of introducing controlling or coercive dynamics into relationships. Thus, other authors suggest caution in the use of one's power resources. For example, Pierce and Page (1986) caution about the risk of dominance and subordination. For Fortune (1989, 1992) and Poling (1991), the ultimate risk is an abuse of power in which others are harmed instead of helped. When it comes to the use of power in ministry partnerships between faith community nurses and faith group leaders, we believe the McGill model of nursing can serve as a framework for interdisciplinary learning and discovery. With its emphasis on assessing strengths and potentials, the McGill model can teach both faith community nurses and faith group leaders how to approach the influence of others in ways that are both empowering and liberating.

Power Differences

Over the past decade, there has been increased public scrutiny given to *power differences* in all forms of personal and professional relationships. Wherever there are power differences, it is possible to identify both persons or groups who have a *power advantage* and those who are in positions of *power disadvantage*. Sources of power imbalance may stem from differences in age, gender, sexual orientation, race, cultural background, office or role, access to information, or life circumstances. Power imbalance, however, does not equate with *power abuse*. One needs to wonder, therefore, why some situations of power imbalance result in exploitation or abuse, even as so many others result in caring and heroic actions, such as advocacy, mentoring, educating, parenting, and healing.

Again, we return to our emphasis on relationship, and our understanding of relationships as outgrowths of association, involvement, or connection. Literature on the topics of caring (Gilligan, 1982; Gilligan, Ward, & Taylor, 1988; Kelsey, 1981; Mayeroff, 1971), responsibility (Mount, 1990; Stiver, 1991), power (Miller, 1991; Poling, 1991, Toffler, 1990), abuse (Fortune, 1989, 1992; Herman, 1992; Hopkins and Laaser, 1995; Rutter, 1989, 1999), and social justice (Meeker-Lowry, 1995; Puleo, 1994) can contribute to one's knowledge base with regard to relationships. From what we have learned over the years, the following reflections may be of assistance to nurses and faith community leaders as they seek colleagueship, while also working with the power differences in their relationships. These ideas need interdisciplinary reflection, feedback, and grounded research (Clark, 1998). At the same time, they are relevant to both the inward-looking and outward-oriented elements of ministry partnership development. These ideas are presented in this section on colleagueship, because a careful assessment of power differences among ministry professionals will support collegial functioning. In addition, this kind of assessment can serve as a foundation on which to build collaborative helping relationships with those who are the focus of one's ministry.

To begin with, we all know from experience that various relationships have parameters. Among these are *professional* vis-à-vis *intimate* and *power imbalanced* vis-à-vis *mutual* ways of relating. These differences are developed in the writings of Fortune (1983, 1989, 1992). Building on her work, Figure 20.2 illustrates four types of power relationships combined in quadrants, and gives examples of each type of resulting relationship.

In this figure, imbalanced power relationships can be studied within both professional and intimate settings. Thus, *relational context* becomes an important factor in looking at power relationships; a person has power advantage or power disadvantage in relationship with another person depending on the context (Fortune, 1992). Thus, parents have a *role power advantage* in relationship with their children, as do teachers with students. Likewise, nurses have a role power advantage in relationship with clients and families, and faith group leaders in relationship with members of their congregations. In addition, when a nurse is employed by a faith community, the hiring person or body has a role power advantage in relationship with the nurse. If the

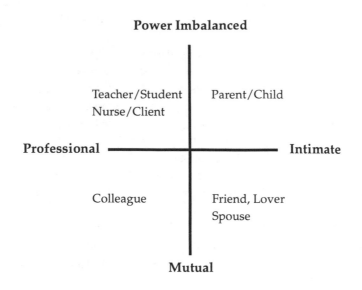

Figure 20.2. Four Types of Power Relationships, With Examples for Each Variance

Source: This figure originally appeared in "Power Imbalance: Evolving Theory in Need of Research," by M. Clark, 1998, *Western Journal of Nursing Research*, 20(5), p. 519.

hiring person is the priest, rabbi, or minister with whom the nurse is seeking to develop a collegial ministry partnership, this element of power imbalance needs to be given explicit consideration. Whatever the circumstance of power imbalance, the established standards for public scrutiny of such relationships include an expectation that the person who is in a position of role power advantage is responsible to ensure that the person with *role power disadvantage* is not at risk of abuse.

In another vein, however, we are all aware of situations where role power disadvantaged persons draw on other power resources to acquire a modicum of power advantage. Thus, a student who is angry with a teacher about an unsatisfactory grade may use power advantages derived from physical force, psychological manipulation, or social and economic pressure to harass the teacher. Indeed, there are distressing examples of teachers being raped or murdered by their students as a result of such power abuse.

What we propose is that each relationship of power imbalance needs to be assessed in two ways. First, reflection is needed in order to discern the presence of various types of power advantage or disadvantage. Some variables worth considering in this regard are age, gender, sexual orientation, race, cultural background, office or role, ordination or professional certification, access to information, and life circumstances. An example of this type of assessment would be to have faith group leaders and faith community nurses sit down together to talk about their relationship in terms of strengths, potentials, limitations, and growth areas. The following process may facilitate their discussion: Begin by writing, at the top of a piece of paper, the three categories of *power advantaged, power disadvantaged,* and *power equal.* Next, along the left side of the page, draw on the suggested variables given earlier and add meaningful new ones to develop a list of power differences that may be operative in the relationship. Once that is done, answer the following question individually: "How do I see myself in our relationship with regard to each of these variables?" Finally, come back together and spend some time discussing how each participant sees the relationship in terms of its power differences. This may lead to further work with the ministry partnership continuum depicted earlier.

The second way to assess each relationship of power imbalance is to weigh the *risk factors* to each member in the relationship with regard to the potential for power abuse. Here, we propose that both role power advantaged and role power disadvantaged persons are capable of a manipulative, oppressive, or predatory use of the power imbalance in a relationship. Furthermore, there may be contextual and relational elements, such as trust, naiveté, preoccupying stress, or lack of experience, that make a person vulnerable to being manipulated, abused, or exploited. Taking stock of one's *power sources* and *vulnerability sources* may enable greater clarity in assessing the true nature of a particular role-defined relationship. This, in turn, can lead to a greater clarification of boundaries in ministry partnerships and relationships.

Figure 20.3 is offered to facilitate the assessment. It depicts the variances of *power advantage* and *power disadvantage* in relationship

Power Advantage

Power advantaged naive or inexperienced person	Power advantaged exploitative or manipulative person

Naive/ 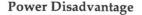 **Exploitation/**
Inexperience   **Manipulation**

Power disadvantaged naive or inexperienced person	Power disadvantaged exploitative or manipulative person

Power Disadvantage

Figure 20.3. Variances of Power Advantage/Disadvantage in Relationship With Power Abuse

Source: This figure originally appeared in "Power Imbalance: Evolving Theory in Need of Research," by M. Clark, 1998, *Western Journal of Nursing Research, 20*(5), p. 520.

with the potential for abuse of power by means of *exploitation and manipulation* or *naiveté and inexperience.* In each quadrant of the diagram, a descriptive phrase summarizes what we suggest are four ways in which the variables can be configured.

As nurses and faith group leaders reflect on this diagram, they will find a number of ways to deepen their communication. For example, a nurse of one faith tradition who ministers in the context of another faith tradition may feel disadvantaged by her or his lack of knowledge about the customs and practices of this faith community. At the same time, however, the nurse is perceived by faith community members to be in a position of role power advantage. What form of support and challenges can be developed collegially by the faith group leader and faith community nurse to deal creatively with this concern? In another vein, the faith community leader may be unaware of the nurse's concerns about professional confidentiality arising when he or she is talking in detailed specifics about the circumstances of a particular congregational member. Furthermore, the faith group leader's directive style of dealing with the congregational member may seem potentially manipulative. How can the nurse and faith group leader work collaboratively, within the power differences of their own relationship, to deal with the issues arising from these perceptions of or differences in leadership style? Once again, in addition to the diagram provided, we recommend the McGill model of nursing as an excellent resource and framework through which to strengthen skills and abilities in promoting inquiry, identifying potentials, and evaluating relational development on the topic of power differences between faith community nurses and faith group leaders.

✍ Elements of Collaboration in Ministry Partnerships

Our discussion of power differences showed some overlap between elements of colleagueship and collaboration in ministry partnership formation. The final section of this chapter focuses attention on *collaboration* as the outward-oriented dimension of ministry partnerships. It includes three elements: *learning*, which we describe as a creative interchange between ministry professionals and those who are the focus of their ministry; *boundaries*, which are places where care and influence encounter both respect and limitations; and *dialogue*, a nuanced and creative integration of insights, words, and ministry actions.

Learning

We believe that collaborative *learning* involves the development of frameworks for shared reflection. In this regard, we have tried to provide a model and a continuum. The McGill model of nursing is a framework that can be used by both nursing prepared and theologically prepared ministers in the fourfold work of promoting inquiry, identifying potentials and strengths, exploring healthy relational development, and evaluating growth areas. Since Moyra Allen (1982a) makes a direct link between learning and collaboration in the nurse-client relationship, we believe a parallel process of learning and collaboration can be manifest in the faith group leader–faith community nurse relationship. Throughout this chapter, we have referred to ways this parallel can be explored. Furthermore, in addition to a model, we have also provided the ministry partnership continuum as a tool that faith group leaders and faith community nurses can use in order to look at issues of learning and power in their relationship.

In another vein, there are a number of resources available on the topic of collaborative ministry that can assist interdisciplinary learning. Sofield and Juliano (1987), for example, share ideas from their experiences in the context of Christian faith communities that we believe have a broader application. They discuss stages in the development of collaborative ministry from a point of no collaboration, along intermediate phases of obsession and ambivalence, to another point of integrated action. These stages are paralleled with varying degrees of motivation. Thus, there are the "we should," "we want to," "we can," and "we will" levels of decision making needed to support the movement from a collusion of dominance and subordinance to a more collaborative sharing of power equity. Faith group leaders and faith community nurses may want to identify their efforts in terms of these stages and degrees of motivation. Additional insights provided by Sofield and Juliano (1987) include learning about beliefs, obstacles, issues of readiness, and kinds of spirituality involved in collaboration. On this latter point of spirituality, they say that "ministry is the embodiment and expression of spirituality" (Sofield & Juliano, 1987, p. 57). They then go on to describe elements needed in a spirituality for it to sustain collaborative ministry. These elements are that a spirituality (a) integrate the whole person, (b) nurture through reflection, (c) include a shared or communal dimension, (d) proceed in balance, and (e) move to compassionate action.

Finally, the book *Models of Collaboration* (Seaburn, Lorenz, Gunn, Gawinski, & Mauksch, 1996), drawing on insights from mental health professionals working with health care practitioners, can give nurses and faith group leaders another type of approach to learning about collaborative work. Here, one finds a discussion of "key ingredients for effective collaboration" and a "spectrum of collaboration" that may prove helpful within a faith community context. The key ingredients outlined in the book are relationship, common purpose, paradigm, communication, location of service, and business arrangement. The spectrum of collaboration includes the approaches of parallel delivery, informal consultation, formal consultation, coprovision of care, and collaborative networking. Although further development of their thoughts is beyond the scope of this chapter, we introduce their ideas to encourage additional exploration and learning through a variety of professional disciplines.

Boundaries

In recent years, a number of books have addressed the topic of *boundaries* from the perspectives of self-care (Katherine, 1991), religious guidance (Cloud & Townsend, 1992), narrative case studies pertinent to pastoral care and counseling (Doehring, 1995), sexual harassment (Rutter, 1997), and in relationship with ministry (Drummond, 1996). Each is helpful, and makes an important contribution. For purposes of this chapter, however, we use Peter Rutter's (1997) definitions. He speaks first of *boundaries in general* as "lines of separation and demarcation" (p. 15). Second, he speaks of *personal boundaries* as "the sometimes-invisible, sometimes-visible lines that separate me from you, what's mine from what's yours, my space from your space" (p. 16). Finally, he suggests that *boundaries* "also have *subtle and complex* [italics added] aspects that can easily lead to misunderstandings because they mark out psychological as well as physical space" (p. 16). It is this comprehensive approach to boundaries that is needed by both nurses and faith community leaders as they pursue collaborative ministry partnerships.

In order to be attentive within any ministry relationship, one must look at not only the temporal and physical dimensions of boundary formation, but also the subtle presence of emotional, sexual, and spiritual boundaries. In these latter realms there is frequently a great deal of ambiguity (Poling, 1991). Although careful consideration of the subtle and complex dimensions of these ambiguities is beyond the scope of this chapter, reference to their existence is important, inasmuch as faith group ministers must be attentive to and respectful of the full scope of boundary manifestation.

According to Peter Rutter (1997), a rich language is beginning to develop around the term *boundary*. He speaks of *boundary events* (p. 35), which can be broken down into the stages of boundary monitoring, boundary testing, and boundary respecting. He also speaks of *boundary crossings* (p. 74), classifying these as minor, major, and egregious. Since the topic of his book is sexual harassment, many of the stories narrated pertain to ways men and women communicate across and between their sexual boundaries. Elements of this communication include giving notice when there is unwelcome boundary crossing, filing formal complaints in the absence of action based on notice, and initiating legal action when this seems warranted.

It is interesting that, early in his book, Rutter (1997) refers to the phenomenon of stereotyping and to the need to move beyond stereotypes. He goes on to list a number of the fixed attitudes and opinions commonly held about cross-gender relationships. Finally, Rutter makes an important assertion when he says, "I believe that we have constructed a world in which all of the [stereotypical] statements are true. I also believe that many of these truths are lamentable—and potentially changeable" (p. 33). With use of the word *lamentable*, Rutter has connected with a powerful concept found in spiritual and religious literature. Theologian Dorothy Soelle (1975), in her reflections on suffering, describes a movement out of helplessness and toward growing personal power that involves public expressions of *lament, complaint,* and *protest* (p. 73). Lament, she says, is the first sound we hear after silence. It is the beginning of having a voice, which, in Rutter (1997), establishes a primary form of boundary notice. Indeed, that which is lamentable about the fixed attitudes and opinions arising within ministry partnerships is potentially changeable when it can be "seen into voice" (Belenky, Clinchy, Goldberger, & Tarule, 1986; Gilligan, 1982); wherever boundaries can be *seen* and given *voice*, there is greater potential for respect and power equity. Needless to say, the positive contributions of Peter Rutter, in giving voice to the significance of boundaries and boundary formation, will need further application within ministry relationships. An important beginning has been made, however, which both nurses and faith community leaders can work with collaboratively as they explore ministry partnerships together.

Dialogue

We have described *dialogue* as a nuanced and creative integration of insights, words, and ministry actions. We believe that every faith community nurse and each faith group leader is the essential "tool" of their ministry practice. In this regard, learning how to speak from the substance of one's being is the foundation on which dialogue can occur. Furthermore, "speaking across" the many differences between self and others is the essential element of dialogue (see *Webster's*, 1989; Vine, 1966).

In a wonderful discussion on the topics of awareness, renewal, and dialogue as pathways for spiritual development, Pope Paul VI (1964) outlines four characteristics of dialogue that are worth sharing here. He says that dialogue is both an attitude and a method. As an attitude, dialogue reveals both rootedness and openness; as a method, it can help individuals and groups to accomplish their sense of purpose or mission. According to Paul VI, the method of dialogue is viewed as a form of spiritual communication that includes the following characteristics. First, dialogue is characterized by clearness. As an outpouring of thought, it is important that each participant in the dialogue review every angle of their language "to guarantee that it be understandable, acceptable, and well-chosen" (Paul VI, 1964, p. 36). Second, dialogue is characterized by meekness. The authority in dialogue, says Paul VI, is intrinsic to the truth it explains, the charity it communicates, and the example it proposes. In this regard, it is not proud, bitter, or offensive; neither does it command or impose. By contrast, in its meekness, dialogue is peaceful, avoids violent methods, is patient, and is generous. Third, dialogue is characterized by trust. Trust promotes confidence and friendship, binds hearts in mutual adherence to the good, and excludes all self-seeking. The fourth and last characteristic of dialogue, according to Paul VI, is its prudence. Prudence esteems the abilities and limitations of one's dialogue partners; thus, it strives to learn about the hearer and to adapt the manner of one's presentation in such a way that it is comprehensible to this hearer.

Although these characteristics of dialogue are demanding, we believe they can foster the qualities of sharing needed for ministry partnerships between faith group leaders and faith community nurses to expand in colleagueship and collaboration. Indeed, Paul VI concludes his comments on the characteristics of dialogue by saying that when dialogue is conducted as spiritual communication, it will achieve a "union of truth and charity, of understanding and love" (p. 36). We believe this union is the heart and soul of ministry partnership.

✧ Summary

The development of collegial and collaborative *ministry partnerships* between nurses and faith community leaders is essential to nursing within faith communities in times of transition. This chapter has looked at ministry partnerships as both inwardly developed and outwardly oriented. It has considered the concepts of *partnership, colleagueship,* and *collaboration* in some depth, in the hope that these considerations will support both faith group leaders and faith community nurses as they sojourn on a path of mutual inquiry that seeks to foster health as integral to faith and faith as integral to health.

21 ✐

Health Promotion and Faith Renewal

*A Ministry Spiral That
Connects and Deepens*

*Margaret B. Clark
Joanne K. Olson*

Our previous chapter emphasized partnership development between faith community nurses and faith group leaders. Our current chapter now looks at the collaborative ministry that grows out of such partnerships. We believe that such a collaborative ministry furthers the integration of faith and health in the lives of individuals, families, groups, and social structures. Think of the richness of serving others through your nursing profession in such a way that you bring a vision of faith to bear on your health-promoting activities! Likewise, imagine being a pastor, rabbi, priest, or imam who serves his or her faith community in such a way that health awareness goes hand in hand with faith awareness! Finally, what about the implications for faith community members, and the broader society surrounding that faith community, when issues of faith and issues of health are considered in relationship to one another? This is the topic we explore in our current chapter.

Just as the colleagueship between nurses and religious leaders relies on a quality of communication that probes professional differences, their collaboration in ministry relies on putting the complementarity of those differences at the service of others. We believe it is service to others, at all stages of health and illness through the life span, that unites both nursing and religious professionals in a shared vision and common purpose. In this chapter, we propose that the shared vision and common purpose are a ministry *spiral*, which professionally connects nurses and faith group leaders while also deepening their health-promoting and faith-renewing service to others.

Previously, we referred to the spiral in describing developmental transitions (Ford, 1988). The spiral, we said, is an ancient symbol (Cirlot, 1962; Walker, 1988), which has received attention in recent decades from scientists, philosophers, nurses, and theologians because it is multidimensional (Laforêt-Fliesser & Ford-Gilboe, 1997; Schillebeeckx, 1984). Philosophical and theological thinkers have developed the "hermeneutic circle" as a paradigm for reflective interpretation, where "the answer is to some extent determined by the question, which is in turn confirmed, extended or corrected by the answer" (Schillebeeckx, 1984, p. 104). Schillebeeckx (1984) points out, however, that this reflective construct has been "given the better title of 'hermeneutic spiral' by the French historian J. Marrou and the American theologian Ray Hart" (p. 109). In this chapter, we look at the hermeneutic spiral as a paradigm that can help faith community nurses and faith group leaders connect their differing knowledge bases, theories, models, skills, and professional tools in a way that deepens their ministry response; that is, their response becomes informed by interdisciplinary resources and enriched with multidimensional points of view. For example, imagine experiencing the loss of a loved one within a faith community: It is often the pastor, priest, or rabbi who is called by the family in order to discuss funeral or burial arrangements. When the compassionate heart of a religious leader enters into relationship with the bereaved family, however, important faith questions, such as "Why me?" and "How can God allow this?" may also be shared. These connections of loss and the questioning of faith can then be responded to by the religious leader through caring support and resources drawn from the religious tradition, such as ritual, sacred texts, and ceremonies. Likewise, the faith community nurse is in a position to be supportive of the bereaved family through her or his whole-person listening skills. In addition to being present at the time of religious ritual, the nurse can also connect the family with resources in both the congregation and broader community, taking into consideration various physical and psychosocial needs linked with their spiritual needs. As a result of this connection and deepening response, those who are the focus of collaborative ministry will be supported and empowered with both health-promoting and faith-renewing benefits.

This chapter develops in two parts. First, we explore the spiral image as a symbol, and develop its potential use as a paradigm for collaborative ministry. Second, we compile a summary table of the resources referred to throughout our book so that it is available to faith community nurses and faith group leaders as they experience shared reflection in ministry collaboration. In our next chapter, we will draw from both the spiral paradigm and summary table of resources in order to apply theory to practice. At that time, we will reflect together on the experiences of interdisciplinary collaboration that have emerged in our health-promoting and faith-renewing ministries.

ـ൸ *The Spiral as Symbol and Paradigm*

Why select a spiral as our paradigm? We live in a world that continually amazes us with the use of lines. Stop for a moment to consider the number of words in popular usage that include linear imagery. There are such terms as *lifeline, family line, flat line, line of scrimmage, battle line,* and *lines of demarcation.* In addition, we use such terms as *lineage* and *linear* in discussing matters of inheritance, measurement, programming, and life span development theory. Linear imagery, represented by these popular words, reflects our various worldviews, paradigms, and filters, which value linear thinking; in this regard, the implications and limits to linear thinking are worth questioning. That is to say, if we think exclusively in linear terms, and restrict our approach to life (including faith- and health-life) through the confines of sequential or chronological perceptions, we miss much of the rich diversity that life, health, and faith have to offer. Think for a moment of the evolution in grief theory over the past 30 years since Kübler-Ross's (1969) book on death and dying was published. An initial response to the stages developed in that book was to think of them in a linear manner. Thus, in applying the theory, many practitioners thought that denial needed to occur before there could be anger, or that acceptance could only happen after all the other stages had been worked through. This approach has been diversified and expanded on through such works as that of Martin and Elder (1991), whose theory describes "pathways through grief" in terms of a "circle of influence" (p. 3). It adds new meaning, depth, and imagery to stage theory in relationship to the grief process.

Beyond linear images, and in addition to them, life patterns are revealed in circles, curves, arcs, and spirals. The presence of such alternative images invites multidimensional visioning. That is, a person's worldview can expand with the inclusion of new experience. Furthermore, out of a broadened worldview, new paradigms can emerge. In this regard, the notion of a hermeneutic spiral has the potential of being informed by the ways in which spirals already exist in symbols, metaphors, natural imagery, and the arts. I (Margaret) remember walking beside some pine trees with my father many years ago in California. As we did so, Dad reached down, picked up a pinecone, and started to examine it. My father, it needs to be said, was a university lecturer in mathematics at the time. "Did you know," he queried, "that the folds of a pinecone and the unfolding of a rose blossom have been mathematically formulated in a type of spiral?" Needless to say, his question has remained with me. It was my first experience of considering the spiral in relationship with both natural beauty and scientific knowledge. Approaching the spiral as symbol and paradigm means that we consider it in such multidimensional ways.

The Spiral as Symbol

From the earliest of times, spirals have signified cycles of living and dying. As such, they have invited reflection and inspired meaning. Sjöö and Mor (1991), for example, noticed that spirals can be oriented both inwardly and outwardly. From this observation, they developed the following cosmic metaphor; they saw "the spiral *involution* [italics added] of energy into matter" as the primary movement of the universe, and the "spiral *evolution* [italics added] of matter into energy" as the movement of created beings back to their source (Sjöö & Mor, 1991,

p. 63). In another vein, the spiral has been used to symbolize many of the complementary rhythms of nature. Thus we read of the spiral representing departure and return, ebb and flow, expansion and contraction, ascent and descent, continuity and change (Gordon, 1993). With regard to its form, we read that the spiral can be found in three main configurations: "expanding (as in the nebula), contracting (like the whirlwind or whirlpool), and ossified (like the snail's shell)" (Cirlot, 1962, p. 305). References to nature in the above quotation invite us to notice the many natural expressions of spiral form that surround us. Think for a moment of the spiral design found in our human ear or in deoxyribonucleic acid (DNA). Notice the spiral in animal horns, the spider's web, conch and clamshells, coiled serpents, or the unfolding fronds of certain ferns and palm branches. Look afresh at the spirals that appear in ancient architectural designs, like those of New Grange in Ireland or the Al Tarxien temple in Malta. Finally, think of some of the ways spirals have been included in the design of musical instruments, dance motifs, paintings, literature, and even such practical items as staircases and bedsprings. All of this underscores the richness of a worldview that includes the spiral as one alternative to linear thinking.

But, one might ask, what does the spiral have to do with faith, health, or the relationship between faith community nurses and faith group leaders? Why choose a spiral as the basis for a collaborative ministry paradigm? Our choice comes from the following reflections.

Does the spiral have anything to do with faith traditions? Yes. The spiral image appears in a number of religiously based cosmologies and in the religious practices of several faith traditions. Chinese thought, for example, includes in its worldview the double-spiraled concept of yin and yang. These two principles are different, but interrelate their differences in ways that are complementary. As one source writes, "yin and yang constantly complement each other, to maintain cosmic harmony" (Sjöö & Mor, 1991, p. 64). Another author points out that yin and yang represent "the ability of the sigmoid [curved] line to express intercommunication between two opposing principles" (Cirlot, 1962, p. 306). From such faith-based applications of the spiral, we draw out its potential to symbolize the values of complementarity and intercommunication.

Does the spiral have anything to do with health traditions? In matters of health, there is the ancient symbol of intertwined snakes with their heads spiraling upward to represent the healing gods within Mesopotamian, Egyptian, Phoenician, East Indian, and Aztec cultures (Walker, 1988). Biblical writers drew on the spiral serpent symbol, giving it a positive value at the time of Moses (Num. 21:9 NRSV), and a negative value during the reign of King Hezekiah of Judah (2 Kings 18:4 NRSV). Within both Jewish and Christian faith traditions, a duality of meaning developed with regard to the spiraling serpent; by contrast, the Greeks adopted the double snake symbol for their medicinal god Asclepius. Likewise, according to Greek and Roman mythology, the "herald's wand" that we have come to know by the name *caduceus* was forged when it was placed between two fighting snakes, causing them to entwine themselves around the wand and face each other in peace. This wand was given to the herald god Mercury, and became a symbol for transforming strife into harmony. It has endured historically as a symbol of homeopathic healing and the medical profession in general. Its prime meaning has to do with "dualism and balance, and the union of opposing forces" (Gibson, 1996, p. 32). From such a health-based application of the spiral, we draw out its potential to symbolize tensions held in balance and dualities that resolve themselves harmoniously.

We chose the spiral in constructing our reflective paradigm for ministry collaboration because it symbolizes the values we have just described: the faith potential of complementarity and intercommunication, as well as the health potential of holding tensions in balance and resolving dualities harmoniously. We believe that nurses and religious leaders who learn to collaborate in ministry will be able to interrelate their educational and professional similarities and differences in ways that are complementary. Likewise, they will be able to foster a quality of communication that transcends and integrates differences by means of harmonious union. It is this evolving union that is offered in service to others. Furthermore, it is from this union that faith community members can learn about, and be empowered by, the integration of faith and health in their individual, family, group, and social lives.

The Spiral as Paradigm

Building on our consideration of the spiral as symbol, we now turn to its potential as a paradigm for use by faith community nurses and faith group leaders. Is there a hermeneutic spiral that can guide collaborative ministry reflection? Just as my worldview expanded when Dad commented on the spiral hidden within pinecones and roses, my awareness of the hermeneutic spiral emerged over a decade ago, when a ministry colleague used this approach during one of our pastoral counseling clinical case conferences. My colleague was presenting her pastoral counseling process in relation to a particular client. She indicated how this client went about exploring relationships with the divine, self, and others in an open-ended manner. Although honoring the client's open-endedness appeared to foster both health and faith for the client, it also gave rise to the following question: How does one trace and order the client's relationships so that they can be assessed professionally? My colleague used a hermeneutic spiral for this purpose. She noticed times in the counseling process when the client referred to God, significant others, and an emerging sense of self. By tracing these points of reference, the counselor recognized the client's deepening levels of awareness about each of the three relationships. As the case review unfolded, the counselor had traced a spiral pattern, and it was clear that significant growth in both faith and health appeared to be underway for the client.

When considering the possibility of using a hermeneutic spiral in faith community nursing, two questions need to be asked: What type of hermeneutic spiral will aid the reflective interpretation being carried forward by faith community nurses and faith group leaders as they explore faith and health issues arising within ministry experience? and, What points of reference need to be traced and ordered by means of spiral design so that faith processes and health processes can be assessed and responded to in a collaborative manner?

The hermeneutic spiral is fueled by continuous inquiry, and questioning is a value held by both theologically educated and nursing educated ministry professionals (Gros & Ezer, 1997; Schillebeeckx, 1984). Likewise, in matters of both health and faith, inquiry is linked with a process of learning (Allen, 1986; Dulles, 1994). Points of reference for the hermeneutic spiral shared by faith community nurses and faith group leaders, therefore, will need to trace an integrative learning process that is guided by open-ended questions.

The specific guiding questions that we suggest are drawn from the McGill model of nursing (Allen, 1986). They consider people within the context of community. The "client," therefore, is always communal in nature. This is true whether working with an individual, family, or group. We like this approach because it rests on a principle of the self in relation to others (Groome, 1991; Jordan, Kaplan, Miller, Stiver, &

Surrey, 1991). It is an approach congruous with what we have been saying in previous chapters about faith, spirituality, theology, religion, health, and health promotion: All of these concepts include reference to community as integral to personal wholeness, and all emphasize the benefits of inquiry as a preferred method for expanding awareness about faith and health. Figure 21.1 provides a listing of the McGill questions that can serve to guide both faith community nurses and faith group leaders in their collaborative inquiry. Since an integration of faith and health is the desired client outcome of ministry collaboration, it is important that both professions draw on a full range of their professional resources and relationships for the enhanced learning benefit of the client or family. Furthermore, in the experience of providing shared ministry, there is the additional bonus of collaborative learning for both the faith community nurse and faith group leader.

By means of these questions, both faith community nurses and faith group leaders, together with those who are the focus of their ministry, participate in processes of learning, boundary formation, and dialogue development. It is a collaborative and integrative learning process through which both faith and health are being learned (Allen, 1982a; Dulles, 1994; Kravitz & Frey, 1989). Thus, in asking the question, "What is the client dealing with?" we can expect nurses to identify health issues, and faith group leaders to explore faith issues. Likewise, when asking about resources, we can expect nurses to draw on their knowledge of health resources, and religious leaders to access a wealth of faith resources. However, it is in the *learning dialogue* of client, faith community nurse, and faith group leader that something new starts to happen. Here, the hermeneutic spiral comes into play, and threads of integrative learning begin to emerge. Through collaborative interdisciplinary learning with those who are the focus of their ministry, both nurses and faith group leaders start exploring ways that health issues and faith issues *connect* for the client. At these points of connection, new questions arise to confirm, expand, or correct the client's deepening level of awareness. Increased awareness, in turn, cycles back around through the integrative learning process to new points of connection, further questioning, and deepened awareness, in what Schillebeeckx (1984) calls "a never ending spiral" (p. 104). Some examples of the new questions that can arise out of this hermeneutic spiral are the following: Where is there evidence of wholeness as the client engages in health-seeking activities that are also faith-seeking? How

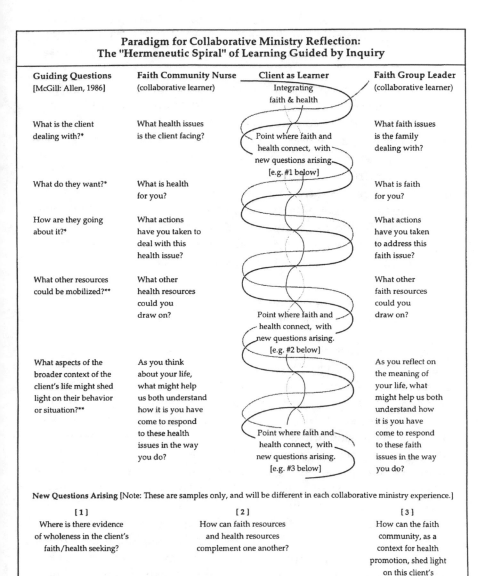

Paradigm for Collaborative Ministry Reflection:
The "Hermeneutic Spiral" of Learning Guided by Inquiry

Guiding Questions [McGill: Allen, 1986]	Faith Community Nurse (collaborative learner)	Client as Learner	Faith Group Leader (collaborative learner)
		Integrating faith & health	
What is the client dealing with?*	What health issues is the client facing?	Point where faith and health connect, with new questions arising. [e.g. #1 below]	What faith issues is the family dealing with?
What do they want?*	What is health for you?		What is faith for you?
How are they going about it?*	What actions have you taken to deal with this health issue?		What actions have you taken to address this faith issue?
What other resources could be mobilized?**	What other health resources could you draw on?	Point where faith and health connect, with new questions arising. [e.g. #2 below]	What other faith resources could you draw on?
What aspects of the broader context of the client's life might shed light on their behavior or situation?**	As you think about your life, what might help us both understand how it is you have come to respond to these health issues in the way you do?	Point where faith and health connect, with new questions arising. [e.g. #3 below]	As you reflect on the meaning of your life, what might help us both understand how it is you have come to respond to these faith issues in the way you do?

New Questions Arising [Note: These are samples only, and will be different in each collaborative ministry experience.]

[1]	[2]	[3]
Where is there evidence of wholeness in the client's faith/health seeking?	How can faith resources and health resources complement one another?	How can the faith community, as a context for health promotion, shed light on this client's present situation?

* Questions that are mainly asked in relation to the client.
** Questions that can be asked of both the client and professional.

Figure 21.1. A Ministry Spiral That Connects and Deepens

can faith resources and health resources complement one another to support and empower the client? How can the faith community, as a context for health promotion, shed light on the client's present situation?

What emerges in this process is a hermeneutic spiral that has multidimensional potential. That is, the inquiry process can lead a client outward, in search of community-based faith and health resources. It can also draw the client inward, in search of the whole-person faith and health resources that arise from one's inner being. In similar fashion, complementary rhythms of expansion and contraction, ascent and descent, may occur for the client. Since the hermeneutic spiral's movement is fueled by continuous inquiry on the part of not only the client, but also the faith community nurse and faith group leader, drawing connections between faith and health is a continual part of the integrative learning process that we call collaborative ministry.

✎ *A Summary Table of Professional Resources for Collaborative Reflection*

Thus far, we have explored the spiral image as both a symbol and paradigm for collaborative ministry. In the final section of this chapter, we turn our attention to the distinct professional backgrounds that inform ministry collaboration between faith community nurses and faith group leaders. Specifically, we want to highlight some of the resources that each profession brings to the integrative learning process undergirding shared ministry provision. By drawing on the wealth of these resources, nursing and religious professionals connect and deepen their learning dialogues with congregational members who are seeking to integrate faith and health.

We mentioned earlier that the guiding questions used in our hermeneutic spiral come from the McGill model of nursing, and are based on a communal approach to faith group members. When nurses and religious leaders use the same set of guiding questions, they will filter their responses to these questions differently. These differences derive from their distinct professional backgrounds. Indeed, divergent filtering processes may, at times, bring about tension and misunderstanding in the collaborative learning endeavor. We believe, however, that perseverance in the process of communication can lead to a breakthrough of consciousness. The positive outcome of such efforts at increased awareness will benefit the faith community in at least three ways. First, differences that are viewed as complementary can expand the range of ministry options available through nurses and religious leaders to the client and faith community. Second, arriving at points of connection in matters of faith and health may trigger the spiraling effect of our hermeneutic paradigm. Third, as spirals of integrated learning deepen, the quality of both health and faith will improve, with wholeness and holiness growing in a meaningful union.

In this section of the chapter, we organize professional resources by means of three major categories (see Figure 21.2). First, we highlight the broad bases of knowledge that inform each profession. For the faith community nurse, this involves a nursing knowledge base. For the faith group leader, this involves a theological knowledge base. In addition, we refer to other knowledge bases that are frequently explored by both professional groups. A second category of resources, that of theories and models, depicts some of the frames of reference used by nurses and religious leaders in their professional practice. Examples of this would be the McGill model of nursing or William Bridges's theory of transitions. In our book, we have used or referred to a number of these resources; at this time, we draw them together in summary form. The third group of resources we discuss is that of professional skills and tools, which often become mainstays in day-to-day professional functioning. Interpersonal skills and process notes would be examples of such resources. Again, our endeavor is to organize and summarize materials that have been discussed in our book.

We are aware that any summary table of resources we may compile for use by faith community nurses and faith group leaders will contain huge gaps of information in all three resource categories. Our objective is not so much to be comprehensive as it is to be suggestive. How would nurses who have been instructed in nursing approaches other than those we have emphasized fill in the details of this table? How would a summary table developed by a Christian faith leader differ from those developed by Muslim, Hindu, Buddhist, or Jewish faith leaders? Likewise, what would it be like for the faith community nurse and faith group leader of a congregation to fill in the details of our summary table by drawing together the unique complement of resources they are using in their collaborative ministry?

Summary of Professional Resources

	Family Community Nurses	Both Professional Groups	Faith Group Leaders
KNOWLEDGE BASE	Anatomy and Physiology Nursing of Individuals Nursing of Families Nursing of Communities The Nursing Profession Health Sciences Health Systems Research and Statistics	History Philosophy Language Arts Social Sciences Behavioral Sciences Physical Sciences Natural Sciences Religious Studies World Religions Multiculturalism	Foundations in Theology Practical Theology Systematic Theology Theology of Scriptures/Texts History of Faith Traditions Spirituality Worship/Liturgy Pastoral Theology
THEORIES and MODELS	Nursing Models (e.g., the McGill Model) Health Promotion Theory Parish Nursing Functions Theory (e.g., Westberg; Solari-Twadell)	Narrative Theory Transition Theory (e.g., Bridges) Spiritual Assessment Theory (e.g., Fitchett's 7x7 Model) Social Analysis Theory Developmental Theories	Faith Development Models (e.g., Ford; Fowler) Theological Reflection Models (e.g., Killen & deBeer) (e.g., Whitehead & Whitehead) Theories of Religious Tradition Models of Ministry

(e.g., Erikson)

Theories of Professional Helping
(e.g., Carkhuff; Rogers; Clinebell)

Theory on Partnership/Collaboration
(e.g., Pierce, Page, & Wagner)

Theories of Power

Learning Theory

		[See NOTE below]		Preaching Tools

SKILLS & TOOLS

Physical Assessment Tools
Nursing Process Notes
Nursing Journals
Parish Nurse Interest Groups
and so forth

[See NOTE below]

Preaching Tools
Worship Guides
Theological Journals
Collegial Interest Groups
and so forth

NOTE: Most of the professional skills and tools we have discussed in our book can be used by both faith community nurses and faith group leaders. These are listed collectively.

SKILLS: Interpersonal communication skills, psychological assessment skills, family assessment skills, spiritual assessment skills, skills in ritual leadership, social skills, skills in self-care, ministry skills, skills in theological reflection, hermeneutic skills, referral skills, group process skills, skills in time management, learning skills, leadership skills, collaborative skills, skills in the use of power, dialogue skills, and boundary clarification skills.

TOOLS: Workshops, journal writing, vision quests, therapy, book or journal study clubs, courses (e.g. Clinical Pastoral Education), annual retreat experiences, questionnaires, conceptual frames of reference and/or diagrams, guided imagery meditation, physical exercise, symbols, genogram and/or sociogram, storytelling, the "ministry partnership continuum," the "hermeneutic spiral of learning guided by inquiry," and so forth.

Figure 21.2. Summary Table of Professional Resources for Collaborative Ministry

Knowledge Bases in Nursing and Theology

In Western society, we usually speak about professional prepared-ness through a language of academic or technical education. We say a person has completed a diploma or degree; we likewise refer to fulfill-ing requirements for professional registration or certification. This is the language of our knowledge base and a person's ability to demon-strate the acquisition of that knowledge base. As we stated previously, we believe that faith community nursing will benefit a wide variety of cultures and faith traditions. At the same time, we are aware that we have been informed by and write out of our Christian religious heri-tage and North American cultural context. As we develop sketches for the knowledge bases that undergird religious and nursing ministry, our language and groupings will betray the limits of our experience. The broader question that can guide a richer development of this topic is, In your culture or faith tradition, what do you need to study or learn in order to be recognized as a nurse or religious leader?

In North America, there are two main types of education that pre-pare students to write a registered nursing licensing examination in their province or state: (a) diploma programs or associate degree pro-grams offered through community colleges, and (b) university pro-grams leading to a baccalaureate degree in nursing. Following a bacca-laureate degree in nursing, some nurses also receive masters and doctoral degrees in nursing. For the faith community nurse, we believe that a baccalaureate degree in nursing best provides the primary knowledge base needed to carry forward this type of ministry. Within baccalaureate nursing degree programs, students may study anatomy, physiology, psychology, sociology, anthropology, and the humanities as a foundation for nursing care of individuals, families, and commu-nities. Likewise, students study the nursing process, including assess-ment, planning, intervention, and evaluation. This process undergirds all types of professional nursing practice. Finally, baccalaureate nurs-ing programs stress the study of healthcare systems, research methods, statistics, nursing trends and issues, as well as professional and ethical standards for nursing.

Building on their present nursing knowledge base, but also expanding beyond it, faith community nurses need to have a clear understanding of the specific functions associated with nursing in a congregational setting. These functions, developed by the International Parish Nurse Resource Center (Holstrom, 1999), can further an understanding of how faith community nursing is a unique ministry resource available to congregations. Parish nurses do not seek to duplicate existing community health services (Solari-Twadell & McDermott, 1999); rather, nursing within a faith community can be seen as a subspecialty of community health nursing, in which faith communities serve as the aggregate, population base, or context for nursing practice. Finally, the contributions of nursing degree programs that include faith community nursing at the master's and doctoral levels will enable professional nurses to integrate their knowledge and experience further. In this regard, ongoing learning about community and population health, family health, advanced nursing practice in health promotion, research development, and an interface of theological studies will both add to the existing knowledge base and contribute to literature available in this important nursing subspecialty.

For the ministry professional, educational preparation is often linked with the question of being *ordained* or *lay*. Among many Christian denominations, the master of divinity and doctor of ministry degrees are becoming a standard theological knowledge base for ordained religious professionals. Lay ministry professionals usually pursue the same, equivalent, or related degrees. Some such master's and doctoral degree programs include those in the areas of theological studies, religious education, sacred theology, and the like. In this regard, theological studies occur in such areas as the history of faith traditions, sacred texts and scriptures, doctrinal and systematic theological topics, spirituality and worship, pastoral theology, and the professional ethics that undergird ministry functioning.

For both religious and nursing professionals, learning at baccalaureate, as well as advanced degree, levels often builds on a shared knowledge base; that is, basic arts and sciences are studied by a variety of professional groups. In this regard, faith community nurses and faith group leaders will bring knowledge from such academic areas as history, philosophy, language arts, the behavioral and social sciences, as well as physical and natural sciences to their ministry collaboration. When we take all of these knowledge bases into consideration, and view them as a potential benefit for the faith community, it is clear that both separately and collaboratively faith community nurses and faith group leaders draw on a broad base of information through which to enrich their ministry practice.

Theories and Models for the Nurse and Faith Group Leader

Our book is arranged in sections that highlight a number of theories and models. We have discussed concepts, such as health and faith, that lie at the foundation of nursing within a faith community. We have considered images, characteristics, and functions of the nurse as health promoter. We have explored the topic of promoting health in times of transition. The book has then gone on to review phases of the nursing process within faith communities in light of the McGill nursing model. Finally, the book has focused on the colleagueship and ministry collaboration that can develop between faith community nurses and faith group leaders as they bring a vision of faith to bear on health for the future. At this point, we would like to draw attention to the kinds of theories and models referred to in our text.

In addition to the McGill nursing model (Chapters 6, 16–19), reference has been made to nursing theories related with definitions of health and health promotion (Chapter 3), images of nursing (Chapter 8), professional practice elements (Chapters 9, 11), and nurse role development (Chapter 10). Furthermore, we have made note of theories that are beginning to surface in the field of parish nursing (Solari-Twadell & McDermott, 1999). The unique functions associated with parish nursing, for example, constitute a forum where subtle nuances in nursing theory can be elaborated on and explored. As the possibilities within faith community nursing expand, there is the promise for ongoing theoretical exploration in areas such as philosophy, education, and practice development. Of particular note in this regard will be theoretical contributions made by registered professional nurses hired to carry forward an intentional health promotion ministry within Buddhist, Hindu, Jewish, Islamic, and numerous other faith traditions.

Drawing from theological knowledge bases, we have discussed several models of faith development. In particular, reference has been made to the work of James Fowler (1981, 1991), and in-depth consideration is given to the spiral faith development model advanced by Iris Ford (1988). With regard to theological reflection theory, the models of James and Evelyn Whitehead (1979/1982, 1986, 1991, 1995), as well as those of Patricia O'Connell Killen and John deBeer (1994), have been highlighted. Finally, models of ministry and theories of religious tradition have been discussed or referred to. These have been drawn from a variety of feminist, liberation, scriptural, and systematic theologians. In particular, we have referred to the works of Crossan (1975), Dulles (1994), Jones (1989, 1992), Kittel and Friedrich (1967), Lonergan (1957, 1972), Schillebeeckx (1984), Soelle (1975), and Thistlethwaite and Engel (1990); in addition, we suggest readers also consult Brueggemann (1978), Chittister (1998), and Metz (1968/1998).

Many theories referred to in our book exist in literature held in common by both faith community nurses and faith group leaders. Here, we include narrative theory in both theology and the behavioral sciences, transition theories (Bridges, 1980, 1991), models of spiritual assessment (Fitchett, 1993a, 1993b), social analysis theory, developmental theories (Erikson, 1963, 1968, 1980, 1982), theories of power, models of professional helping, and theories of partnership or collaboration (Pierce & Page, 1986; Pierce et al., 1998). When viewed through the differing professional filters of nurses and religious leaders, these theories and models can enrich collegial dialogue, and this dialogue can expand the range of possibilities for applying various theories or models to collaborative ministry processes. We note, again, that our book is shaped in keeping with the specific nursing and theological points of view taken by those whom we have used as resources. It leaves open large areas where further theoretical exploration can occur by those who are schooled in other sources or models. What we offer is one example of collaborative theoretical integration. With this offering, we also extend an invitation for others to work toward additional types of synthesis drawn from the wealth of theories and models that exist in both nursing and theology.

Professional Skills and Tools That Nurses and Faith Group Leaders Can Share

Professional ministry knowledge that is theoretically grounded and based in practice will include a variety of skills and tools. For the nurse and faith group leader, these become manifest in day-to-day functioning. For example, the preaching skills of a religious leader are at work during both the preparation phase and proclamation phase of delivering a sermon or textual discourse. Likewise, the assessment skills of a faith community nurse are present while meeting people after worship, engaging in health education or health counseling, and monitoring the outcomes of health-promoting processes. In another vein, a stethoscope is not the only tool used by faith community nurses to listen to the whole-person heartbeat of congregational members. Neither is the tool of religious language the only type of language available to religious leaders in discussing the whole-person issues of faith, spirituality, theology, religion, health, and health promotion.

We recognize the importance of skills and tools that are unique to each profession. Although it is possible for there to be a crossover of ability, it is also realistic to assume that faith communities would hire a religious leader to carry forward faith-renewing activities and a nurse to carry forward health-promoting activities. With this in mind, we include reference to the physical assessment tools and skills provided through nursing professionals. We also highlight the skills and tools provided through religious leaders in developing various kinds of liturgical, ritual, and worship expression. This does not mean that nurses are unable to lead worship or that religious leaders are unable to notice health indicators; it simply means that nurses carry a particular professional responsibility to retain expertise in nursing skills, and will benefit from recourse to physical assessment tools, nursing process notes, nursing journals, a faith community nurse interest group within one's professional association, and so forth. Likewise, for religious leaders, it will mean carrying ongoing professional responsibility for expertise in pastoral assessment skills, worship leadership, and the like through recourse to theological journals, tools, and interest groups within the circle of one's professional association.

Our summary table (Figure 21.2) reflects the fact that most of the professional skills and tools discussed in our book can be used by both faith community nurses and faith group leaders. Again, we note that these skills and tools will be filtered through the differing knowledge bases of each type of profession, and can therefore be used in many forms of ministry provision. What we offer here is a synthesis of skills and tools referred to in our book.

Skills needed by both faith community nurses and faith group leaders include those of interpersonal communication, psychological assessment, family and systems awareness, and spiritual assessment. In another vein, there are social as well as ministry skills; these include theological reflection, hermeneutics (as a form of reflective interpretation), ritual leadership, group process skills, the ability to make appropriate referrals, the ability to draw on diverse learning styles, and the ability to manage time in such a way that dedication to others is balanced by self-care. Finally, in order for nurses and religious leaders to develop colleagueship in their approach to shared ministry, they will benefit from exploring skills related with collaboration, delegation, the use of power, boundary clarification, and shared leadership.

Tools that faith community nurses and faith group leaders may wish to draw on, both separately and in collaborative ways, include the following: For personal reflection and growth, there are the tools of journal writing, therapy, guided imagery meditation, physical exercise, reading, storytelling, and so forth. In community contexts, nurses or religious leaders may find themselves in a role of either participant or leader when it comes to such tools as workshops, vision quests, study clubs, courses, retreat experiences, and similar gatherings. Finally, there are tools that serve to frame one's thinking or provide conceptual clarity in ministry experiences. Some of these tools would be our ministry partnership continuum and hermeneutic spiral of learning guided by inquiry; other such tools would include questionnaires, diagrams, genograms, sociograms, images, and symbols.

Before we conclude this section, we want to underscore the fact that our summary table of resources concentrates on ministry professionals. It leaves out, therefore, specific reference to *client resources*, which are also integral to health promotion and faith renewal within a faith community. In this regard, a description of the resources brought into ministry relationships by congregational members, families, and groups is needed. Thus, both faith community nurses and faith group leaders will need, when they engage themselves in collaborative ministry endeavors, to be attentive to questions such as the following: What life experiences and ways of knowing does the congregational member or client bring into the ministry dialogue? And what learning styles, talents, and abilities does this person, family, or group appear to draw on as resources for collaborating in the ministry process?

✍ Summary

This chapter has looked at two major topic areas. First, we explored the spiral image as both a cultural symbol and ministry paradigm. Second, we compiled a summary table of the knowledge bases, theories and models, and skills and tools available to faith community nurses and faith group leaders. These will assist both groups of professionals in carrying forward the shared reflection needed for ministry collaboration. Now, we turn to a third topic of consideration in collaborative ministry development: Building on our understanding of health promotion and faith promotion as a ministry spiral that connects and deepens, our next chapter will apply theory to practice. In this regard, we will reflect together on the experiences of interdisciplinary collaboration that have emerged within our health-promoting and faith-renewing ministries.

22 ✑

Applying Theory to Practice

Collaborative Ministry Reflections

Margaret B. Clark
Joanne K. Olson

Several years ago, while planning a course for faith community nurses, we began discussing the idea of *mission*. It is a term we have used many times in talking with faith communities about the benefits of having a registered professional nurse as a member of the ministry team. Indeed, we have noticed that a number of faith communities include the concepts of health and healing as part of their congregational vision or mission statements. In our discussion, we arrived at an awareness that there can be personal as well as communal expressions of mission. In this regard, Margaret said to Joanne, "For many years, I have been motivated in my call to ministry by a sense of personal mission. It is as if I can hear God's voice deep within me saying, *Tell the people that I love them.*" Joanne's eyes lit up as she made the parallel connection: "I guess if I were to reframe that for myself, I would say that God's calling in my life as a nurse has been, *Tell the people that I want them to be healthy.*" In each expression of mission, there is a sense of being moved by a source or impetus that is "beyond" one's self. According to the language of some faith traditions, a mission originates with an experience of grace or charism. This charism is then appropriated over the course of one's life through a sense of call or vocation (Bosch, 1996; Bowker, 1997). What does this have to do with faith community nurses and faith group leaders?

Our story about mission comes back to us as we consider applying theory to practice in collaborative ministry reflection. For each of us, there is a dimension of mission within our calls to nursing and faith group ministry. In whatever nurse-related or pastoral activities we find ourselves, our deeper sense of meaning and motivation is derived from transcendent values, such as those of *love* or *health*. For Margaret, it is not enough to offer loving relationship through pastoral ministry; her deeper motivation is that, through her ministry, others may come to know that they are loved by God. Likewise, for Joanne, it is not enough to engage in health-promoting nursing relationships; her deeper motivation is that, through her nursing ministry, others may come to know that it is God who desires their health and wholeness.

By reflecting on our story as it applies to collaborative ministry, we notice that there are at least three layers of motivation operating simultaneously when serving others. Let us call these motivational layers *charism, mission* (or *vision*), and *ministry.*[1] *Charism,* or grace, answers the question, "Why?" Why am I doing this? Why am I here, working in this setting, with these people, and in this endeavor? In the story we have shared, charism is the sound deep within that says, "Tell the people that I love them," and, "Tell the people that I want them to be healthy." *Mission,* or *vision,* brings the transcendent grace and values of charism forward into time and space. As such, mission or vision answers the question, "What?" What do I bring to this ministry experience? What am I trying to accomplish? What can I do to provide service in this setting? Finally, *ministry* answers the question, "How?" It draws on an awareness of both grace and purpose, but it becomes grounded in concrete words and actions. Thus, we ask further questions: How do I get to know this faith community? How do I go about establishing ministry relationships within this context? How do I best respond to the needs of this person, family, or group? We believe it is important for faith community nurses and faith group leaders to have an awareness of these three dimensions of motivation as they approach collaborative ministry reflection. What are the stories in your own experience that bring to light (a) why you are attracted to faith community nursing or congregational leadership, (b) what you are about as you enter into this unique ministry, and (c) how you propose to live out your call both personally and professionally?

In this chapter, we seek to apply the hermeneutic spiral of learning guided by inquiry, developed in Chapter 21, to some actual ministry experiences. The approach we use is to share five different stories of collaborative ministry that illustrate each of the five guiding questions taken from the McGill nursing model. In deciding to address the questions separately and within the context of different clinical vignettes, we are aware that another approach to this chapter could be that of an in-depth consideration of all five questions in relationship with a single ministry story. Since the previous section of this book discussed nursing processes in the McGill model by means of in-depth reflection on the Brown family, we have chosen a different approach here. In Chapters 16 through 19, the point was to highlight the nurse's experience in relationship with family, faith group leader, faith community, and the broader environment. In-depth consideration seemed appropriate to that objective. By contrast, the current chapter looks at both the nurse and the religious leader. Specifically, it looks at how each ministry professional responds differently to the McGill model's guiding questions because of his or her unique background.

The five clinical vignettes we propose to share highlight actual ministry experiences within faith community settings. Names and identifying circumstances have been altered to preserve confidentiality and broaden the clinical perspective. In the terms of our hermeneutic spiral, guiding questions from the McGill model serve to trigger faith questions in the faith group leader, and health questions in the faith community nurse. These questions facilitate assessment and shared reflection. Out of this collaborative ministry reflection, points of connection occur where the learning dialogue gives rise to new questions. These are the points where health promotion and faith renewal intersect in relationship with the client and faith community. The process of collaborative learning that encircles and accompanies the integration of faith and health in those who are being served is what we call a ministry spiral that connects and deepens.

∞ Experiencing Sudden Death

Esther and Yamin, ages 23 and 25, are sister and brother. They recently moved to North America from eastern Europe in order to be reunited with Yamin's fiancée, Rachel. Although he was happy being closer to Rachel, the experience of saying good-bye to his family and home village weighed heavily on Yamin. He struggled with the limits of living in a three-room flat located in the midst of a crowded urban center. One afternoon, as he was walking past a Jewish synagogue, Yamin heard the plaintive song of a cantor: It touched him deeply. After talking with both Rachel and Esther, they decided to attend service at the synagogue. Before long, they received a call from Ruth. She shared that she was working as a registered nurse within the Jewish community affiliated with the synagogue, and would be happy to be of support to them in whatever way they felt might be helpful. Her welcoming outreach to Esther, Rachel, and himself struck Yamin as sincere and trustworthy. He thought about calling back sometime to talk about the heaviness of heart he was feeling; maybe Ruth could offer some suggestions about what to do. Before he had a chance to make the call, however, Yamin's sister Esther was hit by a car on her way home from the grocery store. Although she survived the accident and was treated in hospital, Esther died of complications from her injuries a week later. During the days Esther was in hospital, as he and Rachel waited with uncertainty, Yamin called Ruth.

Guiding Question #1: What Is the Client Dealing With?

What faith issues is the client dealing with? Even before the crisis around Esther's motor vehicle accident and eventual death, there was a faith issue for Yamin related to his estrangement from his homeland. He missed his family in eastern Europe. His heart was burdened with loneliness and a sense of not yet fitting into his new location. A second faith issue had to do with his engagement to Rachel. Together, they were making plans to marry and spend their lives together. This was a time of decision making that was complicated by Yamin's feelings of dislocation. Finally, there was the crisis of Esther's life-threatening injuries followed by death.

Although Yamin's faith connections with Judaism are deep, his experience of attending the local synagogue was very limited. He needed the richness of his faith tradition to make sense out of the tragedy of his loss. He needed the special burial rituals that are familiar to Jewish believers. Likewise, he needed the structure of traditional relationships and prayer practices existing within his faith community to support both him and Rachel at this time of crisis, loss, and grieving. Yamin sought out the faith community nurse as a point of connection with the synagogue. He was hoping, likewise, that Ruth would put him in touch with the rabbi.

What health issues is the client facing? Ruth visited Yamin and Rachel in the hospital. Many health-related issues surfaced as Yamin and Rachel talked with Ruth about the things that had happened to them recently. Shortly after Ruth's visit to the hospital, she received the news that Esther had died of complications from her injuries. New health-related issues emerged for the couple at that time.

During the first visit, Yamin and Rachel explained that they were dealing with the uncertainty that can surround a sudden injury, as had occurred to Yamin's sister. They were trying to go on with their lives as much as possible, but were filled with questions. They were attempting to understand the nature of the injuries, and had not been satisfied with the explanations given to them. Further questions emerged as to what the machines used in the intensive care unit were doing to support Esther's life. Likewise, Yamin and Rachel were struggling to think about the possibility of life without Esther, if indeed the injuries proved fatal.

Once Esther's injuries resulted in death, the couple was dealing with a new set of health issues. It is at such times, when issues related to "customary changes in family size, composition, roles, and relationships" occur (see Chapter 16), that people often turn to professional nurses. Ruth discovered, in talking with Yamin and Rachel, that they were working on the following health issues: learning to live without Esther, planning a meaningful burial service for Esther, and caring for themselves physically and emotionally while entering a period of grief. At times, they sought information about how others have learned to live without significant loved ones and ways to care for themselves in this time of grief. At other times, they simply appreciated Ruth's caring presence as she listened to their plans for a meaningful burial service.

Points of Connection and Deepening in Collaborative Learning

A first significant role Ruth played, immediately following Esther's death, was to join them in the hospital. Ruth spoke with hospital staff in the intensive care unit about the importance of not touching the body until the *chevra kadisha,* the Jewish burial society, arrived to make preparations in keeping with Jewish traditional practices. Ruth facilitated arrangements with staff to have Esther's body moved to a quiet and private location. She then called the burial society leader, and waited with Yamin and Rachel until everything was completed at the hospital. Ruth also contacted the rabbi, so that he could become part of the faith community's support to Yamin and Rachel from the beginning. In preparing for the burial, the rabbi became a focal point for support. He accompanied Yamin and Rachel through each phase of the Jewish mourning rituals, drawing on elements of sacred tradition that nurtured their faith and spiritual connections.

Following the burial, Ruth coordinated resources from within the faith community to continue reaching out to Yamin and Rachel. She kept in mind their health issues of bereavement and self-care. Through collaborative inquiry and learning, she accompanied them in ways that were empowering. Likewise, with their sense of increased belonging to the Jewish community affiliated with the synagogue, Yamin and Rachel found ways to carry on. As part of their long-term health goals, they consulted Ruth on the availability of community resources related with marriage preparation, family planning, and whole-person self-care. In these ways, Ruth served as a point of contact, support, and referral for Yamin and Rachel as they worked through their processes of faith and health integration.

✎ A Family Member Dying at Home

George returned to work after keeping a doctor's appointment during his lunch hour. He had gone alone to the doctor to hear about test results from a liver scan. Nothing could have prepared him for what he heard. Parts of the conversation with the doctor kept playing themselves out in his mind: "George, you have a rapid spreading type of

cancer, which originated in your stomach and has gone into your liver.
. . . I recommend you take a few days to talk this over with your family,
write down any questions or concerns you have, then contact my office
and we can discuss treatment options." George needed someone to talk
with. He was not sure how to share this news with his wife and family.

Although he was not a very religious man, George was on the
Board of Directors for an interdenominational social services co-op. He
had been impressed, on a number of occasions, with both the enthusiasm and compassion of a Baptist minister who was on the board.
George found the list of board members in his file, and called the Baptist Church listed under the Reverend Scott Drew's name. George's call
was put through to Scott's cell phone, and within minutes they were
talking. Scott listened to George's news with an open heart. He communicated his attentiveness and empathy in ways that comforted
George. Since George was not able to leave work without raising questions that he was not yet prepared to discuss, Scott and George agreed
to meet later in the afternoon, before George went home to talk with
his family. In the meantime, George would write down on a piece of
paper anything that came up for him in response to a question Scott
invited him to consider: "What am I dealing with in light of this cancer
diagnosis?" Scott, for his part, received George's permission to discuss
his health situation with Leslie, the parish nurse. Scott knew that
Leslie's health expertise would be of value to George, and wanted her
to become involved as soon as possible.

Later that afternoon, in their meeting together, Scott and George
talked about all the things George felt he was dealing with. There were
financial concerns. And how could he ever say good-bye to his wife of
30 years? Also, there was his youngest son; they were not on good
terms right now. And what about the grandchildren? Would he ever
see them again? The list of concerns was complex and multifaceted.
For the time being, Scott focused on George's immediate concern of
telling his wife Martha about the cancer diagnosis. Scott could hear
George's feelings of guilt as he talked about causing Martha grief and
distress because of this illness. By the caring way Scott was able to
acknowledge George's feelings, George was able to reconnect with the
strength of his love for Martha, and regain some of his confidence
about being so physically vulnerable. They had made it through tough
times before, and he knew he could count on Martha's faithful companionship now. As they parted, George said to Scott, "I'm not a reli-

gious man, but I thank you for what you have given me today. And maybe you could say a word to the 'Man Upstairs' for me." Scott acknowledged this trust, and said, "I'd be honored to do that, George. Also, if its all right with you, I'd like to give you a call tomorrow afternoon just to see how things have gone. Then, sometime in the not too distant future, I'd like you to meet Leslie, our parish nurse. She's part of our staff, and I believe she can be a real help to you and your family at this time." George was fine with that suggestion.

Guiding Question #2: What Does the Client Want?

What is health for you? No one had ever asked George such a question before. He thought for a long time, and then responded, "I guess health always meant before that the doctor told me my test results were negative or that my medications were doing what they were supposed to, but I think now health is something different. The doctor has told me that I have a very serious condition, and that I may not have much time with my family. Now, I think health is what I do with the time I have left. I want to die 'healthy,' with no regrets about how I lived my life. I also think that health is feeling somewhat in control of what happens to me in the future regarding treatments, where I am as I become more ill, and that sort of thing."

The nurse heard in George's answer the health goals toward which he was working, even at this early stage of getting the serious diagnosis. George desired to use his remaining time having good relationships with the people in his life. Furthermore, he desired to know as much as he could about what was available to him in terms of treatment. He wanted to feel part of the decision-making process, rather than be someone who had no control over his situation. With these two goals in mind, the faith community nurse formulated ideas about possible interventions that could be helpful as she continued to work with George, his family, and the faith community leader over the next months.

What is faith for you? Although George referred to himself as "not a religious man," he had some sense about "saying a word to the 'Man Upstairs.'" Faced with the imminence of his death, George began to take stock of his life. He asked Scott to accompany him in this process. Together, they explored the network of relationships in George's life story; they looked at the events and relationships he felt good about, as well as those he felt bad about. Occasionally, Scott would raise the question, "How would you like that relationship to be by the time you die, George?" As a final phase in this sharing, Scott invited George to work through a form of life review called a "healing of memories." It was an opportunity for George to talk more deeply about some of his most important relationships in the light of what he wanted them to be like before his death. This process was very important in leading George to a place of reconciliation with his youngest son, and to a time of shared planning with Martha about his death and funeral.

Points of Connection and Deepening in Collaborative Learning

In this ministry experience, the faith group leader and faith community nurse were intentional in their collaborative work with George and his family. They each approached the activity of a life review in different ways, but these differences empowered George to take charge of the process, and draw others into it at times and in ways that were meaningful. Of special note in this regard was George's decision to write a "legacy of love" to his family. In this document, he expressed his cares and concerns for each family member. He bequeathed to them a number of "affirmations," in which he pointed out strengths and potentials that he saw in them. Then, he gathered his family around him for a reading of this legacy. It was a powerful time of preparation for his death and consideration of what life might be like after his passing.

In another vein, both Scott and Leslie were attentive to George's wife and children. They coordinated their team approach to this family by serving as both primary and backup contacts for Martha and the children. Leslie provided Martha and George with resources where they could learn more about writing a will, as well as spousal health benefits for widows. Although Scott took lead responsibility in working with George and Martha on funeral plans, he and Leslie worked collaboratively in the matter of listening to input from each child regarding this process. They were aware that each member of the family would need to approach George's death in his or her own way, grieving and sharing in their own unique rhythms of time. Finally, both Leslie and Scott consulted together to anticipate faith and health concerns that might arise following George's death. In these ways, they were a steady supporting presence for this family.

✍ The Experience of Impending Surgery

Anita Moresby is a middle-aged professional woman who lives alone. She works as an accountant with a large telecommunications network, and, despite her 26 years with the same company, there has been talk of downsizing. Anita realized that her position was vulnerable. Although her family lives at a distance, she had a close circle of friends and colleagues who shared a number of her personal and professional interests. Two months ago, Anita was tested for an eye condition that she had been monitoring for several years. The results indicated that Anita needed cataract surgery. In three weeks, she was to go into the hospital for the operation. Although she did not need to stay overnight in the hospital, she would need to be off work for three weeks. Anita was unsure about how best to prepare for the surgery and the time off from work. Even though she talked things over with her friends and colleagues, she was hearing a number of different opinions. Also, people were asking Anita questions about approaches to the surgery with which she was unfamiliar. Consequently, she was becoming increasingly confused and anxious.

Anita's next-door neighbor is a nurse named Veronica, who works in the same church that Anita attends for worship. After talking briefly on the telephone, Anita asked to meet Veronica at the church. Her intention was to acquire information about the surgery. What Anita discovered was that Veronica, in her role as a faith community nurse, not only had a wealth of information, but could also provide helpful referrals and follow-up support. Although Anita knew that she was dealing with a health condition not commonly seen in people her age, and that it could affect her ability to work, she had not stopped to consider how important her work was as a source of meaning and purpose in her life. In follow-up appointments with Veronica, Anita discussed how the impending surgery was triggering not only health questions, but also faith questions. Veronica invited Anita to consider what she had already done to prepare for the surgery, and to look at how these preparations were helping her address both faith and health concerns. Having done this, an important new question emerged quite spontaneously, when Veronica asked Anita, "What do you need to know to feel prepared for this surgery?" It was as if a frame had been placed around the picture. The question provided a touch point that Anita could return to in every aspect of her surgery preparation. She applied the question in exploring various types of medical procedures related with cataract surgery. She also applied it to negotiating time away from work, drawing on her circle of friends for practical support and companionship, securing enough food and household supplies to see her through the days immediately after surgery, and arranging for the minister at the church to visit her just prior to the surgery for prayer and spiritual support.

Guiding Question #3: How Is the Client Going About Achieving What She or He Wants?

What actions have been taken to deal with this health issue? Anita was working on the health goal of feeling prepared for surgery and for the recovery period to follow. The nurse, Veronica, asked what Anita had done toward achieving this goal. Anita explained that she had sought out information about the actual surgery from the surgeon and the nurse at the physician's office. In addition, she had purchased several books about how the eye looks and works, so she could understand exactly what was going to be done during the cataract surgery. With Veronica's suggestion that she think about her needs after she gets home from surgery, Anita reported during a later visit that she had enlisted several close friends to take turns staying with her during her first week at home. In addition, she had anticipated basic needs, such that her cupboards and refrigerator were filled with easy-to-prepare food. She had even thought ahead enough to anticipate the bills that needed to be paid in the week or two after surgery, and paid them ahead of time. To make her recovery time at home something to look forward to rather than dread, Anita had purchased new pajamas, several new compact discs, and the cassette-taped version of some current novels.

What actions have been taken to address this faith issue? For Anita, needing cataract surgery triggered faith concerns related with the meaning and purpose of her life. Since she already feared loosing her job through downsizing, the thought of being off work for three weeks made her feel extremely vulnerable. Likewise, there was a sense of being betrayed by her body. If God was supposed to be loving and providential, why were her eyes being afflicted? Without good eyesight, Anita could not do her accounting job. Out of control, disempowered, and feeling angry with God, Anita clung to the question raised by the faith community nurse, because it gave her some sense of dignity in the midst of so much confusion. As she returned time and time again to the words "What do you need to know to feel prepared," Anita discovered that a lot of people were there to support her. She began to feel deeply loved and valued in ways she had not previously known. This renewed her sense of worth, and broadened her perspective on the meaning of her life. In the final stages of preparation for surgery, Anita realized that she needed to let go of her anger with God. Having the minister visit and pray with her provided one final way of being prepared. Going into the hospital, Anita felt a sense of peace. She knew she would be okay.

Points of Connection and Deepening in Collaborative Learning

Given the support she experienced from the faith community nurse's inquiring approach to preparing for her surgery, Anita came through her experience with improved health. Her unexpected need to relate with others from her place of vulnerability and dependence had an impact on her sense of self. Likewise, the loving support of friends and colleagues positively expanded the sense of meaning life had for her. What began as a crisis of health and faith evolved into a period of renewed belief in the goodness of God, her circle of support, and her own purpose in this world.

✍ Caring for a Down's Syndrome Child

Mark works in construction. His wife Helen, a dental hygienist, delivered their third child two weeks ago. Soon after the birth, a number of concerns were raised regarding baby Jimmy's health, and it had subsequently been determined that their son has Down's syndrome. News of this congenital condition came as a shock to both Mark and Helen; as yet, they were unable to make sense of it. Furthermore, Mark believed that it is a man's gene that carries the condition. In light of this belief, he began to feel guilty, and blamed himself.

Since Mark is a religious man with many links to the church, he turned to his faith community for support. After talking over his sense of guilt and self-blame with Pastor Wilkinson, he felt some relief. He was especially impressed by the pastor's ability to listen to his mixed-up words, thoughts, and occasional emotional outbursts. He was encouraged when Pastor Wilkinson told him about a nurse who was working in the parish to support people at such times as this. With the understanding that his wife Helen was agnostic and might not be comfortable with church-related outreach, Mark gave the pastor permission to talk with the faith community nurse about their baby's condition.

Several evenings later, after talking by telephone with both Mark and Helen, the parish nurse came to their home for an initial visit. Evangeline, the faith community nurse, prepared for the meeting with Mark and Helen by familiarizing herself with details of the medical condition, compiling a list of local resources and support networks for parents with Down's syndrome children, and consulting with Pastor Wilkinson about what he would like his ongoing involvement to be. In the course of their conversation, Evangeline was able to draw on a great deal of the information collected. Her approach, however, was open-ended, and this made both Helen and Mark feel as if they were intimately involved in every aspect of the discussion.

Guiding Question #4: What Other Resources Could Be Mobilized?

What other health resources could be drawn on? When meeting with Helen and Mark, the faith community nurse offered a number of possible resources that they had not considered in their search for ways to learn to live with the fact that their son has Down's syndrome. The couple was unaware, for example, that at least one other couple in the congregation had a child with Down's syndrome. They were unaware, as well, of the early childhood education programs available within the community for children with Down's syndrome. In planning for future children, Helen and Mark expressed much fear and concern, and had some misinformation regarding the congenital nature of Down's syndrome. In this regard, they were not aware of the excellent genetic counseling services available at the local university hospital. Finally, the couple was unaware of the support groups available to parents with children who have genetic abnormalities. The faith community nurse was able to assist the family in accessing the resources that they decided to seek out and to "walk beside them" as they made difficult decisions about whether or not to try to have more children.

What other faith resources could be drawn on? Mark's initial recourse to his faith community was for crisis intervention. His guilt and shame prevented him from relating with both Helen and his new son, Jimmy. After coming through that crisis, he was open to ongoing contact with his faith community through meetings with the faith community nurse, Evangeline. It was in this relationship that additional faith resources opened up for both Mark and Helen. For years, Mark had practiced his religion alone. Likewise, he and Helen had an understanding that the children could attend church with Mark, but would not be formally initiated until they were adults and could make their own choice. As a nurse, Evangeline posed no threat to Helen's sensitivity regarding religion. Although Evangeline was from Mark's faith community, Helen saw her strictly as a healthcare worker. As the relationship developed, opportunities arose to celebrate special health-related events in Jimmy's life. Some of these were rites of passage, others were achievements, and still others addressed feelings of discouragement or fatigue. At first Evangeline offered, and then was regularly asked, to lead the rituals honoring these events. As the value of ritual grew for this family, they found a number of ways to create and participate in events that took Jimmy into the broader community. Thus, they regularly attended parades, public ceremonies, treasure hunts, and similar activities. In these ways, rituals contributed to Jimmy's widening social integration and to the family's ability to face both good times and bad in a spirit of solidarity.

Points of Connection and Deepening in Collaborative Learning

In light of Jimmy's health condition, Pastor Wilkinson and Evangeline knew that a long-term process of accompaniment would be called for. With Mark and Helen's permission, they began to involve the broader faith community in supportive ways. First, there was a need to educate the congregation regarding the abilities and limitations experienced by those with Down's syndrome. Mark and Helen met the other couple in the faith community who had a Down's syndrome child. Together, this child's parents and Mark decided to bring their children with them to church, just as Mark was in the habit of doing with his other children. The modeling of the two families stimulated a wonderful response of inclusiveness among other members of the congregation. They were touched by the loving presence communicated by these two young Down's syndrome persons. They became valued members of the faith community, and contributed to its mission of outreach. Evangeline included this sense of Jimmy's outreach role in her ritual connections with the family.

As he grew through various age periods, Jimmy's family found ways for him to "go to school" and "go to work." That is, anytime he was discovering some new task or capability, they called it school. They also acknowledged Jimmy's capacity to express love and affection as a strength that was parallel to a job skill. When Jimmy was asked to take a turn cuddling infants in the congregation's day care center, he said he was going to work with his "loving skills."

There were times through the years when Mark, Helen, and their family experienced doubt, discouragement, and frustration. At these times, they wrestled with the questions, "Why did this congenital condition occur in our family?" and "Why do *we* have a child with a condition that asks so much of us all the time?" In this regard, both Evangeline and Pastor Wilkinson accompanied them, suggesting resources for self-care and family support. On one occasion, Pastor Wilkinson told them about the writings of Jean Vanier and the L'Arche communities he founded.[2] It is a belief within these communities that people with limited mental abilities have something special to teach us. In particular, they have something to teach us about what it means to love and to be loved. Learning more about Vanier and L'Arche opened both Mark and Helen to a sort of spiritual bond that was new for them. They read and discussed the writings of Vanier and others affected by the L'Arche philosophy. In its own peculiar way, the questioning process carried forward by Mark and Helen over the course of many years enabled faithfulness and respect to be the mainstay in parenting Jimmy. Having access to the collaborative support of Evangeline and Pastor Wilkinson, as well as the inclusive consciousness of Mark's faith community, gave them deep grounding in their faith and health integration.

◄ Coping With Depression

Five years ago, Sayyid Kassam, a man in his mid-30s, immigrated to Canada from Egypt to pursue specialized research in biomedical engineering. Within six months of his arrival, Sayyid was feeling discouraged in his work, and was questioning its worth. He was having a difficult time concentrating, and felt tired most of the day. Over the last several weeks, his eating patterns were fluctuating, and he was having trouble sleeping. He felt bad about everything, and could not get beyond a sense of overwhelming gloom. When thoughts of suicide began to enter his mind, he knew he needed help. A first recourse was his Muslim faith community. He learned that a prayer room had been set up for Muslims in the work site, and he began joining others at their daily prayer times. It helped Sayyid to feel connected with traditions from his home country. In conversation with his coworkers, Sayyid also learned about a Muslim health clinic that operated in conjunction with the Islamic Center on the south side of the city. He decided to see if there was any help to be found at that clinic. Corrine is a registered professional nurse who had been hired by the Islamic Center to work in the clinic. Sayyid made an appointment to meet with her for an assessment of his sadness and lack of energy.

Guiding Question #5: What in the Broader Context
Can Shed Light on the Situation?

As you reflect on the meaning of your life, what might help us both understand how you have come to respond to these faith issues in the way you do? From the information available, it would appear as though Sayyid's research work was a source of life meaning for him; it is what motivated him to leave Egypt and immigrate to Canada. What he discovered was how closely related his work had been to a number of previously unnamed cultural and religious factors. Without these, Sayyid gradually lost touch with himself, and became depressed. Although there was a psychological reality to this depression, there were also spiritual and cultural considerations. In Egypt, his days regularly included the sounds of a call to prayer and the movement of coworkers as they sought out places for *salat*, the obligatory prayer in Islam that occurs five times a day. Likewise missing were the familiar smells and tastes of foods cooked in traditional ways for Muslim dietary practices. Finally, the fast of Ramadan, which had commenced several weeks earlier, was difficult to carry out in Canada without the spiritual and cultural ties he had always felt with his family. The sense of isolation was more than Sayyid could bear. This was when the depression set in. Having recourse to the Muslim prayer room at his work site was an important connection between Sayyid and his faith tradition. It opened doors for him to enter more fully into the local Muslim faith community and to seek out health resources at the Islamic Center. What Sayyid learned in this experience was how closely his culture and faith were tied to his sense of purpose and life meaning.

As you think about your life, what might help us both understand how it is you have come to respond to these health issues in the way you do? Since Corrine, the faith community nurse, was not of the Muslim faith, she approached her work with new clients in an exploratory manner. Over the course of several weeks, Corrine came to know more about not only Sayyid, but also his immediate family and extended family background. Included was information about family development; family type; family structure; family processes; cultural influences on family beliefs, attitudes, and lifestyle; family lifestyle patterns; family role models; and family religious beliefs (Bomar, 1996). The nurse learned that Sayyid was married, and the father of four school-age children. This situated him and his family in the school-age stage of development. At the same time, having learned that Sayyid's mother was living with him, Corrine recognized that there was also a multigenerational dimension to this family's structure. In the area of family processes, the nurse learned more about how Sayyid and his wife communicated, and how decisions were made within the family. Likewise, more was learned about the health issues arising from value struggles occurring for Sayyid in Canada as he tried to adapt his cultural and religious practices to a very strange living environment. Of special note here was information provided to Corrine about the history of depression in Sayyid's family.

Points of Connection and Deepening in Collaborative Learning

In her role as a faith community nurse, Corrine was in a position to learn about a faith tradition with which she was only somewhat familiar. The imam was happy to respond to her questions about religious and cultural traditions. He also put her in touch with members of the community who were recognized for healing abilities. The imam's wife occasionally invited Corrine into their home to learn more about dietary and cleansing practices. Issues of gender separation factored strongly into the topics of communication processes, decision making, and health care practices. Corrine used what she learned to serve as a liaison between Islamic families, such as Sayyid's, and various options within the healthcare system that might be compatible with Muslim health needs. On a number of occasions, she found that faith and health integration occurred as diet, ritual, and spiritual teachings were approached holistically.

∽ Summary

In this chapter, we have addressed the idea of *mission* as it relates to the three layers of motivation in service orientation. The terms *charism, mission*, and *ministry* were used to distinguish these layers of inner urging. Charism explains *why* we are moved toward service of others, mission describes *what* our purpose is, and ministry spells out *how* we carry forward our service orientation toward others. These dimensions of motivation are important when entering into collaborative ministry in that they provide insight into the vocational uniqueness of both nurses and religious leaders. Optimizing these uniquenesses will maximize the ministry benefits to faith community members.

The chapter went on to discuss five clinical vignettes in light of the hermeneutic spiral of learning guided by inquiry designed in Chapter 21. Each of the five guiding questions taken from the McGill nursing model was featured in a different ministry story. Faith and health inquiry was developed around the stories in order to explore issues, strengths, potentials, resources, and possibilities for faith group members.

As we draw this section of the book to a close, we hope there will be further use and development of the theoretical foundations, conceptual explorations, clinical tools, and narrative applications that have been developed. Likewise, we believe that a number of courses, workshops, and retreats for both faith community nurses and faith group leaders could easily grow out of the broad-based approach we have taken. Our hope is that we have entered into the topic of faith community nursing with enough theoretical content to stir deeper levels of reflection and dialogue in the minds and hearts of others. We trust that, having read this book, front line faith community nurses, congregational leaders, nurse educators, and theological educators will have their curiosity stimulated, differing points of view evoked, and professional convictions awakened. In this regard, we look forward to seeing further developments in the literature related to the important fields of faith community nursing and interdisciplinary collaboration in ministry.

Notes

1. The terms *charism, mission,* and *ministry,* as well as the related questions "Why?" "What?" and "How?" used in this chapter were originally learned during a workshop presentation many years ago. The name of the Roman Catholic sister who led that workshop has been forgotten. It feels important to give her credit, however, for inspiring insights that have long endured.

2. L'Arche is an international federation of communities in which people with a developmental disability and their assistants live, work, pray, and share their lives together. Founded in 1964 in France by Jean Vanier (1995) and Fr. Thomas Philippe, there are now over 100 L'Arche communities around the world. See the web page at http://www.dsuper.net/~jcpas/aaccueil.html for more information.

PART VII

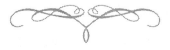

CONCLUSION

23

Bringing a Vision of Faith and Health Into the Future

Margaret B. Clark
Joanne K. Olson

Throughout the pages of this book, we have spoken about faith community nurses as registered professional nurses hired or recognized by faith communities, within diverse spiritual and religious traditions, to carry forward an intentional health-promotion ministry. In the various sections of our text, we have introduced guiding concepts, historical perspectives, theories, models, considerations about change and transition, narrative studies, and in-depth reflections on a number of approaches to nursing within faith community settings. Our explorative descriptions reflect the belief that health is an integral dimension of living, behaving, and developing. Likewise, faith involves discovering what it means to be in holistic relationships with the divine, the self, and others. Now, we wonder if, in their emergence at the crossroads of faith and health, faith community nurses are not only historically rooted, but also a "new" manifestation of ancient and essential linkages between faith and health. Put another way, is it possible that faith community nurses are integral to bringing a vision of health and faith into the future? The final chapter of our book explores this possibility, and provides concluding remarks on the rich potential within faith communities for visioning the ongoing integration of faith and health.

There are four important aspects to our consideration of bringing *vision* into the future. First, what does it mean for individuals, families, groups, and communities to generate "vision"? Second, what role can faith communities have in bringing a vision of faith to health? Third, what role can healthcare systems have in bringing a vision of health to faith? Finally, what contributions can faith community nurses make in bringing visions of faith and health into the future?

∽ The Role of "Visioning"

Vision is intimately linked with the concepts of worldview, paradigm, and filter. Rather than dichotomizing this notion in such a way that some are considered to have vision and others are considered to be without vision, let us assume that every person has vision. The question then shifts from "Who has, or does not have, vision?" to "What is my, or our, vision?" Gaining greater clarity about the particularities surrounding one's vision is an ongoing task and responsibility that arises from within our humanity and social consciousness (Dulles, 1994; Freire, 1970/1993; Lonergan, 1972). During times of change and transition, it is to be expected that visioning, vision statements, and questioning a vision will come to the fore of human consciousness. Let us examine these ideas further.

Visioning begins with the simple, but also profound, question: "What do I see?" It is a question each individual, family, group, and community might want to ask as we stand in our many places of seeking. What we notice is that answers arising in response to this question are multidimensional. Furthermore, what we see implies that there are also things we do not see. Likewise, there may be things that we want to see, but are prevented from seeing by limits and obstacles to our vision. Thus, visioning is a complex concept that can lead to deepening and expanding realms of awareness. This can have implications for the ways that we choose to be in relationship with the divine, self, and others.

In faith communities, as in other social groupings, it is not uncommon to see members gather for the purpose of developing a vision, or *mission, statement*. Here, the question is no longer "What do I see?" but rather, "How do we 'write the vision down and make it plain?'" (Hab. 2:2 NRSV). Something we encounter when trying to articulate a vision is that it shifts from a place of ambiguity to a place of specificity. It gets rooted, structured, and can be evaluated.

Although vision statements are needed to concretize the multidimensional perceptions of visioning, they are not intended to be rigid or absolute. Vision is deeper than the vision statement. A vision statement, therefore, will need ongoing renewal and reconstruction as new aspects of a vision's meaning rise to consciousness and are explored through diverse principles of interpretation. This is where the idea of *questioning a vision* becomes important. The focus of attention shifts away from "How do we write the vision down and make it plain?" to "Where did this vision come from?" It is a search for sources. That is, although we have already said that vision is deeper than a vision statement, there are additional depths to pursue; questioning a vision is an opportunity to remember, contextualize, and rediscover origins. Furthermore, it is an opportunity to probe for the vision's sources. These sources of vision can be found in the enduring and unifying assumptions, values, and beliefs that undergird the vision's current form. The Universal Declaration of Human Rights of the United Nations, for example, communicates a vision "of freedom, justice and peace in the world" (quoted in Multifaith Calendar, 1999). This vision, however, rests on the enduring and unifying values "of the inherent dignity and of the equal and inalienable rights of all members of the human family" (quoted in Multifaith Calendar, 1999). Although questioning a vision is no small task, it helps individuals and groups assess whether or not the vision is healthy and viable. It queries whether the enduring assumptions, values, and beliefs undergirding the vision are in evidence. Questioning a vision, then, is a type of inquiry that can promote renewal, exploration, and discovery in thought, word, and deed.

Visioning for the future involves looking at the present, drawing from the past, and moving forward into what is yet unknown. It involves reclaiming, reconstructing, and being sustained by enduring and unifying values. The role of visioning is especially important during times of transition and uncertainty. When individuals, families, and groups within faith communities spend time with the questions, "What do I see?" "How do we write the vision down and make it plain?" and "Where did this vision come from?" they will discover future possibilities. In short, for vision to take hold, there is a need for openness, inquiry, practical rootedness, risk, courage, and perseverance. We now bring these understandings of vision into the context of faith communities as they consider linkages between faith and health.

✧ *Bringing a Vision of Faith to Health*

In Chapter 4, we reflected on the topic of local faith communities as places of seeking. We spoke of an adaptive quality within religious groups that has enabled them to draw on geography, social structure, cultural symbols, and significant events in order to be able to say, "We are here" to the people whom they seek to serve. We also pointed to evidence that the values that have given shape to our existing physical and attitudinal structures are in a process of shifting. In this regard, we suggested that faith communities position themselves to listen deeply for indicators, within both their ancient traditions and contemporary cultures, that may be giving rise to a new sense of place for the future. With this in mind, we believe that faith communities are in a position to *bring a vision of faith to health* through the activities of remembering and imagining.

Remembering is an ancient activity. It explores story, and discovers relational and insightful treasures among lost or forgotten events. Furthermore, remembering reawakens primitive curiosities and probes living traditions. To remember is to gather up pieces of the journey of one's life into words, symbols, songs, rituals, and the like. For individuals, families, and groups within faith communities, there is much that needs to be remembered so that a vision for the future can be fashioned. Faith group leaders and faith community nurses, therefore, are in a position to encourage remembering, and to foster the various forms of collaborative learning that can flow out of this intentional remembrance. This may involve stepping back from one's immersion in current realities to ask the question "What do I see?" It may also involve conversing with today's social structures, dictums, headlines, and global events with the question "Where did these visions come from?" Activities of remembering can lead people into places of seeking and deep listening. This quality of deep listening allows for the probing of sources. That is, within diverse faith traditions, seekers of faith and health will be attracted by the allure of originating values, graces, and insights hidden as treasures within sacred texts, healing practices, symbols, and mythic narratives. These are the ancient, enduring, and unifying threads of meaning that need to be carried from the past, through the present, and into the future. Sogyal Rinpoche, in *The Tibetan Book of Living and Dying* (1993), captures this process of remembering as an ancient activity when he says, "Gradually, as we listen to the teachings, certain passages and insights in them will strike a strange chord in us, memories of our true nature will start to trickle back, and a deep feeling of something homely and uncannily familiar will slowly awaken" (p. 121).

In addition to remembering, faith communities are in a position to bring a vision of faith to health through *imagining*. There are three approaches to imagination we would like to suggest. First, Walter Brueggemann (1978) has written about "prophetic imagination." He says that this form of community-based imagination commences when people wake up from what he calls the sleep of "royal consciousness," or a total immersion in one's social location. For Brueggemann, "the task of prophetic imagination and ministry is to bring people to engage the promise of newness that is at work in our history with God" (p. 62). Imagination, in this sense, is compatible with giving voice (Belenky et al., 1986; Gilligan, 1982) to both *faith* as health seeking, and *health* as faith seeking.

A second understanding of imagination is what Kwok Pui-Lan (1990) calls "dialogical imagination" (p. 275). She says that dialogue, in Chinese, means talking with each other. It implies mutuality, active listening, and openness to what the other has to say. She draws on the German word for imagination, *Einbildungskraft*, as the power of shaping into one. Kwok then goes on to describe her use of dialogical imagination as an "attempt to bridge the gap of time and space, to create new horizons, and to connect the disparate elements of our lives into a meaningful whole" (p. 276). For faith communities and health care systems, this may mean talking with each other in a spirit of mutuality, active listening, and openness so that the power of unifying and enduring values can be stimulated collaboratively.

Finally, faith communities are invited to imagine themselves looking and acting differently. According to Patrick Brennan in *Re-imagining the Parish* (1994), it can be said that "the parish many of us knew and loved as we grew up is inadequate to meet the evangelical needs of believers in the future" (p. ix). He advocates that faith communities, as they move into the future, filter self-perception through three new lenses: (a) small intentional communities, (b) an emphasis on adult faith formation, and (c) an expanded family consciousness. In his book, Brennan discusses such topics as the basic ecclesial communities in Latin America, the RCIA (Rite of Christian Initiation of Adults) as a model for adult faith formation, andragogy as an adult learning praxis,[1] and the faith community as a training center for parenting. The notion of faith communities as centers for expanded family consciousness is further developed in Gerald Foley's *Family-Centered Church* (1995). This book takes note of the fact that in local faith communities the family has many faces. Thus, Foley says that multicultural and multiracial families, interdenominational marriages, dual-career families, mobile families, single parent families, blended families, childless marriages, multigenerational families, and single persons will all pursue the activities of faith seeking and health seeking in unique and diverse ways. Such diversity needs to be included as integral to the way faith communities imagine themselves in the future.

To summarize this section, then, we underscore the importance of bringing a vision of faith to health through remembering and imagining. Indeed, this task is one in which faith communities need to play a key role. Bringing faith to health is the task of probing faith traditions for the spiritual health resources that emanate from deeply rooted, enduring, and unifying religious values. Such core, embedded, healing values, and the spiritual health resources they give rise to, will foster wholeness for today and for the future.

৵ Bringing a Vision of Health to Faith

Just as we have identified faith communities, in all their diversity, as playing a key role in the process of bringing a vision of faith to health, we believe it is important to consider key players in the complementary task of bringing a vision of health to faith. Previous chapters of this book have identified that we are living in significant times of personal, as well as societal, transition. In this regard, some of what we see when we look around us is the turbulence of shifting values and a climate of unending cultural change. Innovations of the second millennium (Friedman, 1997), together with technological breakthroughs of the twentieth century, have had profound consequences regarding health as an integral dimension of living, behaving, and developing. For health to bear witness to faith, therefore, everyone needs to recognize, accept, and take seriously his or her unique role as an agent of health promotion. We are *all* key players when it comes to health. Health is a social phenomenon, with family and community as the primary contexts within which health is learned (Allen, 1981). Whether a person is identified as a health professional or not, it is the responsibility of every individual, family, group, and community to foster life qualities that promote wholeness. With this in mind, we believe that families and communities are in a position to *bring a vision of health to faith* through the activities of connecting and embodying.

With spiritual hunger in such great evidence, and the need for *connection* as a recognized dimension of this hunger (Clinebell, 1992), it is lamentable that faith communities are only little known for their connective function. Health issues, on the other hand, connect people in every walk of life and in every population base around the world. Writing about community health nursing in the future, Miriam Stewart (1995a) says that health reform in Canada is intimately linked with the unpredictable economic, environmental, technological, and social challenges that are in evidence. She goes on to connect health in Canada with health issues around the globe by listing a number of the health challenges we are facing today. Included in this list are the following:

- The continued escalation of total health costs
- The growing population of seniors
- New health problems arising from environmental pollutants
- The reemergence of communicable diseases
- The treatment of resistant strains of bacteria and viruses
- Increases in sexually transmitted illness and HIV infection
- The continuing costs of cancer, cardiovascular illness, and other chronic diseases

- Persistent maternal and infant health challenges
- The prolongation of physical function by technology

One would be hard pressed to find oneself excluded from such a list. By their very nature, health, health issues, and health challenges are connecting. This is the vision health brings to religious traditions and faith communities. Put another way, just as health and illness are innate to every human community, they are innate to every faith community. Including an awareness of health as integral to faith in our living, behaving, and developing, therefore, needs to become a new *sine qua non* within our world's religious traditions and faith communities.

In addition to connecting, bringing a vision of health to faith occurs through *embodying*. Previous chapters of this book have drawn attention to historical, philosophical, and attitudinal processes that have resulted in artificial separations. Dichotomies and dualisms, for example, can create some unhealthy forms of differentiation. Without going into the rich depth of theological and philosophical literature on this topic, it can be said that Christianity incorporated an unhealthy dichotomy in the formulation of its theological anthropology. On the side of wholeness promotion, Pauline literature reveals a theocentric or God-centered approach to the human person. The letter 1 Thessalonians, for instance, draws to a close with the words, "May the God of peace make you perfect and holy; and may you all be kept safe and blameless, spirit, soul and body" (1 Thess. 5:23 NRSV). This image of humanity conveys a holistic theological anthropology, and, although there are differentiations within the Pauline texts, they maintain a theocentric focus on wholeness.

By contrast, within a few centuries' time, Christianity was using language derived from Greek philosophy. In that cultural context, tensions between spirit/matter and body/spirit were in evidence. These tensions became linked with Christian theological anthropology in patristic literature (Cross & Livingstone, 1974). There, a significant shift toward anthropocentric or human-centered consciousness is noticeable. Likewise in evidence is a tendency away from *embodiment*. There has been a call in recent years to reconnect the body, mind, and spirit within Christian theology (Brock, 1988; Ferder & Heagle, 1992; Goergen, 1974; Heyward, 1982, 1989; Nelson, 1976). In contrast, there is no questioning of the importance of the body in the arena of health. It is simply understood, as a matter of fact, that the body is important and deserving of care. Embodying health is a positive objective. Furthermore, the orientation to embody health through one's living, behaving, and developing is an orientation that has parallels in faith communities. Faith, like health, is something oriented to embodiment, inasmuch as it is through our bodies that we learn about our faith, appropriate the meaning of our faith, and express the values of our faith. Indeed, the enduring and unifying values embedded in diverse faith traditions, as referred to in the previous section of this chapter, need to become connected and embodied in concrete ways. Examples of this might be (a) learning more, within the context of local faith communities, about the determinants of health, (b) visualizing local congregations as community health centers, and (c) developing health initiatives within local faith communities that impact the health of broader realms of society.

✑ Faith Community Nurses at the Crossroads of Faith and Health

This book has discussed various topics about nursing within the context of a faith community. It offers theoretical underpinnings drawn from the two disciplines of theology and nursing. Furthermore, the book focuses on faith community nurses as agents of health promotion in times of transition. In this final section of our final chapter, we draw attention to faith community nurses at the crossroads of faith and health. Since the unique functions developed within parish nursing (Holstrom, 1999) are foundational to our understanding of faith community nursing, we repeat once again what we have shared previously: At the same time that it is historically rooted, faith community nursing is also "new." It is being formed out of, and will embody, values of today that hold promises for health and faith integration for the future. Thus, faith community nursing is a unique health resource that can be made available through local faith communities to the larger society. Faith community nurses, therefore, will want to explore the *mediating* and *transforming* potential of their social location at the crossroads of faith and health.

Earlier, when discussing the idea of bringing a vision of faith to health through imagination, we wrote about the value of family-centered faith communities. In our current discussion, we return to this focus on families, and reiterate what we have been saying throughout our book about the McGill model of nursing. Specifically, the McGill model derives from a family-based approach to health promotion. Furthermore, it rests on the core concepts of health, family, learning, and collaboration. It is thus a health model with the potential to interact with faith models. In Chapter 21, by means of the hermeneutic spiral of learning guided by inquiry, we demonstrated one possible way through which this interaction can occur. In our spiral of learning, the McGill nursing model serves in a *mediating* capacity. That is, with the assistance of guiding questions derived from the model, faith leaders and faith community nurses can foster integrative learning about faith and health in the lives of those they serve. This example raises the possibility that there are additional ways to imagine family-centered faith communities using nursing models and holistic community health approaches as they bring visions of faith to health, and health to faith, for the future. We look forward to hearing more from others on this topic.

In addition to introducing the McGill nursing model as a mediating resource for faith community nurses, we also presented two mediating images of nursing. These are the health-promoting images of nurse as *confidant*, found in Chapter 9, and faith community nurse as *broker*, found in Chapter 15. We believe each of these images reflects the mediating function of the nurse as referral agent and liaison with congregational and community resources (Holstrom, 1999). The nurse as confidante is emotionally and spiritually mature, clear about the scope and boundaries of her or his nursing practice within the faith community context, sincere and caring in relating with others, and views nursing work as a ministry. The nurse as broker serves as a middle person or agent in connecting people, in their times of transition, with health, healing, and health-promoting resources found in both faith community and broader community contexts. Thus, faith community nurses are in a position to be continually mediating or brokering health resources. That is, as a ministry professional who works in collaboration with other faith group leaders, the faith community nurse is free to go out from the local congregation to meet, sojourn with, and accompany those who are awakening to health issues that are also faith issues. Likewise, as a health professional, the nurse is also free to bring into the local faith community health resources that can also foster spiritual growth. It is a pivotal position.

In closing, we draw attention to the *transforming* potential of faith community nursing in its location at the crossroads of faith and health. In this regard, we turn to the insights of Leland Kaiser (1993), who discusses leaders creating healthier communities. He describes seven types of transformational leadership, and we propose applying Kaiser's leadership types as follows. First, bringing faith visions to health involves leadership that "invokes the void of infinite possibilities" through the activities of remembering and imagining. Likewise, bringing health visions to faith can involve connecting and embodying by "crystallizing" ideas about health and faith from vague notions to concrete blueprints, "seeding" ideas regarding the integration of faith and health into consciousness, and "incarnating" ideas into form. Furthermore, faith community nurse leaders are "perfecting the form" of the identified functions associated with this new nursing specialty, "deepening the idea" of faith community nursing in such a way that it can move into its full potential, and "evolving the form" of faith community nursing by creating ever better manifestations of its effectiveness, in making the idea work in a real world. These seven leadership roles are what it means to be *transforming*. That is, faith community nursing is a journey that takes the nurse into a metamorphic condition; like the caterpillar yielding itself to the cocoon and beginning to spin the chrysalis of transformation, faith community nurses surrender to a process of conversion and permutation. Although their identity as nurses remains constant, they are opening themselves to a form that has not yet achieved its full potential. Faith community nursing, in other words, is still an evolving phenomenon at the crossroads of faith and health.

Nursing within a faith community in times of transition is transformative through the medium of health promotion. It is a ministry profession sustained through inquiry and collaboration. It constantly learns by means of skilled compassion, disciplined exploration, and careful discovery. Seen in this light, we believe it is more valuable to speak of faith community nursing as a question about the integration of faith and health, than to refer to it as an answer for integrating faith with health. We believe faith community nurses, as question-raising and question-accompanying confidantes, will *transform* their environments by promoting inquiry within the context of faith communities that represent a broad diversity of faith traditions. Our invitation is "to love the *questions themselves*," and let the living of questions about this valuable health resource within faith communities proceed gradually, so that it can "live along some distant day into the answer" (Rilke, 1934, p. 35).

∽ Summary

In this chapter, we have looked at bringing a vision of faith and health into the future with an exploration of four topic areas. First, we discussed *visioning* by means of three questions: Vision is generated by asking "What do I see?" Moving vision forward from ambiguity to specific form involves asking "How do we write the vision down and make it plain?" Finally, in order to keep vision current and viable, it is important to question the vision by asking "Where did this vision come from?" For vision to take hold, there is need for openness, inquiry, practical rootedness, risk, courage, and perseverance.

The second and third topics in this chapter were *bringing a vision of faith to health* and *bringing a vision of health to faith*. In this regard, we said that faith visioning engages health through remembering and imagining; likewise, health visioning engages faith through connecting and embodying. Our final topic was *faith community nursing at the crossroads of faith and health*. Here, we discussed the mediating and transforming potential of faith community nursing in its social location at the crossroads where faith and health are being integrated in the lives of individuals, families, groups, and communities.

Now, we draw our book to a close by returning to the T. S. Eliot poem used to introduce our first chapter. In light of all that has been shared from that point to this, we repeat the words already shared, and add further verses, to convey the sense of hope and encouragement we feel in relationship with the emerging field of faith community nursing.

> With the drawing of this Love and the voice of this Calling
> We shall not cease from exploration
> And the end of all our exploring
> Will be to arrive where we started
> And know the place for the first time.
> Through the unknown, remembered gate
> When the last of earth left to discover

Is that which was the beginning;

. . . .

But heard, half-heard, in the stillness

. . . .

A condition of complete simplicity
(Costing not less than everything)
And all shall be well and
All manner of thing shall be well. . . .

(Eliot, 1943/1971)

Note

1. The person in North America credited with focusing on adult learning praxis is Malcolm Knowles (1980). *Pedagogy*, in Knowles, refers to child learning praxis; *andragogy* to adult learning praxis. The roots for both words are in the Greek words for child (*paidos*) and adult (*andros*). Although Knowles' approached andragogy from a secular perspective, Paulo Freire (1970/1993) has adapted similar principles for spiritual formation and political action. Leon McKenzie (1982), Nancy Foltz (1986), and Thomas Groome (1991) have adapted similar principles for religious education.

References

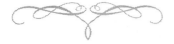

Achterberg, J. (1985). *Imagery in healing: Shamanism and modern medicine.* Boston: Shambhala.

Achterberg, J. (1990). *Woman as healer.* Boston: Shambhala.

Alberta Association of Registered Nurses. (1997). *Professional boundaries: A discussion paper on expectations for nurse-client relationships.* Edmonton, Alberta: Author.

Allemang, M. (1985). Development of community health nursing in Canada. In M. Stewart, J. Innes, S. Searl, & C. Smillie (Eds.), *Community health nursing in Canada* (pp. 3-29). Toronto, Ontario: Gage.

Allen, M. (1977). Comparative theories of the expanded role in nursing and implications for nursing practice: A working paper. *Nursing Papers, 9,* 38-45.

Allen, M. (1979). Viewpoint: Notes on the contribution of nursing to health care. *Nursing Papers, 11,* 3.

Allen, M. (1981). The health dimension in nursing practice: Notes on nursing in primary health care. *Journal of Advanced Nursing, 6,* 153-154.

Allen, M. (1982a). A model of nursing: A plan for research and development. In *Research—A base for the future: Proceedings of the international conference on nursing research.* Edinburgh, Scotland: University of Edinburgh.

Allen, M. (1982b, May). *Shaping health potential: The cutting edge of practice in nursing.* Paper presented at the Rozella M. Scholfeldt Lectureship, Frances Payne Bolton School of Nursing, Case Western Reserve University, Cleveland, OH.

Allen, M. (1986). A developmental health model—Nursing as continuous inquiry [Cassette recording]. In *Nursing theory congress: Theoretical pluralism: Directions for a practice discipline.* Markham, Ontario: Audio Archives of Canada.

Allen, M. (1997a). Comparative theories of the expanded role in nursing and implications for nursing practice: A working paper. In L. Gottlieb & H. Ezer (Eds.), *A perspective on health, family, learning and collaborative nursing: A collection of writing on the McGill model of nursing* (pp. 10-15). Montreal, Quebec: McGill University School of Nursing.

Allen, M. (1997b). Primary care nursing: Research in action. In L. Gottlieb & H. Ezer (Eds.), *A perspective on health, family, learning and collaborative nursing: A collection of writing on the McGill model of nursing* (pp. 164-190). Montreal, Quebec: McGill University School of Nursing.

American college dictionary. (1970). New York: Random House.

Amundsen, D. W., & Ferngren, G. B. (1986). The early Christian tradition. In R. L. Numbers & D. W. Amundsen (Eds.), *Caring and curing: Health and medicine in the Western religious traditions* (pp. 40-64). New York: Macmillan.

Anderson, E., & McFarlane, J. (1988). *Community as client: Application of the nursing process.* Philadelphia: J. B. Lippincott.

Ashbrook, J. B. (1955). Not by bread alone. *American Journal of Nursing, 55*(2), 164-168.

Astedt-Kurki, P. (1995). Religiosity as a dimension of well-being. *Clinical Nursing Research, 4*(4), 387-396.

Attridge, C., Ezer, H., & Macdonald, J. P. (1981). Implementing program philosophy through curricular decisions. *Nursing Papers, 13*(1), 59-69.

Barker, J. (1992). *Paradigms: The business of discovering the future.* New York: HarperCollins.

Barnum, B. S. (1996). *Spirituality in nursing: From traditional to new age.* New York: Springer.

Becker, A. (1985). *The compassionate visitor.* Minneapolis, MN: Augsburg.

Belcher, A. E., Dettmore, D., & Holzemer, S. P. (1989). Spirituality and sense of well-being in persons with AIDS. *Holistic Nursing Practice, 3*(4), 16-25.

Belenky, M., Clinchy, B., Goldberger, N., & Tarule, J. (1986). *Women's ways of knowing: The development of self, voice and mind.* New York: Basic Books.

Bellingham, R., Cohen, B., Jones, T., & Spaniol, L. (1989). Connectedness: Some skills for spiritual health. *American Journal of Health Promotion, 4*(1), 18-24, 31.

Berger, P., & Luckmann, T. (1966). *The social construction of reality.* Garden City, NY: Doubleday.

Berggren-Thomas, P., & Griggs, M. J. (1995, March). Spirituality in aging: Spiritual need or spiritual journey? *Journal of Gerontological Nursing,* pp. 5-9.

Bergquist, S., & King, J. (1994). Parish nursing: A conceptual framework. *Journal of Holistic Nursing, 12*(2), 155-170.

Bibby, R. (1993). *Unknown gods: The ongoing story of religion in Canada.* Toronto, Ontario: Stoddart.

Bibby, R. (1995). *There's got to be more!* Winfield, British Columbia: Woodlake Books.

Blattner, B. (1981). *Holistic nursing.* Englewood Cliffs, NJ: Prentice Hall.

Bolton, R. (1979). *People skills.* Englewood Cliffs, NJ: Prentice Hall.

Bomar, P. J. (1996). Family health promotion. In S. Hanson & S. Boyd (Eds.), *Family health care nursing: Theory, practice, and research* (pp. 175-199). Philadelphia: F. A. Davis.

Booty, J. E. (1986). The Anglican tradition. In R. L. Numbers & D. W. Amundsen (Eds.), *Caring and curing: Health and medicine in the Western religious traditions* (pp. 240-270). New York: Macmillan.

Bosch, D. (1996). *Transforming mission: Paradigm shifts in theology of mission.* Maryknoll, NY: Orbis Books.

Boschma, G. (1994). The meaning of holism in nursing: Historical shifts in holistic nursing ideas. *Public Health Nursing, 11*(5), 324-330.

Boss, J. G., & Corbett, J. (1990). The developing practice of the parish nurse: An inner-city experience. In P. A. Solari-Twadell, A. M. Djupe, & M. A. McDermott (Eds.), *Parish nursing: The developing practice* (pp. 77-103). Park Ridge, IL: National Parish Nurse Resource Center.

Boutell, K. A., & Bozett, F. W. (1990). Nurses' assessment of patients' spirituality: Continuing education implications. *Journal of Continuing Education in Nursing, 21*(4), 172-176.

Bowker, J. (Ed.). (1997). *The Oxford dictionary of world religions.* New York: Oxford University Press.

Boyd, C. (1952). *Tithes and parishes in medieval Italy: The historical roots of a modern problem.* Ithaca, NY: Cornell University Press.

Bradley, J., & Edinberg, M. (1982). *Communication in the nursing context.* Englewood Cliffs, NJ: Prentice Hall.

Brammer, L. M. (1979). *The helping relationship: Process and skills.* Englewood Cliffs, NJ. Prentice Hall.

Brennan, P. (1994). *Re-imagining the parish.* New York: Crossroad.

Bridges, W. (1980). *Transitions.* Reading, MA: Addison-Wesley.

Bridges, W. (1991). *Managing transitions: Making the most of change.* Reading, MA: Addison-Wesley.

Briggs, J. S. (1987). Volunteer qualities: A survey of hospice volunteers. *Oncology Nursing Forum, 14*(1), 27-31.

Brittain, J. N. (1986). Theological foundations for spiritual care. *Journal of Religion and Health, 25*(2), 107-121.

Brittain, J. N., & Boozer, J. (1987). Spiritual care: Integration into collegiate nursing curriculum. *Journal of Nursing Education, 26*(4), 155-160.

Brock, R. N. (1988). *Journeys by heart.* New York: Crossroad.

Brown, E. L. (1948). *Nursing for the future.* New York: Russell Sage Foundation.

Browne, A. (1993). Conceptual clarification of respect. *Journal of Advanced Nursing, 18,* 211-217.

Brueggemann, W. (1978). *The prophetic imagination.* Philadelphia: Fortress.

Bunkers, S. (1998). A nursing theory—Guided model of health ministry: Human becoming in parish nursing. *Nursing Science Quarterly, 11*(1), 7-8.

Bunkers, S. (1999). Translating nursing conceptual frameworks and theory for nursing practice. In P. A. Solari-Twadell & M. A. McDermott (Eds.), *Parish* nursing: Promoting whole person health within faith communities (pp. 205-214). Thousand Oaks, CA: Sage.

Burgener, S. C., Jivovec, M., Murrel, L., & Barton, D. (1992). Caregiver and environmental variables related to difficult behaviors in institutionalized, demented elderly persons. *Journal of Gerontology: Psychological Sciences, 47*(4), 242-249.

Burgener, S. C., Shimer, R., & Murrel, L. (1993). Expressions of individuality in cognitively impaired elders. *Journal of Gerontological Nursing, 19*(4), 13-22.

Burkhardt, M. A. (1989). Spirituality: An analysis of the concept. *Holistic Nursing Practice, 3*(3), 69-77.

Burkhardt, M. A., & Nagai-Jacobson, M. G. (1985). Dealing with spiritual concerns of clients in the community. *Journal of Community Health Nursing, 2*(4), 191-198.

Burley-Allen, M. (1995). *Listening, the forgotten skill.* New York: John Wiley.

Burnard, P. (1987). Spiritual distress and the nursing response: Theoretical considerations and counseling skills. *Journal of Advanced Nursing, 12*, 377-382.

Buttitta, P. (1995). Theological reflection in health ministry: A strategy for parish nurses. In J. D. Whitehead & E. E. Whitehead, *Method in ministry* (pp. 112-122). Kansas City, MO: Sheed & Ward.

Buttrick, G. A. (Ed.). (1962). *The interpreter's dictionary of the bible.* Nashville, TN: Abingdon.

Cada, L., Fitz, R., Foley, G., Giardino, T., & Lichtenberg, C. (1979). *Shaping the coming age of religious life.* New York: Seabury.

Campbell, J. (1968). *The hero with a thousand faces.* Princeton, NJ: Princeton University Press.

Campbell, J. (1988). *The power of myth.* Garden City, NY: Doubleday.

Caplow, T. (1954). *The sociology of work.* Minneapolis, MN: University of Minnesota Press.

Capra, F., & Steindl-Rast, D. (1991). *Belonging to the universe.* New York: HarperCollins.

Carkhuff, R. (1983). *The art of helping.* Amherst, MA: Human Resource Development.

Carpenito, L. J. (1989). *Nursing diagnosis, application to clinical practice.* Philadelphia: J. B. Lippincott.

Carson, V. B. (1980). Meeting the spiritual needs of hospitalized psychiatric patients. *Perspectives in Psychiatric Care, 8*(1), 17-20.

Carson, V. B. (1989). *Spiritual dimensions of nursing practice.* Philadelphia: W. B. Saunders.

Catholic Health Association of Canada. (1996). *Spirituality and health: What's good for the soul can be good for the body, too.* Ottawa, Ontario: Author.

Chandler, C. K., Holden, J. M., & Kolander, C. A. (1992). Counseling for spiritual wellness: Theory and practice. *Journal of Counseling and Development, 71*, 168-175.

Chevier, F., Steuer, R., & MacKenzie, J. (1994, July/August). Factors affecting satisfaction among community-based hospice volunteer visitors. *American Journal of Hospice and Palliative Care*, pp. 30-37.

Chittister, J. (1998). *Heart of flesh.* Grand Rapids, MI: W. B. Eerdmans.

Christensen, P. J. (1986a). Assessment: Overview of data collection. In J. W. Griffith-Kenney & P. J. Christensen (Eds.), *Nursing process: Application of theories, frameworks, and models* (2nd ed., pp. 57-67). St. Louis, MO: C. V. Mosby.

Christensen, P. J. (1986b). Planning: Priorities, goals, and objectives. In J. W. Griffith-Kenney & P. J. Christensen (Eds.), *Nursing process: Application of theories, frameworks, and models* (2nd. ed., pp. 169-182). St. Louis, MO: C. V. Mosby

Cirlot, J. E. (1962). *A dictionary of symbols.* New York: Philosophical Library.

Clark, C. C., Cross, J. R., Deane, D. M., & Lowry, L. W. (1991). Spirituality: Integral to quality care. *Holistic Nursing Practice, 5*(3), 67-76.

Clark, M. (1998). Power imbalance: Evolving theory in need of research. *Western Journal of Nursing Research, 20*(5), 517-520.

Clark, M., & Brink, P. (1996). *Toward the definition of a spiritual need.* Unpublished research feasibility project presented to St. Stephen's College, Edmonton, Alberta.

Clinebell, H. (1984). *Basic types of pastoral care and counseling.* Nashville, TN: Abingdon.

Clinebell, H. (1992). *Well being.* New York: HarperCollins.

Cloud, H., & Townsend, J. (1992). *Boundaries.* Grand Rapids, MI: Zondervan.

Cobb, M., & Robshaw, V. (1998). *The spiritual challenge of health care.* London: Churchill Livingstone.

Cohen, D. (1991). *The circle of life: Rituals from the human family album.* New York: HarperCollins.

Colgrove, M., Bloomfield, H., & McWilliams, P. (1991). *How to survive the loss of a love.* Los Angeles: Prelude.

Combs, A., Avila, D., & Purkey, W. (1971). *Helping relationships: Basic concepts for the helping professionals.* Boston: Allyn & Bacon.

Conrad, N. L. (1985). Spiritual support for the dying. *Nursing Clinics of North America, 20*(2), 415-426.

Covey, S. R. (1994). *First things first.* New York: Simon & Schuster.

Cross, F. L., & Livingstone, E. A. (Eds.). (1974). *The Oxford dictionary of the Christian church.* New York: Oxford University Press.

Crossan, J. (1975). *The dark interval: Towards a theology of story.* Allen, TX: Argus Communications.

Cutrona, C. (1990). Stress and social support: In search of optimal matching. *Journal of Social and Clinical Psychology, 9*(1), 3-14.

Deloughery, G. L. (1995). History of the nursing profession. In G. L. Deloughery (Ed.), *Issues and trends in nursing* (2nd ed., pp. 1-52). St. Louis, MO: C. V. Mosby.

Dickinson, C. (1975). The search for spiritual meaning. *American Journal of Nursing, 75*(10), 1789-1793.

Djupe, A. M., Olson, H., & Ryan, J. A. (1994). *Reaching out: Parish nursing services.* Park Ridge, IL: National Parish Nurse Resource Center.

Doehring, C. (1995). *Taking care: Monitoring power dynamics and relational-boundaries in pastoral care and counseling*. Nashville, TN: Abingdon.

Doka, K. (1996). *Living with grief after sudden loss*. Washington, DC: Hospice Foundation of America.

Dolan, J. A., Fitzpatrick, M. L., & Hermann, E. K. (1983). *Nursing in society: A historical perspective* (5th ed.). Philadelphia: W. B. Saunders.

Donahue, M. P. (1985). *Nursing: The finest art*. St. Louis, MO: C. V. Mosby.

Doyle, A. (1929a). Nursing by religious orders in the United States. Part 2—1841–1870. *American Journal of Nursing, 29*(8), 959-969.

Doyle, A. (1929b). Nursing by religious orders in the United States. Part 4—Lutheran Deaconesses, 1849–1928. *American Journal of Nursing, 29*(10), 1197-1207.

Doyle, A. (1929c). Nursing by religious orders in the United States. Part 6—Episcopal Sisterhood, 1845–1928. *American Journal of Nursing, 29*(12), 1466-1481.

Draper, E. (1965). *Psychiatry and pastoral care*. Englewood Cliffs, NJ: Prentice Hall.

Droege, T. A. (1995). Congregations as communities of health and healing. *Interpretation: A Journal of Bible and Theology, 49*(2), 117-129.

Drummond, T. (1996). *The ministerial counseling role*. Carson City, NV: The Plains Group.

Dulles, A. (1994). *The assurance of things hoped for*. New York: Oxford University Press.

Edelman, J., & Crain, M. (1993). *The tao of negotiation*. New York: HarperCollins.

Egan, G. (1982). *The skilled helper: Model, skills, and methods for effective helping* (2nd ed.). Belmont, CA: Brooks/Cole.

Eisler, R. (1987). *The chalice and the blade: Our history, our future*. New York: Harper & Row.

Eisler, R., & Loye, D. (1990). *The partnership way*. New York: HarperCollins.

Eliot, A. (1976). *The universal myths, heroes, gods, tricksters and others*. New York: Penguin.

Eliot, T. S. (1971). "Little Gidding." *The four quartets*. New York: Harcourt Brace Jovanovich. (Original work published in 1943)

Ellis, D. (1980). Whatever happened to the spiritual dimension? *Canadian Nurse, 76*(8), 42-43.

Ellison, C. W. (1983). Spiritual well-being: Conceptualization and measurement. *Journal of Psychology and Theology, 11*(4), 330-340.

Ellison, C. W., & Smith, J. (1991). Toward an integrative measure of health and well-being. *Journal of Psychology and Theology, 19*(1), 35-48.

El-Sanabary, N. (1993). The education and contributions of women health care professionals in Saudi-Arabia: The case of nursing. *Social Science and Medicine, 37*(11), 1331-1343.

Emblen, J. D. (1992). Religion and spirituality defined according to current use in nursing literature. *Journal of Professional Nursing, 8*(1), 41-47.

Emblen, J. D., & Halstead, L. (1993). Spiritual needs and interventions: Comparing the views of patients, nurses and chaplains. *Clinical Nurse Specialist, 7*(4), 175-182.

Erikson, E. (1963). *Childhood and society.* New York: Norton.

Erikson, E. (1968). *Identity: Youth and crisis.* New York: Norton.

Erikson, E. (1980). *Identity and the life cycle.* New York: Norton.

Erikson, E. (1982). *The life cycle completed.* New York: Norton.

Evans, A. R. (1995). The church as an institution of healing. *Interpretations: A Journal of Bible and Theology, 49*(2), 158-171.

Evans, A. R. (1998, September). *Prescription for health: Healthy living, holy lives.* Paper presented at the 12th Annual Westberg Parish Nurse Symposium, Itasca, IL.

Everett, D. (1996). *Forget me not: The spiritual care of people with Alzheimer's.* Edmonton, Alberta: Inkwell.

Ezer, H., Bray, C., & Gros, C. (1997). Families' descriptions of the nursing interventions in a randomized control trial. In L. Gottlieb & H. Ezer (Eds.), *A perspective on health, family, learning and collaborative nursing: A collection of writing on the McGill model of nursing* (pp. 362-368). Montreal, Quebec: McGill University School of Nursing.

Fawcett, J. (1993). *Analysis and evaluation of nursing theories.* Philadelphia: F. A. Davis.

Fawcett, J. (1995). *Analysis and evaluation of conceptual models of nursing* (3rd ed.). Philadelphia: F. A. Davis.

Fayram, E. S. (1986). Implementation. In J. W. Griffith-Kenney & P. J. Christensen (Eds.), *Nursing process: Application of theories, frameworks, and models* (2nd ed., pp. 212-218). St. Louis, MO: C. V. Mosby.

Federal Provincial and Territorial Advisory Committee on Population Health. (1994). *Strategies for population health.* Ottawa, Ontario: Health Canada.

Feeley, N., & Gerez-Lirette, T. (1997). Development of professional practice based on the McGill model of nursing in an ambulatory care setting. In L. Gottlieb & H. Ezer (Eds.), *A perspective on health, family, learning and collaborative nursing: A collection of writing on the McGill model of nursing* (pp. 296-307). Montreal, Quebec: McGill University School of Nursing.

Fehring, R. J., Brennan, P. F., & Keller, M. L. (1987). Psychological and spiritual well-being in college students. *Research in Nursing and Health, 10,* 391-398.

Ferder, F., & Heagle, J. (1989). *Partnership: Women and men in ministry.* Notre Dame, IN: Ave Maria Press.

Ferder, F., & Heagle, J. (1992). *Your sexual self.* Notre Dame, IN: Ave Maria Press.

Feucht, O. E. (1974). *Everyone a minister.* St. Louis, MO: Concordia.

Fitchett, G. (1993a). *Assessing spiritual needs.* Minneapolis, MN: Augsburg.

Fitchett, G. (1993b). *Spiritual assessment in pastoral care: A guide to selected resources.* Decatur, GA: Journal of Pastoral Care Publications.

Flexner, A. (1910). Is social work a profession? *Medical education in the United States and Canada: A report to the Carnegie Foundation for the Advancement of Teaching* (Vol. 4). New York: Carnegie Foundation for the Advancement of Teaching.

Foley, G. (1995). *Family-centered church.* Kansas City, MO: Sheed & Ward.

Foltz, N. (1986). *Handbook of adult religious education.* Birmingham, AL: Religious Education.

Ford, I. M. (1988). *Life spirals: The faith journey.* Burlington, Ontario: Welch.

Ford-Gilboe, M. (1994). A comparison of two nursing models: Allen's developmental health model and Newman's theory of health as expanding consciousness. *Nursing Science Quarterly, 7*(3), 113-118.

Fortune, M. (1983). *Sexual violence: The unmentionable sin.* New York: Pilgrim Press.

Fortune, M. (1989). *Is nothing sacred?* New York: HarperCollins.

Fortune, M. (1992). *Clergy misconduct: Sexual abuse in the ministerial relationship.* Seattle, WA: Center for the Prevention of Sexual and Domestic Violence.

Fowler, J. W. (1981). *Stages in faith.* New York: Harper & Row.

Fowler, J. W. (1991). *Weaving the new creation.* New York: HarperCollins.

Frankl, V. (1984). *Man's search for meaning.* Boston: Beacon. (Original work published in 1959)

Freire, P. (1993). *Pedagogy of the oppressed.* New York: Continuum. (Original work published in 1970)

Freud, S. (1953-1974). *The standard edition of the complete psychological writings of Sigmund Freud* (Vols. 1-24). (J. Strachey, Ed. and Trans.) London: Hogarth Press.

Friedman, E. (1985). *Generation to generation: Family process in church and synagogue.* New York: Guilford.

Friedman, M. (1986). *Family nursing: Theory and assessment.* Norwalk, CT: Appleton-Century-Crofts.

Friedman, R. (Ed.). (1997, Fall). *Life Magazine: The millennium* [Special issue].

Gass, R. (1992). The song of Chief Seattle. *Medicine wheel* [Cassette recording]. Boulder, CO: Spring Hill Music.

Germain, C. P. (1992). Cultural care: A bridge between sickness, illness, and disease. *Holistic Nursing Practice, 6*(3), 1-9.

Gerrard, B., Boniface, W., & Love, B. (1980). *Interpersonal skills for health professionals.* Reston, VA: Reston.

Ghai, S., & Ghai, C. M. (1997). The ancient origin of nursing in India. *Nursing Journal of India, 88*(6), 131-132.

Gibbon, J., & Mathewson, M. (1947). *Three centuries of Canadian nursing.* Toronto, Ontario: Macmillan.

Gibson, C. (1996). *Signs and symbols.* Rowayton, CT: Saraband.

Gilligan, C. (1982). *In a different voice.* Cambridge, MA: Harvard University Press.

Gilligan, C., Ward, J., & Taylor, J. (1988). *Mapping the moral domain: A contribution of women's thinking to psychological theory and education.* Cambridge, MA: Harvard Graduate School of Education, Center for the Study of Gender, Education, and Human Development.

Giovannetti, P. (1990). News release. *AARN Newsletter, 46*(1), 7.

Goddard, N. (1995a). *The fourth dimension: Conceptualizations of spirituality.* Unpublished master's thesis, University of Alberta, Edmonton, Alberta.

Goddard, N. (1995b). Spirituality as "integrative energy": A philosophical analysis as precursor to wholistic nursing practice. *Journal of Advanced Nursing, 22*, 808-815.

Goergen, D. (1974). *The sexual celibate.* New York: Seabury.

Gold, V. (1989, June). Shalom. Paper presented at ELCA Churchwide Leadership Conference on Health and Wholeness in the Church, Berkeley, CA.

Goleman, D., & Speeth, K. R. (1982). *The essential psychotherapies.* New York: New American Library.

Gordon, S. (1993). *The encyclopedia of myths and legends.* London: Headline.

Gordon, T. (1970). *Parent effectiveness training.* New York: Wyden.

Gottlieb, L. (1997). Health promoters: Two contrasting styles in community nursing. In L. Gottlieb & H. Ezer (Eds.), *A perspective on health, family, learning and collaborative nursing: A collection of writing on the McGill model of nursing* (pp. 98-112). Montreal, Quebec: McGill University School of Nursing.

Gottlieb, L., & Allen, M. (1997). Developing a classification system to examine a model of nursing in primary care settings. In L. Gottlieb & H. Ezer (Eds.), *A perspective on health, family, learning and collaborative nursing: A collection of writing on the McGill model of nursing* (pp. 18-31). Montreal, Quebec: McGill University School of Nursing.

Gottlieb, L., & Ezer, H. (1997). Preface. In L. Gottlieb & H. Ezer (Eds.), *A perspective on health, family, learning and collaborative nursing: A collection of writing on the McGill model of nursing* (pp. xi-xiii). Montreal, Quebec: McGill University School of Nursing.

Gottlieb, L., & Rowat, K. (1987). The McGill model of nursing: A practice-derived model. *Advances in Nursing Science, 9*(4), 51-61.

Gould, M. (1994). Volunteerism: A method of self-renewal. *ANNA Journal, 21*(5), 297.

Graham, L. K. (1992). *Care of persons, care of worlds.* Nashville, TN: Abingdon.

Griffith-Kenney, J. W. (1986). Evaluation. In J. W. Griffith-Kenney & P. J. Christensen (Eds.), *Nursing process: Application of theories, frameworks, and models* (2nd. ed., pp. 219-230.). St. Louis, MO: C. V. Mosby.

Groer, M. W., O'Connor, B., & Droppleman, P. G. (1996). A course in health care spirituality. *Journal of Nursing Education, 35*(8), 375-377.

Groome, T. (1991). *Sharing faith.* New York: HarperCollins.

Gros, C., & Ezer, H. (1997). Promoting inquiry and nurse-client collaboration: A unique approach to teaching and learning. In L. Gottlieb & H. Ezer (Eds.), *A perspective on health, family, learning and collaborative nursing: A collection of writings on the McGill model of nursing* (pp. 219-235). Montreal, Quebec: McGill University School of Nursing.

Grossman-Schulz, M., & Feeley, N. (1997). A working model of support. In L. Gottlieb & H. Ezer (Eds.), *A perspective on health, family, learning and collaborative nursing: A collection of writing on the McGill model of nursing* (pp. 277-286). Montreal, Quebec: McGill University School of Nursing.

Haase, J. E., Britt, T., Coward, D. D., Leidy, N. K., & Penn, P. E. (1992). Simultaneous concept analysis of spiritual perspective, hope, acceptance and self-transcendence. *Image: Journal of Nursing Scholarship, 24*(2), 141-147.

Hall, B. P. (1982). *Shepherds and lovers: A guide to spiritual leadership and Christian ministry.* New York: Paulist Press.

Hall, B. P. (1986). *The genesis effect.* New York: Paulist Press.

Hall, B. P. (1991). *Spiritual connections.* Dayton, OH: Values Technology.

Hall, G. R., & Buckwalter, K. C. (1987). Progressively lowered stress threshold: A conceptual model for care of adults with Alzheimer's disease. *Archives of Psychiatric Nursing, 1*, 399-406.

Hamilton, E. (1940). *Mythology: Timeless tales of gods and heroes.* New York: Penguin.

Harakas, S. S. (1986). The eastern tradition. In R. L. Numbers & D. W. Amundsen (Eds.), *Caring and curing: Health and medicine in the Western religious traditions* (pp. 146-172). New York: Macmillan.

Heliker, D. (1992). Re-evaluation of a nursing diagnosis: Spiritual distress. *Nursing Forum, 27*(4), 15-20.

Hellwig, M. (1992). *Theology at the service of spirituality. The Anthony Jordan Lectures* [Cassette recording]. Edmonton, Alberta: Newman Theological College.

Herink, R. (1980). *The psychotherapy handbook.* New York: New American Library.

Herman, J. (1992). *Trauma and recovery.* New York: Basic Books.

Hermani, H. (1996). *The history of nursing in Pakistan: A struggle for professional recognition.* Unpublished master's thesis, University of Alberta, Edmonton, Alberta.

Heyward, C. (1982). *The redemption of God.* Lanham, MD: University Press of America.

Heyward, C. (1989). *Touching our strength.* New York: HarperCollins.

Highfield, M. F., & Cason, C. (1983, June). Spiritual needs of patients: Are they recognized? *Cancer Nursing,* pp. 187-192.

Holland, J., & Henriot, P. (1986). *Social analysis: Linking faith and justice.* Washington, DC: Center for Concern.

Holstrom, S. (1999). Perspectives on a suburban parish nursing practice. In P. A. Solari-Twadell & M. A. McDermott (Eds.), *Parish nursing: Promoting whole person health within faith communities* (pp. 67-74). Thousand Oaks, CA: Sage.

Hopkins, N. M., & Laaser, M. (1995). *Restoring the soul of a church: Healing congregations wounded by clergy sexual misconduct.* Bethesda, MD: Alban Institute.

Hungelmann, J., Kenkel-Rossi, E., Klassen, L., & Stollenwerk, R. M. (1985). Spiritual well-being in older adults: Harmonious interconnectedness. *Journal of Religion and Health, 24*(2), 147-153.

International Parish Nurse Resource Center. (1997/1998). *Basic preparation course for parish nurses.* Park Ridge, IL: Author.

International Parish Nurse Resource Center. (1998). Functions of the parish nurse role [Bookmark]. Park Ridge, IL: Author.

Irons, R. (1991). *The sexually exploitive professional: An addition sensitive model for assessment.* Paper presented at the 2nd Annual Conference on Addictions Prevention, Recognition and Treatment.

Iwasiw, C., & Olson, J. (1995). Nonprofessional staff-patient interaction analysis in long-term care facilities. *Clinical Nursing Research, 4*(4), 411-424.

James, W. (1961). *Varieties of religious experience.* New York: Collier.

Jensen, L., & Allen, M. (1993). Wellness: The dialectic of illness. *Image: Journal of Nursing Scholarship, 25*(3), 220-224.

Johnson, D. E. (1980). The behavioral system model for nursing. In J. P. Riehl &
C. Roy (Eds.), *Conceptual models for nursing practice* (2nd ed., pp. 207-216).
Norwalk, CT: Appleton-Century-Crofts.

Jones, A. (1985). *Soulmaking: The desert way of spirituality.* New York: Harper & Row.

Jones, W. P. (1989). *Theological worlds.* Nashville, TN: Abingdon.

Jones, W. P. (1992). *Trumpet at full moon.* Louisville, KY: Westminster/John Knox.

Jordan, J., Kaplan, A., Miller, J. B., Stiver, I., & Surrey, J. (1991). *Women's growth in
connection.* New York: Guildford.

Juchereau de Sainte-Ignace, J. F., & Duplessis, M. A. Regnard. (1989). *Les
Annales de l'Hôtel-Dieu de Québec, 1636–1716.* Quebec, Quebec: Hôtel-Dieu de
Québec. (Original work published in 1939)

Jung, C. G. (1961). *Memories, dreams and reflections.* New York: Random House.

Kaiser, L. (1993). *Leaders creating healthier communities* [Cassette recording].
Millersville, MD: Recorded Resources.

Kalisch, P. A., & Kalisch, B. J. (1982). Anatomy of the image of the nurse: Disso-
nant and ideal models. In C. Williams (Ed.), *Image-making in nursing*
(pp. 3-23). Kansas City, MO: American Academy of Nursing.

Kalisch, P. A., & Kalisch, B. J. (1987). *The changing image of the nurse.* Menlo Park,
CA: Addison-Wesley.

Katherine, A. (1991). *Boundaries: Where you end and I begin.* New York: Simon &
Schuster.

Kegan, R. (1982). *The evolving self: Problem and process in human development.*
Cambridge, MA: Harvard University Press.

Kelsey, M. (1981). *Caring: How can we love one another?* New York: Paulist Press.

Kidd, S. M. (1990). *When the heart waits.* New York: HarperCollins.

Killen, P. O., & deBeer, J. (1994). *The art of theological reflection.* New York:
Crossroad.

Kim, M., McFarland, G., & McLane, A. (1989). *Pocket guide to nursing diagnosis.*
St. Louis, MO: C. V. Mosby.

King, I. M. (1981). *A theory for nursing: Systems, concepts, process.* New York: John
Wiley.

Kittel, G., & Friedrich, G. (Eds.). (1967). *Theological dictionary of the New Testament* (Vol. 5). Grand Rapids, MI: W. B. Eerdmans.

Kleinman, A. (1980). *Patients and healers in the context of culture.* Berkeley: University of California Press.

Knowles, M. (1980). *The modern practice of adult education: From pedagogy to
andragogy.* Chicago: Follett.

Kohlberg, L. (1969). Stage and sequence: The cognitive developmental
approach to socialization. In D. Goslin (Ed.), *Handbook of socialization: Theory
and research* (pp. 347-480). Chicago: Rand McNally.

Kohlberg, L. (1976). *Collected papers on moral development and moral education.*
Cambridge, MA: Center for Moral Education.

Kosik, S. (1972). Patient advocacy or fighting the system. *American Journal of
Nursing, 72*(4), 694-698.

Krauss, P., & Goldfischer, M. (1990). *Why me? Coping with grief, loss, and change.*
New York: Bantam.

Kravitz, M., & Frey, M. (1989). The Allen nursing model. In J. Fitzpatrick & A. Whall (Eds.), *Conceptual models of nursing: Analysis and application* (pp. 313-329). Norwalk, CT: Appleton & Lange.

Kübler-Ross, E. (1969). *On death and dying.* New York: Macmillan.

Kuhn, T. (1970). *The structure of scientific revolutions.* Chicago: University of Chicago Press.

Kwok, P. (1990). Discovering the Bible in the non-biblical world. In S. B. Thistlethwaite & M. P. Engel (Eds.), *Lift every voice* (pp. 270-282). New York: Harper & Row.

Labonte, R. (1993). *Health promotion and empowerment: Practice frameworks* [Issues in health promotion series #3]. Toronto, Ontario: Centre for Health Promotion, University of Toronto & ParticipACTION.

Labonte, R. (1994). Death of program, birth of metaphor: The development of health promotion in Canada. In A. Peterson, M. O'Neill, & I. Rootman (Eds.), *Health promotion in Canada: Provincial, national and international perspectives* (pp. 72-90). Philadelphia: W. B. Saunders.

Labonte, R., & Penfold, S. (1981). *Health promotion philosophy: From victim blaming to social responsibility.* Vancouver, British Columbia: Health Promotion Directorate.

Labun, E. (1988). Spiritual care: An element in nursing care planning. *Journal of Advanced Nursing, 13,* 314-320.

Laforêt-Fliesser, Y., & Ford-Gilboe, M. (1997). Learning to nurse families using the developmental health model: Educational strategies for undergraduate students. In L. Gottlieb & H. Ezer (Eds.), *A perspective on health, family, learning and collaborative nursing: A collection of writing on the McGill model of nursing* (pp. 236-247). Montreal, Quebec: McGill University School of Nursing.

Lalonde, M. (1974). *A new perspective on the health of Canadians.* Ottawa, Ontario: Health and Welfare Canada.

Lane, J. A. (1987, November/December). The care of the human spirit. *Journal of Professional Nursing,* pp. 332-337.

Latourette, K. (1953). *A history of Christianity.* New York: Harper & Brothers.

Leeming, D. A. (1990). *The world of myth.* New York: Oxford University Press.

Leetun, M. C. (1996). Wellness spirituality in the older adult: Assessment and intervention protocol. *Nurse Practitioner, 20*(8), 60-70.

Legal, E. (1916). *Reglements concernant courvents et hopitaux. Entraits des reglements, usages, et discipline de l'Archidiocese d'Edmonton* [Brochure]. Quebec.

Levine, M. E. (1969). The pursuit of wholeness. *American Journal of Nursing, 69,* 93-98.

Levine, M. E. (1971). Holistic nursing. *Nursing Clinics of North America, 6,* 253-264.

Levine, S. (1982). *Who dies? An investigation of conscious living and conscious dying.* New York: Anchor.

Lewis, C. S. (1961). *A grief observed.* New York: Bantam.

Ley, D. C., & Corless, I. B. (1988). Spirituality and hospice care. *Death Studies, 12,* 101-110.

Lindberg, C. (1986). The Lutheran tradition. In R. L. Numbers & D. W. Amundsen (Eds.), *Caring and curing health and medicine in the Western religious traditions* (pp. 173-203). New York: Macmillan.

Lippman, D. T., & Ponton, K. S. (1989). *Attitudes, values and beliefs of the public in Indiana toward nursing as a career: A study to enhance recruitment into nursing.* Indianapolis, IN: Sigma Theta Tau International Honor Society of Nursing.

Lonergan, B. (1957). *Insight: A study of human understanding.* New York: Philosophical Library.

Lonergan, B. (1972). *Method in theology.* New York: Herder & Herder.

MacPhail, J. (1996). The professional image: Impact and strategies for change. In J. Ross Kerr & J. MacPhail (Eds.), *Canadian nursing: Issues and perspectives* (3rd ed., pp. 54-66). St. Louis, MO: C. V. Mosby.

Macrae, J. (1995). Nightingale's spiritual philosophy and its significance for modern nursing. *Image: Journal of Nursing Scholarship, 27*(1), 8-10.

Main, J. (1982). *Communitas II: The first series* [Cassette recording]. Montreal, Quebec: The Benedictine Priory.

Maley, M. (1995). *Living in the question.* Minneapolis, MN: Bodysmart.

Martin, K., & Elder, S. (1991, May). *Pathways through grief: A model of the process.* Unpublished manuscript. Available from Karen Martin, 6803-111 Street, Edmonton, Alberta, Canada, T6H 3G2.

May, R. (1977). *The meaning of anxiety.* New York: Washington Square. (Original work published in 1950)

Mayeroff, M. (1971). *On caring.* New York: Harper & Row.

McBrien, R. P. (1981). *Catholicism.* Minneapolis, MN: Winston.

McBrien, R. P. (1987). *Ministry: A theological, pastoral handbook.* New York: Harper & Row.

McDougall, M., Lasswell, H., & Chen, L. (1980). *Human rights and world public order: The basic policies of an international law of human dignity.* New Haven, CT: Yale University Press.

McGoldrick, M., & Gerson, R. (1985). *Genograms in family assessment.* New York: Norton.

McKenzie, L. (1982). *The religious education of adults.* Birmingham, AL: Religious Education.

McPherson, K. (1996). *Bedside matters: The transformation of Canadian nursing, 1900–1990.* New York: Oxford University Press.

McSherry, E. (1983, Fall). The spiritual dimension of elder health care. *Generations,* pp. 18-21.

Meeker-Lowry, S. (1995). *Invested in the common good.* Philadelphia: New Society.

Meili, D. (1991). *Those who know: Profiles of Alberta's native elders.* Edmonton, Alberta: NeWest.

Meleis, A. (1990). Being and becoming healthy: The core of nursing knowledge. *Nursing Science Quarterly, 3*(3), 107-114.

Metz, J. (1998). *Poverty of spirit.* New York: Paulist Press. (Original work published in 1968)

Mickley, J. R., Carson, V., & Soeken, K. L. (1995). Religion and adult mental health: State of the science of nursing. *Issues in Mental Health Nursing, 16,* 345-360.

Miles, M. R. (1985). *Image as insight*. Boston: Beacon.

Milgrom, J. (5750/1990). The "ger" (Numbers 15:27-29). In *The JPS Torah Commentary* (pp. 398-402). Philadelphia: Jewish Publication Society.

Miller, C. (1995). *Nursing care of older adults* (2nd ed.). Philadelphia: J. B. Lippincott.

Miller, J. B. (1991). Women and power. In J. Jordan, A. Kaplan, J. B. Miller, I. Stiver, & J. Surrey (Eds.), *Women's growth in connection* (pp. 197-205). New York: Guilford.

Moffatt, B. (1996). *A soulworker's companion: A year of spiritual discovery*. Berkeley, CA: Wildcat Canyon.

Montuori, A., & Conti, I. (1993). *From power to partnership*. New York: HarperCollins.

Morris, L. E. (1996). A spiritual well-being model: Use with older women who experience depression. *Issues in Mental Health Nursing, 17*, 439-455.

Mount, E. (1990). *Professional ethics in context*. Louisville, KY: Westminster/John Knox.

Multifaith Calendar Committee. (1999). *Multifaith calendar*. Port Moody, British Columbia: Multifaith Action Society.

Mura, P., & Mura, A. (1995). Cyclical evolution of nursing education and profession in Iran: Religious, cultural, and political influences. *Journal of Professional Nursing, 11*(1), 58-64.

Murphy, F. (1997). A staff development programme to support the incorporation of the McGill model of nursing into an out-patient clinic department. In L. Gottlieb & H. Ezer (Eds.), *A perspective on health, family, learning and collaborative nursing: A collection of writings on the McGill model of nursing* (pp. 287-295). Montreal, Quebec: McGill University School of Nursing.

Murrant, G., & Strathdee, S. (1995). Motivations for service volunteer involvement at Casey House AIDS hospice. *Hospice Journal, 10*(3), 27-38.

Nagai-Jacobson, M. G., & Burkhardt, M. A. (1989). Spirituality: Cornerstone of holistic nursing practice. *Holistic Nursing Practice, 3*(3), 18-26.

Neeld, E. (1990). *Seven choices*. New York: Bantam Doubleday.

Nel, M. J. (1998, May). *A theological framework for parish nursing*. Paper presented at the Parish Nursing as a Church Ministry Workshop, Trinity Western University, Langley, British Columbia.

Nelson, J. (1976). *Embodiment*. New York: Pilgrim Press.

New revised standard version of the Holy Bible. (1989). Nashville, TN: Division of Christian Education of the National Council of the Churches of Christ.

Newman, M. A. (1989). The spirit of nursing. *Holistic Nursing Practice, 3*(3), 1-6.

Newton, G. (1984). Self-help groups: Can they help? *Journal of Psychosocial Nursing, 22*(7), 27-31.

Niklas, G. (1981). *The making of a pastoral person*. New York: Alba House.

Noer, D. (1993). *Healing the wounds: Overcoming the trauma of layoffs and revitalizing downsized organizations*. San Francisco: Jossey-Bass.

North American Liturgy Resources. (1977). Amazing grace. *Glory and praise*. Phoenix, AZ: North American Liturgy Resources.

Nouwen, H. (1995). *With open hands*. Notre Dame, IN: Ave Maria Press.

Nutting, M. A., & Dock, L. (1907). *A history of nursing*. New York: Putnam.

Oldnall, A. S. (1995). On the absence of spirituality in nursing theories and models. *Journal of Advanced Nursing, 21*, 417-418.

Oldnall, A. S. (1996). A critical analysis of nursing: Meeting the spiritual needs of patients. *Journal of Advanced Nursing, 23,* 138-144.

Olson, J. (1995). Relationships between nurse-expressed empathy, patient-perceived empathy, and patient distress. *Image: Journal of Nursing Scholarship, 27*(4), 317-320.

Olson, J., & Clark, M. (1999, Spring). What is parish nursing? *Exchange,* pp. 13-16.

Olson, J., Clark, M., & Simington, J. (1999). The Canadian experience. In P. A. Solari-Twadell & M. A. McDermott (Eds.), *Parish nursing: Promoting whole person health within faith communities* (pp. 277-286). Thousand Oaks, CA: Sage.

Olson, J., & Hanchett, E. (1997). Nurse-expressed empathy, patient outcomes, and development of a middle range theory. *Image: Journal of Nursing Scholarship, 29*(1), 71-76.

Olson, J., Simington, J., & Douglass, L. (1995, November). *The feasibility of parish nursing in a reformed health care system.* Paper presented at the Sigma Theta Tau International Biennial Convention, Detroit, MI.

Omoto, A. (1995). Sustained helping without obligation: Motivation, longevity of service, and perceived attitude change among AIDS volunteers. *Journal of Personality and Social Psychology, 68*(4), 671-686.

Ontario Multifaith Council on Spiritual and Religious Care. (1995). *Multifaith information manual.* Toronto, Ontario: Author.

Orem, D. E. (1980). *Nursing: Concepts of practice* (2nd ed.). New York: McGraw-Hill.

Orem, D. E. (1985). *Nursing: Concepts of practice* (3rd ed.). New York: McGraw-Hill.

Orlando, I. J. (1961). *The dynamic nurse-patient relationship.* New York: Putnam.

Orlando, I. J. (1972). *The discipline and teaching of nursing process.* New York: Putnam.

Panikkar, R. (1971). Faith, a constitutive dimension of man. *Journal of Ecumenical Studies, 8*(2), 223-254.

Parse, R. R. (1981). *Man-Living-Health: A theory of nursing.* New York: John Wiley.

Parse, R. R. (1987). *Nursing science: Major paradigms, theories, and critiques.* Philadelphia: W. B. Saunders.

Parse, R. R. (1990a). Health: A personal commitment. *Nursing Science Quarterly, 3*(3), 136-140.

Parse, R. R. (1990b). Promotion and prevention: Two distinct categories. *Nursing Science Quarterly, 3*(3), 101.

Patterson, J. G., & Zderad, L. T. (1976). *Humanistic nursing.* New York: Wiley.

Paul VI. (1964). *Paths of the church.* Boston: Daughters of St. Paul.

Payne, Cook, & Associates. (1990). *Insight: The 1989 provincial public opinion study of nursing in Alberta.* Edmonton. (Available from the Alberta Association of Registered Nurses, 11620-168th Street, Edmonton, Alberta, T5M 4A6)

Pender, N. J. (1987). *Health promotion in nursing practice* (2nd ed.). Norwalk, CT: Appleton & Lange.

Pender, N. J. (1990). Expressing health through lifestyle patterns. *Nursing Science Quarterly, 3*(3), 115-122.

Peri, T. C. (1995). Promoting spirituality in persons with acquired immunodeficiency syndrome: A nursing intervention. *Holistic Nursing Practice, 10*(1), 68-76.

Petitat, A. (1989). *Les infirmières de la vocation ô la profession.* Montréal, Quebec: Boréal.

Phillips, D., Howes, E., & Nixon, L. (1975). *The choice is always ours.* Wheaton, IL: Request. (Original work published in 1948)

Piaget, J. (1952). *The origins of intelligence in children.* New York: International Universities Press.

Piaget, J. (1954). *The construction of reality in the child.* New York: Basic Books.

Pierce, C., & Page, B. (1986). *A male/female continuum: Paths to colleagueship.* Laconia, NH: New Dynamics.

Pierce, C., Page, B., & Wagner, D. (1998). *A male/female continuum: Paths to colleagueship* (Expanded ed.). Laconia, NH: New Dynamics.

Pietroni, P. C. (1987). The meaning of illness-holism dissected: Discussion paper. *Journal of the Royal Society of Medicine, 80,* 357-360.

Piles, C. L. (1990). Providing spiritual care. *Nurse Educator, 15*(1), 36-41.

Poling, J. (1991). *The abuse of power.* Nashville, TN: Abingdon.

Poulet, C. (1934). *A history of the Catholic church.* St. Louis, MO: Herder.

Pruyser, P. (1976). *The minister as diagnostician.* Philadelphia: Westminster.

Puleo, M. (1994). *The struggle is one: Voices and visions of liberation.* Albany: State University of New York Press.

Rahner, K., & Vorgrimler, H. (1965). *Theological dictionary.* New York: Herder & Herder.

Reed, P. (1998). The re-enchantment of health care: A paradigm of spirituality. In M. Cobb & V. Robshaw (Eds.), *The spiritual challenge of health care* (pp. 35-55). London: Harcourt Brace.

Reichelt, P. A. (1988). Public perceptions of nursing and strategy formation. *Western Journal of Nursing Research, 10*(4), 472-476.

Reilly, D. E. (1975). Why a conceptual framework? *Nursing Outlook, 23,* 566-569.

Reutter, L., & Harrison, M. (1996). Primary health care and the health of families. In J. Ross Kerr & J. MacPhail (Eds.), *Concepts in Canadian nursing* (pp. 72-84). St. Louis, MO: C. V. Mosby.

Reverby, S. M. (1982). *The nursing disorder: A critical history of the hospital-nursing relationship, 1860–1945.* Unpublished doctoral dissertation, Boston University, Boston, MA.

Rew, L. (1996). *Awareness in healing.* Toronto, Ontario: Delmar.

Reynolds, C. (1988). The measurement of health in nursing research. *Advances in Nursing Science, 10*(4), 23-31.

Reynolds, R., & Lynn, D. (1992). *Losses and changes: Finding hope in life's difficult times.* Grand Rapids, MI: Zondervan.

Rice, J. (1994, December). Assessing community health. *Trustee,* pp. 16-17.

Richardson, R. (1996). *Creating a healthier church.* Minneapolis, MN: Augsburg Fortress.

Rilke, R. M. (1934). *Letters to a young poet.* New York: Norton.

Rinpoche, S. (1993). *The Tibetan book of living and dying.* New York: HarperCollins.

Roach, M. S. (1997). *Caring from the heart: The convergence of caring and spirituality.* New York: Paulist Press.

Rodwell, C. M. (1996). An analysis of the concept of empowerment. *Journal of Advanced Nursing, 23,* 305-313.

Rogers, C. (1951). *Client centered therapy.* Boston: Houghton Mifflin.

Rogers, C. (1961). *On becoming a person.* Boston: Houghton Mifflin.

Rogers, M. (1970). *An introduction to the theoretical basis of nursing.* Philadelphia: F. A. Davis.

Roget's pocket thesaurus: A treasury of synonyms and antonyms. (1982). New York: Simon & Schuster.

Rosenberg, C. E. (1987). *The care of strangers: The rise of the American hospital system.* New York: Basic Books.

Rosner, D. (1982). *A once charitable enterprise: Hospitals and healthcare in Brooklyn and New York.* Cambridge, MA: Cambridge University Press.

Ross, L. (1995). The spiritual dimension: Its importance to patients' health, well-being and quality of life and its implications for nursing practice. *International Journal of Nursing Studies, 32*(5), 457-468.

Ross Kerr, J. (1996a). The origins of nursing education in Canada: An overview of the emergence and growth of diploma programs: 1874 to 1974. In J. Ross Kerr & J. MacPhail (Eds.), *Canadian nursing: Issues and perspectives* (3rd ed., pp. 291-305). St. Louis, MO: C. V. Mosby.

Ross Kerr, J. (1996b). Professionalization of Canadian nursing. In J. Ross Kerr & J. MacPhail (Eds.), *Canadian nursing: Issues and perspectives* (3rd ed., pp. 23-30). St. Louis, MO: C. V. Mosby.

Ross Kerr, J. (1998) *Prepared to care: Nurses and nursing in Alberta.* Edmonton, Alberta: University of Alberta Press.

Ross Kerr, J., & MacPhail, J. (Eds.). (1996). *Canadian nursing: Issues and perspectives* (3rd ed.). St. Louis, MO: C. V. Mosby.

Roy, C. (1976). *Introduction to nursing: An adaptation model.* Englewood Cliffs, NJ: Prentice Hall.

Roy, C. (1984). *Introduction to nursing: An adaptation model* (2nd ed.). Englewood Cliffs, NJ: Prentice Hall.

Russell, L. (1974). *Human liberation in a feminist perspective: A theology.* Philadelphia: Westminster.

Russell, L. (1981). *Growth in partnership.* Philadelphia: Westminster.

Rutter, P. (1989). *Sex in the forbidden zone.* New York: Fawcett Crest.

Rutter, P. (1997). *Understanding and preventing sexual harassment.* New York: Bantam. (Also published in hard cover under the title *Sex, power and boundaries,* 1996, New York: Bantam.)

Rutter, V. B. (1993). *Woman changing woman.* New York: HarperCollins.

Ryan, J. A. (1990). Society, the parish and the parish nurse. In P. A. Solari-Twadell, A. M. Djupe, & M. A. McDermott (Eds.), *Parish nursing: The developing practice* (pp. 41-53). Park Ridge, IL: National Parish Nurse Resource Center.

Sampson, C. (1982). *The neglected ethic: Religious and cultural factors in the care of patients.* London: McGraw-Hill.

Sanford, J. (1977). *Healing and wholeness.* New York: Paulist Press.

Sanford, J. (1980). *The invisible partners.* New York: Paulist Press.

Sardana, R. (1990, May). Spiritual care of the elderly: An integral part of the nursing process. *Nursing Homes*, pp. 30-31.

Satir, V. (1976). *Making contact.* Millbrae, CA: Celestial Arts.

Satir, V. (1988). *The new peoplemaking.* Palo Alto, CA: Science and Behavior Books.

Schillebeeckx, E. (1984). *The Schillebeeckx reader.* New York: Crossroad.

Schumacher, M. E. (1964). The Christian nurse's role. *Canadian Nurse, 60*(8), 774-775.

Seaburn, D., Lorenz, A., Gunn, W., Gawinski, B., & Mauksch, L. (1996). *Models of collaboration.* New York: Basic Books.

Sellner, E. (1990). *Mentoring: The ministry of spiritual kinship.* Notre Dame, IN: Ave Maria Press.

Shaffer, J. L. (1991). Spiritual distress and critical illness. *Critical Care Nurse, 11*(1), 42-45.

Shaw Sorensen, E. (1998). "For Zion's sake": The emergence of Mormon nursing. *Nursing History Review, 6,* 51-69.

Shea, J. (1997). *The art of theological reflection: Connecting faith and life* [Cassette recordings, tapes 1-6]. Chicago: Acta.

Shelly, J. A., & Fish, S. (1988). *Spiritual care: The nurse's role.* Downers Grove, IL: Intervarsity.

Sjöö, M., & Mor, B. (1991). *The great cosmic mother: Rediscovering the religion of the earth.* New York: HarperCollins.

Smith, J. (1982). Letter to the editor. *Advances in Nursing Science, 4*(3), xi.

Smith, M. C. (1990). Nursing's unique focus on health promotion. *Nursing Science Quarterly, 3*(3), 105-106.

Soeken, K. L. (1987). Responding to the spiritual needs of the chronically ill. *Nursing Clinics of North America, 22*(3), 603-611.

Soelle, D. (1975). *Suffering.* Philadelphia: Fortress.

Sofield, L., & Juliano, C. (1987). *Collaborative ministry.* Notre Dame, IN: Ave Maria Press.

Solari-Twadell, P. A., & McDermott, M. A. (Eds.). (1999). *Parish nursing: Promoting whole person health within faith communities.* Thousand Oaks, CA: Sage.

Solari-Twadell, P. A., McDermott, M. A., Ryan, J. A., & Djupe, A. M. (1994). *Assuring viability for the future: Guideline development for parish nursing-education programs.* Park Ridge, IL: National Parish Nurse Resource Center.

Starck, P. L. (1992). The human spirit: The search for meaning and purpose through suffering. *Humane Medicine, 8*(2), 132-137.

Starhawk. (1989). *Spiral dance: A rebirth of the ancient religion of the great goddess.* New York: Harper & Row.

Stepnick, A., & Perry, T. (1992). Preventing spiritual distress in the dying client. *Journal of Psychosocial Nursing, 30*(1), 17-24.

Stevens, B. J. (1979). *Nursing theory: Analysis, application, and evaluation.* Boston: Little, Brown.

Stewart, M. (1995a). Community health nursing in the future. In M. Stewart (Ed.), *Community nursing: Promoting Canadians' health* (pp. 62-78). Toronto, Ontario: W. B. Saunders.

Stewart, M. (1995b). Social support, coping and self-care: Public participation concepts. In M. Stewart (Ed.), *Community nursing: Promoting Canadians' health* (pp. 89-124). Toronto, Ontario: W. B. Saunders.

Stiles, M. K. (1990). The shining stranger: Nurse-family spiritual relationship. *Cancer Nursing, 13*(4), 235-245.

Stiver, I. P. (1991). The meaning of care: Reframing treatment models. In J. Jordan, A. Kaplan, J. B. Miller, I. Stiver, & J. Surrey (Eds.), *Women's growth in connection* (pp. 250-267). New York: Guilford.

Stokes, K. (1989). *Faith is a verb.* Mystic, CT: Twenty-Third Publishers.

Stoll, R. (1979, September). Guidelines for spiritual assessment. *American Journal of Nursing,* pp. 1574-1577.

Striepe, J. (1993, Winter). Reclaiming the church's healing role. *Journal of Christian Nursing,* pp. 4-7.

Striepe, J., King, J., & Scott, L. (1993, Winter). Nurses in the church: Profiles of caring. *Journal of Christian Nursing,* pp. 8-11.

Stuart, E., Deckro, J., & Mandle, C. (1989). Spirituality in health and healing: A clinical program. *Holistic Nursing Practice, 3*(3), 35-46.

Sullivan, L. (1989). *Health and restoring: Health and medicine in the world's religious traditions.* New York: MacMillan.

Sullivan, P. F. (1991). *The mystery of my story.* New York: Paulist Press.

Swimme, B. (1984). *The universe is a green dragon: A cosmic creation story.* Santa Fe, NM: Bear & Company.

Thistlethwaite, S. B., & Engel, M. P. (1990). *Lift every voice.* New York: Harper.

Thomas, L., & Pierce, C. (1999). *Journeys of race and culture* [Graphic chart]. Laconia, NH: New Dynamics.

Toffler, A. (1990). *Powershift.* New York: Bantam.

Tournier, P. (1987). *A listening ear: Reflections on Christian care.* Minneapolis, MN: Augsburg.

Travelbee, J. (1971). *Interpersonal aspects of nursing* (2nd ed.). Philadelphia: F. A. Davis.

Trocchio, J. (1994, March). The hows and whys of conducting a community needs assessment. *Trustee,* pp. 6-7.

Tubesing, D. (1977). *History of the wholistic health centers project, 1970–1976.* Hinsdale, IL: Society for Wholistic Medicine.

Turner, B. K. (1995). *Multifaith information manual.* Toronto, Canada: Ontario Multifaith Council on Spiritual and Religious Care.

Tyler, L. (1997). The McGill model of nursing in a hospital ambulatory setting. In L. Gottlieb & H. Ezer (Eds.), *A perspective on health, family, learning and collaborative nursing: A collection of writings on the McGill model of nursing* (pp. 327-332). Montreal, Quebec: McGill University School of Nursing.

Underhill, E. (1961). *Mysticism.* New York: E. P. Dutton. (Original work published in 1911)

University of Rochester, School of Nursing. (1998). *The Woodhull study on nursing and the media: Health care's invisible partner.* Indianapolis, IN: Center Nursing.

Valvarde, C. (1991). *Critical theory in health education* [Mimeograph]. Montreal, Quebec: Départemente de Santé Communautaire.

Vanauken, S. (1977). *A severe mercy.* New York: Harper.

Van Biema, D. (1991, October). The journey of our lives. *Life Magazine,* pp. 5-92.

van Gennep, A. (1960). *Rites of passage.* Chicago: University of Chicago Press.

Vanier, J. (1995). *An ark for the poor: The story of l'Arche.* New York: Crossroad.

Vanier, J. (1988). *Becoming human.* Toronto, Ontario: Anansi.

Van Loon, A. M. (1999). The Australian concept of faith community. P. A. Solari-Twadell & M. A. McDermott (Eds.), *Parish nursing: Promoting whole person health within faith communities* (pp. 287-297). Thousand Oaks, CA: Sage.

Vaughan, R. (1987). *Basic skills for Christian counselors.* New York: Paulist Press.

Vine, W. E. (1966). *An expository dictionary of New Testament words.* Old Tappan, NJ: Fleming H. Revell.

Wake, R. (1998). *The Nightingale training school, 1860–1996.* London: Haggerston.

Wald, F. S., & Bailey, S. S. (1990, November). Nurturing the spiritual component in care for the terminally ill. *Caring Magazine,* pp. 64-68.

Walker, B. (1988). *The woman's dictionary of symbols and sacred objects.* New York: HarperCollins.

Wallace, R. (1967). New image for the hospital chaplain. *Canadian Nurse, 63*(8), 29-31.

Walton, J. (1996). Spiritual relationships. *Journal of Holistic Nursing, 14*(3) 237-250.

Warner, M. (1981). Health and nursing: Evolving one concept by involving the other. *Nursing Papers, 13*(1), 10-17.

Warner, M. (1997). Learning to be healthy: The workshop approach. In L. Gottlieb & H. Ezer (Eds.), *A perspective on health, family, learning and collaborative nursing: A collection of writing on the McGill model of nursing* (pp. 146-154). Montreal, Quebec: McGill University School of Nursing.

Webster's encyclopedic unabridged dictionary of the English language. (1989). Avenel, NJ: Gramercy Books.

Webster's ninth new collegiate dictionary. (1991). Markham, Ontario: Thomas Allen.

Wells-Federman, C. L. (1996). Awakening the nurse healer within. *Holistic Nursing Practice, 10*(2), 13-29.

Wenger, A. (1993). Cultural meaning of symptoms. *Holistic Nursing Practice, 7*(2), 22-35.

Westberg, G. E. (1984, October). Churches are joining the health care team. *Urban Health,* pp. 34-36.

Westberg, G. E. (1987). *The parish nurse: How to start a parish nurse program in your church.* Park Ridge, IL: Parish Nurse Resource Center.

Westberg, G. E. (1990a). A historical perspective: Wholistic health and the parish nurse. In P. A. Solari-Twadell, A. M. Djupe, & M. A. McDermott (Eds.), *Parish nursing: The developing practice* (pp. 27-39). Park Ridge, IL: National Parish Nurse Resource Center.

Westberg, G. E. (1990b). *The parish nurse: Providing a minister of health for your congregation.* Minneapolis, MN: Augsburg Fortress.

Westberg, G. E. (1999). A personal historical perspective of whole person health and the congregation. In P. A. Solari-Twadell & M. A. McDermott (Eds.), *Parish nursing: Promoting whole person health within faith communities* (pp. 35-41). Thousand Oaks, CA: Sage.

Westerhoff, J. (1976). *Will our children have faith?* New York: Seabury.

Whitehead, J. D., & Whitehead, E. E. (1982). *Christian life patterns.* Garden City, NY: Doubleday. (Original work published in 1979)

Whitehead, J. D., & Whitehead, E. E. (1986). *The emerging laity.* Garden City, NY: Doubleday.

Whitehead, J. D., & Whitehead, E. E. (1991). *The promise of partnership.* Philadelphia: Westminster.

Whitehead, J. D., & Whitehead, E. E. (1995). *Method in ministry.* Kansas City, MO: Sheed & Ward.

Wicks, G. (1987). Improving nursing's public image and impact. *American Nephrology Nurses Association, 14*(4), 243-244.

Wicks, R., Parsons, R., & Capps, D. (1985). *Clinical handbook of pastoral counseling.* New York: Paulist Press.

Widerquist, J., & Davidhizer, R. (1994). The ministry of nursing. *Journal of Advanced Nursing, 19,* 647-652.

Wiedenbach, E. (1963). The helping art of nursing. *American Journal of Nursing, 63*(11), 54-57.

Wilkinson, T. (1996). *Persephone returns.* Berkeley, CA: Pagemill.

Wink, W. (1984). *Naming the powers: The language of power in the new testament.* Philadelphia: Fortress.

Wishik, H., & Pierce, C. (1994). *Sexual orientation and identity.* Laconia, NH: New Dynamics.

Woodham-Smith, C. (1950). *Florence Nightingale, 1820–1910.* London: Constable.

World Health Organization. (1978). *Primary health care: Report of the International Conference on Primary Health Care,* Alma Ata, USSR. Geneva: Author.

World Health Organization, Health and Welfare Canada, & Canadian Public Health Association. (1986). *Ottawa charter for health promotion.* Ottawa, Ontario: Author.

Wright, L., & Leahy, M. (1984). *Nurses and families: A guide to family assessment.* Philadelphia: F. A. Davis.

Wylie, J. (1990). The mission of health and the congregation. In P. A. Solari-Twadell, A. M. Djupe, & M. A. McDermott (Eds.), *Parish nursing: The developing practice* (pp. 11-26). Park Ridge, IL: National Parish Nurse Resource Center.

Yura, H., & Walsh, M. B. (1983). *The nursing process: Assessing, planning, implementing, evaluating* (4th ed.). Norwalk, CT: Appleton-Century-Crofts.

INDEX

About the Authors

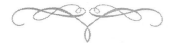

Margaret B. Clark, M.C.Sp., D.Min., is a Teaching Chaplain in Pastoral Care Services at the University of Alberta Hospital, Edmonton, Alberta. She holds a baccalaureate degree in sociology from Trinity College, Washington, D.C.; a master's degree in Christian spirituality from Creighton University in Omaha, Nebraska; and has completed graduate theological studies at Newman Theological College in Edmonton, Alberta. She recently completed her doctor of ministry program at St. Stephen's College in Edmonton. She is certified as a teaching supervisor in clinical pastoral education (CPE) with the Canadian Association for Pastoral Practice and Education/Association Canadienne Pour la Practique et l'Éducation Pastorales (CAPPE/ACPEP). She ministered for 12 years in Roman Catholic parishes in Montana and California, and for the past 16 years has been doing hospital ministry in Montana, Utah, and Alberta. She has held positions in the following ministry locations: Holy Family Parish, Great Falls, Montana; Angela Center, Santa Rosa, California; Ursuline Centre, Great Falls, Montana; Foothills Hospital, Calgary, Alberta; Royal Alexandra Hospital, Edmonton, Alberta; Pastoral Institute of Edmonton, Edmonton, Alberta; Holy Cross Hospital, Salt Lake City, Utah. She codeveloped and has cotaught both theoretical and clinical faith community nursing courses offered at the University of Alberta, and offers CPE courses for faith community nurses through the University of Alberta Hospital.

Joanne K. Olson, R.N., Ph.D., is Associate Professor in the Faculty of
Nursing and Associate Faculty in the Centre for Health Promotion
Studies at the University of Alberta, Edmonton. She holds a baccalaureate degree in nursing from Augustana College, Sioux Falls, South
Dakota, and a master's degree in public health from the University of
Minnesota. At Wayne State University, in Detroit, Michigan, she
focused her nursing doctoral research on empathic nurse-client interactions. She has held positions as a community health nurse, community health nursing supervisor, and nurse educator in Minnesota, Missouri, Ontario, and Alberta. Prior to her move to Alberta, she held
positions in the following agencies: the Kandiyohi County Nursing
Service, Willmar, Minnesota; Anoka County Health Department,
Anoka, Minnesota; Ramsey County Nursing Service, St. Paul, Minnesota; St. Louis Health Department, St. Louis, Missouri; Maryville University, St. Louis, Missouri; and the University of Western Ontario,
London, Ontario. Her teaching, research, and writing interests are in
the areas of community and family health, nursing education,
nurse-client interaction, spiritual aspects of nursing care, and faith
community nursing. She has served on the Board of Directors and in
multiple other positions within the Sigma Theta Tau International
Nursing Honor Society. She has codeveloped and cotaught both theoretical and clinical faith community nursing courses offered at the
University of Alberta.

About the Contributor

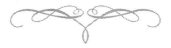

Pauline Paul, R.N., Ph.D., obtained a baccalaureate degree in nursing at the Université de Montréal, a master's of science in nursing from McGill University, and a doctorate in nursing, with a focus on the history of nursing, at the University of Alberta, Edmonton. Her research has primarily been related to the history of nursing in Canada, and she is currently studying the social history of tuberculosis in Alberta. She is an Assistant Professor in the Faculty of Nursing and an Associate of the Centre for Health Promotion Studies at the University of Alberta. For the last two years, she has been teaching Web-based courses in the graduate program offered by this centre. Being bilingual, Pauline Paul publishes in English and French, the two official languages of Canada. She is a member of the Canadian Association for the History of Nursing and past president of the Mu Sigma Chapter of Sigma Theta Tau International.

DATE DUE

			Printed in USA

HIGHSMITH #45230